Skin Cancer: Pathogenesis and Diagnosis

Ashish Dwivedi • Anurag Tripathi •
Ratan Singh Ray • Abhishek Kumar Singh
Editors

Skin Cancer: Pathogenesis and Diagnosis

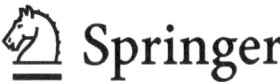 Springer

Editors
Ashish Dwivedi
Food, Drug & Chemical Toxicology
CSIR-IITR
Lucknow, Uttar Pradesh, India

Anurag Tripathi
Food, Drug & Chemical Toxicology
Indian Institute of Toxicology Research
Lucknow, Uttar Pradesh, India

Ratan Singh Ray
Photobiology Division
Indian Institute of Toxicology Research
Lucknow, Uttar Pradesh, India

Abhishek Kumar Singh
Amity Institute of Neuropsychology and
Neurosciences
Amity University
Noida, Uttar Pradesh, India

ISBN 978-981-16-0366-2   ISBN 978-981-16-0364-8   (eBook)
https://doi.org/10.1007/978-981-16-0364-8

This Springer imprint is published by the registered company Springer Nature Singapore Pte Ltd.
The registered company address is: 152 Beach Road, #21-01/04 Gateway East, Singapore 189721, Singapore

Contents

About the Editors

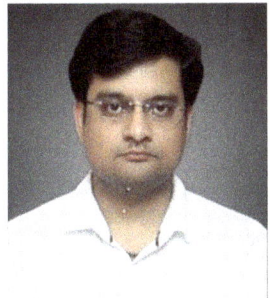

Ashish Dwivedi is a Scientist in the Division of Food, Drug & Chemical Toxicology, CSIR-IITR, a premier Institute of Toxicology Research in India. He has done his post-doctoral research from the Israel Institute of Technology (IIT), Israel and Colorado University, US on cancer therapy. He has also been awarded a prestigious Dr. D.S Kothari Post-Doctoral Fellowship by UGC. He has done his Doctoral Research from Photobiology Division, Indian Institute of Toxicology Research (IITR), Lucknow. His Doctorate research work was focused on phototoxicity/photosafety assessment of therapeutic drugs, environmental pollutants and nanotized phytochemicals at ambient UV-R exposure. He has more than ten years of research experience in Photo & Dermal Toxicology and published several articles in reputed journals of Photochemistry & Photobiology, Toxicology, Biomaterials, and Hazardous materials.

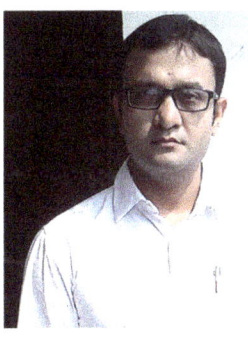

Anurag Tripathi is working as a Senior Scientist in the Department of Food, Drug and Chemical Toxicology at CSIR-Indian Institute of Toxicology Research. He did his Ph.D. from the School of Biotechnology, Banaras Hindu University. He has 16 years of research experience and published more than 50 research articles in peer-reviewed international journals such as Immunology, Molecular Immunology, Molecular Aspects of Medicine, Toxicology Letters, ACS Nano, Toxicology, and Applied Pharmacology. He is a life member of the Indian Nanoscience Society and serves as an editorial board member in several prestigious international journals such as Journal of Immunology & Serum Biology, SM Journal of Nanotechnology and Nanomedicine, Journal of Toxicology and Forensic cases and Austin Immunology.

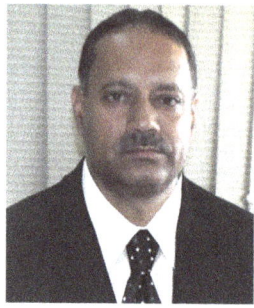

Ratan Singh Ray is a Senior Principal Scientist & Head, Photobiology Division, CSIR-Indian Institute of Toxicology Research, Lucknow. He has twenty-nine years of research experience in the area of Photobiology. He is an active member of various scientific societies including, the Bureau of Indian Standards (Cosmetics Sectional Committee PCD 19), India, American Society for Photobiology, USA, Indian Photobiology Society, India, Society of Toxicology, India. He has published many research articles in reputed journals of Photochemistry & Photobiology, and Toxicology.

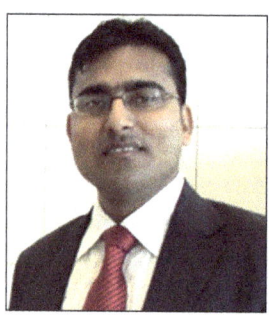

Abhishek Kumar Singh is an Assistant Professor at Amity University, Noida. He earned his PhD from CSIR-Indian Institute of Toxicology Research, Lucknow, in 2013. Then, he joined Guru Ghasidas Central University, Bilaspur, as an Assistant Professor in the Department of Biotechnology. His major research interest is to investigate the interplay between autophagy and pro-survival pathways during aging of the brain and aging-induced neurodegenerative disorders. Dr. Singh has more published more than 50 research articles in international journals of high repute and ten book chapters. He is a member of the Indian Academy of Neuroscience, the International Society of Neurochemistry, and the Society of Toxicology India.

Cancer of the Skin: Types and Etiology

1

Shiv Poojan and Ruchi Pandey

Abstract

Skin, the largest organ system in the human body, plays an important role in making a porous barrier to detach internal organs from external stimuli. Genetic or natural mutations in skin cells can cause cutaneous tissue hypethrophic and inflammatory condition or malignant transformation, that accounting for a big number of ailment in human skin which leads to skin cancer developement in the skin cells. Here in this chapter, we are describing the recent details on skin cancer types and their etiology. It also gives a brief idea of skin growth and how mutations or misregulations of these are elaborated in the pathogenesis of skin cancer development.

Keywords

Skin cancer · Basal cell carcinoma · Melanoma · Nonmelanoma keratinocytes · Wounding · Skin tumor · Skin blistering

Abbreviations

AFX	Atypical fibroxanthoma
AK	Actinic keratoses
AS	Angiosarcoma

S. Poojan (✉)
Department of Dermatology & Cutaneous Biology, Sidney Kimmel Cancer Center, Thomas Jefferson University, Philadelphia, PA, USA
e-mail: shiv.poojan@jefferson.edu

R. Pandey
Center for Translational Medicine, Thomas Jefferson University, Philadelphia, PA, USA

1

BCC	Basal cell carcinoma
DFSP	Dermatofibrosarcoma protuberans
DTS	Digital transcriptome subtraction
EB	Epidermolysis bullosa
EMPD	Extramammary Paget disease
HIV	Human immunodeficiency virus
HPV	Human papilloma virus
LAS	Lymphedema-associated angiosarcoma
MAC	Microcystic adnexal carcinoma
MCC	Merkel cell carcinoma
NBCCS	Nevoid BCC syndrome
NMSC	Nonmelanoma skin cancer
OS	Overall survival
PUVA	Psoralen plus UVA
RDEB-SCC	Recessive dystrophic epidermolysis bullosa squamous cell carcinoma
SC	Sebaceous carcinoma
SCC	Squamous cell carcinoma
SEER	Surveillance, epidemiology, and end results
STS	Stewart-Treves syndrome
UPS	Undifferentiated pleomorphic sarcoma
UV	Ultraviolet
WHO	World Health Organization

1.1 Nonmelanoma Skin Cancer

Nonmelanoma skin cancer (NMSC) develops in one out of five Americans throughout their lifetime. It is the most common human cancer; an annual rate assessed more than three million as recorded in 2006 in the USA. It is relatively higher than the frequency of breast cancer, colon cancer, lung cancer, and prostate cancer collectively [1–3]. The recent trends showed more number of NMSC in Australia, Northern America, and Western Europe, due to holidays in sunny places and outdoor activities. Even then incidence is continuing to rise instead of public awareness of the harmful effect of ultraviolet (UV) exposure from the sunlight. Age shift, high ambient solar irradiance and artificial UV exposure are responsible for the increasing frequency of NMSC. Using tanning beds or sunlamps too much can also cause it. It also derives from exposure to different sources of UV, such as artificial tanning. Light skinned people are more susceptible to get skin cancer and people over 40 are at higher risk. Even risk is higher if any in family have had it or had it before. It may also be more possible to get it if you have been exposed often to X-rays, to toxic chemicals (such as arsenic, coal tar, and creosote), or to radioactive substances [4] (Fig. 1.1).

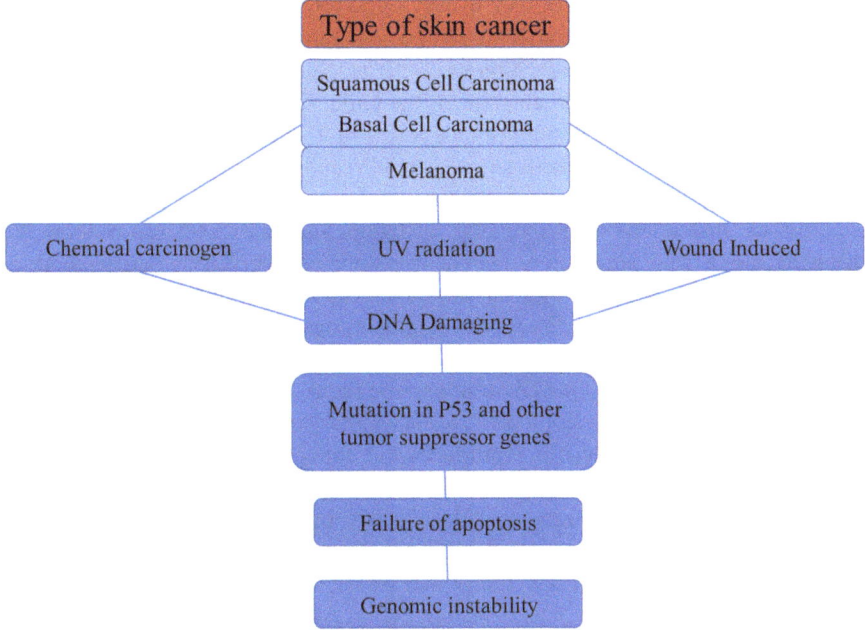

Fig. 1.1 Mechanisms involved in cancer pathogenesis

1.2   Actinic Keratoses

Actinic keratoses (AK) cancer is a very common cancer type that is frequently linked to sun-exposed areas, it affects mostly blond or red-haired, fair-skinned people with green or blue eyes phenotype. AKs signify the initial intraepidermal feature of abnormal growth of keratinocytes and possess the canonical mutations in tumor suppressor genes such as p53, PTCH (Drosophila patched gene) seen in SCC. AK is the earliest lesions with the chance of progression to SCCIS and invasive SCC [4]. Clinically, there are three main patterns seen in AKs: unprompted relapse, perseverance, or progression to invasive SCC [5]. The risk of AK development to SCC has been calculated between 0.025% and 16% per year, and the estimated total risk of malignant transformation for a patient with AKs surveyed for a period of 10 years ranges from 6.1% to 10.2% [6]. AKs are responsible to rise approximately 60–65% of SCCs. Over a period of 12 months, impulsive relapse has been stated in as high as 25.9% of AKs and even 15% relapse rate was distinguished at continuation [4]. Both individual and environmental factors are involved in the etiology of actinic keratoses [4]. Extreme exposure to UV radiation which acts as a complete carcinogen is the main reason for both enhancing and promoting tumor growth [6–8]. Activation of molecular signaling pathways, which are contribted in modifications of regulatory cytokines levels, immunosuppressive properties, faulty cell differentiation, and apoptosis are mainly caused by UV radiation [7]. Along with the formation of proinflammatory cytokines and initiation of mast cells with the inhibitory factor of macrophage migration, the arachidonic acid pathway mediates the inflammatory process. The outcome of the initiation of these mediators contains lipid peroxidation, growth in intralesional levels of T lymphocytes and Langerhans cells, rise of p53 Bcl-2, and decrease in Fas (cd95) and Fas-ligand, which are crucial early factors in the apoptosis progression of UV-mutated cells [7]. Activation, suppression, and removal of apoptotic mediators such as CD95 cause apoptotic disorders along with some other factors like apoptosis driven by tumor necrosis factor and of pro-apoptotic tumor suppressor genes, or by regulation of p53 apoptotic signal activity [9, 10]. In disease development, important risk factors are related to age, sex, phototypes I and II, previous history of cutaneous neoplasms, prolonged sun exposure and occupational environment are the reasons, that play an important role in actinic keratoses development [11]. The history of previous skin neoplasms is also very significant because it reproduces the connotation of individual genetic factors, which may affect the understanding of UV radiation and the level of exposure of chronic UV radiation during the life of a particular individual [11, 12]. While assessing the impact of occupational sun exposure for the development of actinic keratoses, it was found that workers from outside area are at 2–3 times the higher risk and they were also at higher risk for all cutaneous neoplasms [13, 14]. Subsequently, both condition acute exposure and chronic UV radiation can lead to mutations in the p53 gene and following clonal keratinocyte growth therefore, the incidence of painful sunburn before 20 years of age may represent the beginning events of the carcinogenesis progression and it enhances even more when arsenic or other heavy metal toxicity is present. It is reported, arsenic exposure disrupts the homeostasis of the skin stem cell population in the mice during carcinogenesis [15, 16]. As a result of the carcinogenic effects of UV radiation, patients with prolonged use of general immunosuppressive drugs are a particular risk group for developing cutaneous neoplasias and dysplasias [17]. NMSC is the most prevalent neoplasm observed in 27% population of solid organ transplant patients [17, 18]. Likewise, higher risk of progression in the immunosuppressed patients due to the prevalence of actinic keratoses developed lesions to SCC [19]. Additional features such as facial telangiectasias, ephelides, solar lentigos, cutis rhomboidalis nuchae, solar elastosis, and around ten melanoses on the dorsa of the hands are also considered as a risk phenotype for actinic keratoses development [20, 21].

1.3   Basal Cell Carcinoma

The most common cancer in humans is basal cell carcinoma (BCC), previously known as basal cell epithelioma and mostly arises on sun-damaged skin and rarely develops on the palms and soles or mucous membranes. BCC is usually a slow-growing tumor for which metastases are rare. Although BCC is rarely fatal, in case of inadequate or delayed treatment it can be extremely critical and mutilate niche tissues. Clinical inspection of BCC typically looks as flesh or pink colored shining papules with covering ulceration or telangiectatic vessels. BCC occurs on the head or neck in majority of cases [22–24]. BCCs are described in the literature with different subtypes and most dermatologists agree on these major, identifiable, clinicopathologic type nodular, superficial, morpheaform, and fibroepithelial structure. Whereas, the occurrence of combinations of these clinical features in patient is also observed with other type of nodular formation in BCC. Variable amounts of melanin may be present within these tumors but otherwise, in majority of cases, BCCs are amelanotic [25]. Typically, lighter-skinned individuals are more prone to BCC and particularly on sun-exposed parts. Mainly nose acquires approximately 30% lesions of BCC. However, BCC can occur anywhere, even without UV exposure by the sun, its occurrence has been observed even on the penis, vulva, scrotum, and perianal areas Effect of BCC is somewhat more observed in men in comparison to women. The younger generation are more vulnerable to the BCC, especially in childhood and adolescence sporadic frivolous sun exposure. Exposure to UVR (UVB has a greater risk than UVA) and overexposure to sun heat (i.e., sunburns) shows substantial risk to develop BCC. Additional aspects such as mutations in regulatory tumor suppressor gene, experiencing ionic radiation, chemicals (arsenic, and PAHs), Psoralen plus ultraviolet A (PUVA) photochemotherapy, and modifications in immune reconnaissance (i.e., organ transplantation, primary hematologic malignancy, immunosuppressive medications, or HIV infection) are involved in the pathogenesis. BCC is considerably more common among childhood cancer survivors, primarily due to prior ionizing radiation treatment with or chemotherapy combination. BCC occurrence found between 20 and 39 years of age in individuals with a history of childhood cancer, and it is more common in cancer survivors, who had received ≥35 Gy versus individuals who did not have radiation therapy [26]. The development of BCC can be due to genetic conditions. Comprised within the nevoid BCC syndrome (NBCCS), Bazex syndrome (X-linked dominant; characterized clinically by follicular atrophoderma, hypotrichosis, hypohidrosis, milia, epidermoid cysts, and facial BCCs), Rombo syndrome (structures like to individuals of Bazex syndrome with marginal vasodilation with cyanosis), xeroderma pigmentosum (an autosomal recessive disorder in spontaneous DNA repair, clinically categorized by numerous NMSCs and melanomas), and individual basal cell nevus syndrome, NBCCS has more prevalence in group of BCC disease. NBCCS is a sporadic autosomal leading disorder defined by a mutation in the patched gene (PTCH1) and tendency to numerous BCC and additional tumors, besides a wide range of developmental abnormalities. In this condition, individuals may develop a broad nasal root, marginal intellect, calcification of the falx cerebri, medulloblastomas, odontogenic keratocysts of the jaw, palmar and plantar pits, and several skeletal abnormalities in addition to a few to thousands of BCCs [27]. As BCCs develop most commonly in sun-exposed areas, it shows sun exposure plays a role in tumor development in patients with NBCCS. Usually, the clinical course is benign before puberty; however, lesions may gradually raise and ulcerate after puberty. Individuals with NBCCS are extremely sensitive to ionizing radiation. Several cases of BCCs were reported in children who have gone through treatment with radiation therapy for medulloblastoma. To understand the molecular signature to the pathogenesis of BCC, a patient with NBCCS has gone through sequencing analysis. This information leads to the behavior of neoplasms in the NBCCS and it confirms a model of carcinogenesis—tumors that develop in cells sustaining two genetic alterations [28]. The first mutational pattern in a TSG is by inheritance, and the second is based on random genetic rearrangement due to inactivation of the normal homologue by environmental mutagenesis factors. Inactivation of the NBCCS, TSG, and PTCH1 is measured and observed main cause of the origin of Intermittent BCCs because of underwent two somatic mutational events. Mutational association with the PTCH1 regulatory gene, which maps to chromosome 9q22.3 was observed with the BCCs studies [29]. In both the sporadic and the hereditary BCCs the loss of heterozygosity at this site is observed. For BCC formation the PTCH1 gene inactivation probably plays a necessary role. The PTCH1 protein is a part of a receptor complex that regulates hedgehog signaling pathway and is a very important regulator of embryonic development and cellular proliferation. Smoothened, a transmembrane receptor for the secreted molecule hedgehog is bound and inhibited by the PTCH1 protein. The inhibitory effects of PTCH1 release Smoothened on the hedgehog binding site and also converts a stimulating signal via GLI transcription factors [20, 30]. Unopposed Smoothened activity and cellular proliferation are permitted by PTCH1 after the loss of function mutation. Therefore, this knowledge of the molecular pathogenesis gives us a ground to develop targeted therapy for BCC with small molecule inhibitors of Smoothened. Some of UV-induced mutations have also been reported in up to 60% of BCCs at the p53 gene [31]. UV light exposure is the prime etiological factor in developing basal cell carcinoma, especially the UVB wavelengths but also the UVA wavelengths. Outdoor workers are significantly at higher risk observed in meta-analysis and sensitivity analysis studies, with an opposite relationship among occupational UV exposure and BCC risk with autonomy. The Fitzpatrick skin type is a suitable marker of the comparative risk of BCC between Whites [25, 32]. UV exposure duration and its intensity also play a role in BCC development along with cumulative UV dose and skin type. Recreational sunlight exposure, use of indoor tanning salons, and UV light therapy may also lead to BCC occurrence. Some other risk factors are obsereved such as intermittent intense sun exposure, sunburning (skin types I or II), blistering in childhood BCC, a fair complexion, ionizing radiation, arsenic exposure, immunosuppression, and genetic predisposition [24]. Some genetic syndromes such as xeroderma pigmentosum, Gorlin Syndrome or basal cell nevus syndrome, Bazex–Dupre–Christol syndrome, and Rombo syndrome are also found to be linked with an increased risk of BCCs. There is no association with diet but smoking also appears to be a risk factor in females [25, 32].

1.4   Squamous Cell Carcinoma

Cutaneous squamous cell carcinoma (SCC) is the second most common nonmelanoma skin cancer (NMSC) after BCC. Neoplasm of keratinizing cells is the main cause of SCC that shows malignant characteristics, including anaplasia, rapid growth, local invasion, and metastatic potential. A recent study of cases of SCC in the USA population on the basis of age-weight incidence ratio is 1.4:1, that predicted high number of SCC burden [33]. Every year in the USA more than 200,000 cases of SCC are diagnosed [34]. And also, a very high number of cases reported in a recent study, the age-standardized incidence rate of SCC in the UK population is 77 cases per 100,000 person-years (PY) [35]. The risk of developing SCC increases more and more with patient age and is highly affected by the amount of ultraviolet (UV) irradiation, exposure based on country latitude and skin phototype of individuals, and is growing with time, expected because of worldwide population aging and improved diagnosis procedures [35, 36]. People of Celtic descent, and same as BCC people with fair complexions, with deprived tanning capability and sensitivity against sunburn, are at increased risk for developing SCC. Conversely, in Blacks SCC most often arises on preexisting inflammatory sites such as scars, burn injuries, or trauma [37]. Patients treated with Psoralen and ultraviolet A radiation (PUVA) or undergoing immunosuppressive therapy following solid-organ transplantation and human papillomavirus (HPV) infections are at increased risk of SCC [36]. Nevertheless, UV exposure for a prolonged period is certainly the main driver of SCC, as observed in the diagnosis and shown at an epidemiologic and molecular level. Mutational signature enrichment shown for $C > T$ transitions at dipyrimidine-sites is related to UVB radiation. In SCC patients, most frequent mutations are in the tumor suppressor gene TP53, but chromosomal rearrangements and as well as genetic alterations have been observed in some other cancer-related genes, such as cyclin-dependent kinase inhibitor 2A (CDKN2A), NOTCH1/2, and RAS [38]. Due to cumulative UV exposure and from a multi-series procedure of accumulation of genetic hits SCC formation occurs. In SCC development another group of genetic disorders is severely observed. Another heterogeneous group of the inherited disorder known as epidermolysis bullosa (EB) is determined by mutations in genes encoding for a building block for cutaneous basement membrane. And during EB skin becomes more fragile and constant blistering shows disease symptoms. Even then defective wound healing is a verse kind of symptoms shown in most EB (sub)types, with fibrosis and inflammation at lesional skin. These features are a way towards serious disease complications, including cutaneous squamous cell carcinomas (SCCs) occurrence. Early and extremely aggressive SCCs (RDEB-SCC) are observed in almost all patients affected with severe recessive dystrophic EB (RDEB) subtype, which is known as the first cause of death in these patients. Less information and the crucial genetic determinants of RDEB-SCC do not thoroughly justify its inimitable behavior as associated with low-risk, ultraviolet-induced SCCs in the population [39, 40].

1.5 Angiosarcoma

Angiosarcoma (AS) is a very rare and extremely aggressive malignant tumor which is also known as malignant hemangioendothelioma, hemangiosarcoma, and lymphangiosarcoma. It originates from lymphatic or vascular endothelial-cell and makes up less than 2% of all soft tissue sarcomas in humans and mainly affects adult and elderly patients [41–43]. Angiosarcoma is a clinically and genetically heterogeneous subgroup of sarcomas that can occur anywhere in the body [44] with an overall incidence of approximately 0.1 per million/year. Cutaneous lesions are the most common site of angiosarcomas (about 60% of cases), especially the head and neck, and can also found within the soft tissues, bone, visceral organs, and retroperitoneum [41–44]. Currently, four variants of cutaneous AS are recognized including AS of the "head and neck" (also known as idiopathic AS) that accounts for 50–60% of all cases, AS in the context of lymphedema (lymphedema-associated AS [LAS]; Stewart-Treves syndrome), radiation-induced AS, and epithelioid AS. However, these variants are different in presentation but share crucial features, like the clinical appearance of primary lesions, a biologically aggressive nature, and, ultimately poor outcomes [41, 44, 45]. According to the studies, the rates of advanced/metastatic disease at presentation differ from 16 to 44%, and the overall survival (OS) range is from 6 to 16 months [46]. Angiosarcoma can occur at any age and has a similar distribution between males and females. However, cutaneous angiosarcoma has been found preferentially in older male individuals, with a reported median age between 60 and 71 years [47]. While the pathogenesis is often unknown in the majority of developing angiosarcoma cases. Several etiological factors, like radiation, environmental carcinogens, chronic lymphoedema, and genetic syndromes are well known for playing an important role in this disease.

1.5.1 Radiation

Radiation is a defined risk factor for benign and malignant tumor development. In retrospective studies, radiation has been associated with the heightened risk of tumors via radiation-induced gene mutation and concurrent chronic lymphoedema [48, 49]. According to an epidemiology survey, the common sources of radiation are occupational exposure, diagnostic, and therapeutic radiation in patients [50]. As radiotherapy is a significant treatment in early-stage sarcomas, particularly for breast sarcomas, therefore, radiation-induced sarcomas are known as the main subtype of secondary sarcomas [51, 52]. Some studies reported breast sarcomas, induced because of radiation have a long latency period after radiation, the median disease-free interval of which was 5–10 years [51, 53, 54]. Hence, beyond the conventional 5-year oncological follow-up, a long-term follow-up is needed to attain the efficient detection of recurrence [53]. The direct relation between angiosarcoma and radiotherapy has not been fully confirmed, but multiple studies outcomes show that with the increased use of radiotherapy for the treatment of angiosarcoma, the risk of radiation-induced angiosarcoma also increases [55, 56]. The high dose of radiotherapy and the incidences of angiosarcoma are also correlated [57]. However, the overall risk of radiation-induced angiosarcoma is little or negligible as compared to the underlying benefit of radiotherapy.

1.5.2 Chronic Lymphoedema

Chronic lymphoedema is another risk factor for angiosarcoma. Chronic lymphoedema and angiosarcoma have been confirmed for having correlation and called Stewart-Treves syndrome (STS) [58]. The Stewart-Treves syndrome is a very sporadic and fatal thing, which is distinct as angiosarcoma rising in the location of chronic lymphedema. It characteristically presents in women after breast conservative surgery followed by adjuvant radiotherapy. The adjuvant radiotherapy in the treatment of early disease is thought to cause the development of STS [50, 58–60]. Some other potential causes are parasitic infections such as filariasis or Milroy's disease, idiopathic, congenital, traumatic, and filarial lymphedema [61]. Approximately 5% of angiosarcomas comprise STS, and it occurs after 5–15 years of local treatment with radiotherapy and surgery [60]. The prediction of STS is unsatisfying, with approximately 10 months survival rate [59]. There is still an argument about the mechanism between secondary angiosarcoma and some forms of chronic lymphedema. In some cases, the mutation of tumor genes, such as p53 and MYC, was thought to be a feasible cofactor [59, 62].

1.5.3 Environmental Carcinogens

Although a major portion around 75% of hepatic angiosarcomas does not exhibit definite etiology [63]. Environmental carcinogens are well known and common factors to induce cancer in many organs in the body. Skin is the most affected organ from environmental polutant due to open exposure from industrial materials such as vinyl chloride monomer and iatrogenic exposure of colloidal thorium dioxides for the radiological examinations, chronic arsenic ingestion [64, 65]. Occupational exposure is the main risk for this disease and most cases are caused by the same [66].

1.5.4 Genetic Syndromes

Approximately 3% of angiosarcomas are gene-induced, gene-associated diseases such as bilateral retinoblastoma, xeroderma pigmentosa, ollier disease, maffucci disease, recklinghausen neurofibromatosis, and Klippel-Trenaunay syndrome. Familial syndromes are associated with angiosarcoma [67]. Some recent genomic studies showed that the dysregulation of angiogenic pathways played a significant role in etiology of angiosarcomas and some other tumor suppressor genes were found to be associated with angiosarcomas, whereas the clinical significance of these findings still should be elucidated [68].

1.6   Dermatofibrosarcoma Protuberans

Dermatofibrosarcoma protuberans (DFSP) is a rare, cutaneous fibrohistiocytic neoplasm that was first defined by Darier and Ferrand in 1924 and the name DFSP was introduced by Hoffman in 1925. With an annual occurrence of 0.8–5 cases/million population, it consists of approximately 1% of all soft tissue sarcomas. DFSP also constitutes approximately 1% of all sarcomas and <0.1% of all malignancies [69]. The vast majority, about 90% of DFSPs are low-grade sarcomas, whereas the rest are classified as intermediate or high grade due to the existence of a high-grade fibrosarcomatous component (DFSP-FS) [70]. Most commonly DFSP affects patients in their mid-to-late 30s; however, people of any age can be affected. DFSP has also been reported in congenital and childhood cases [71]. A comparative higher incidence has been observed in Blacks than Whites. Gender wide also both men and women are equally affected [72]. DFSP rates are highest among Blacks, with a male-to-female ratio of 1:1 and a 5-year relative survival rate of 99% [2–4]. There are no particular risk factors related to DFSP; it can arise in chronically damaged areas or even on healthy skin. With a high rate of local recurrence DFSP typically follows an indolent clinical course because of its infiltrative behavior, but low metastatic potential. Chromosomal translocation is also associated with DFSP tumorigenesis and leads to the fusion of collagen type 1 alpha 1 (COL1A1) and platelet-derived growth factor subunit b (PDGFB) genes. This fusion protein origins a nonstop beginning of the receptor PDGF receptor b (PDGFRB) tyrosine kinase, which indorses DFSP cell growth [73].

1.7   Merkel Cell Carcinoma

Merkel cell carcinoma (MCC) disease is scarce, originated from the neuroendocrine cell, and has a very aggressive tumor showing similarity with mechanoreceptor Merkel cells. In the USA, MCC is an annual incidence with an estimated rate of 3 people per million of the population [74]. Normally MCC is present in men than women, and it increases in White individuals than Black, MCC average diagnosis rate is 70 years [75]. Neural crest is the driving source of Merkel cells, and it differentiates as a part of the amine precursor uptake and decarboxylation system and it also functions as slowly adapting type I mechanoreceptors [75]. Merkel cell tumor is evident in two distinct forms. First, a virus called Merkel cell polyomavirus participates in the pathogenesis of one form of Merkel tumors, and the second is driven by ultraviolet (UV)-linked mutations [73]. MCC is a primary, cutaneous, and neuroendocrine neoplasm associated with a poor prognosis [76–78]. The mortality rate for MCC disease is greater than 40%, significantly higher than that of melanoma and other cutaneous cancers [77, 79]. Some factors as loss of immune competence, prolonged ultraviolet exposure, and advanced age constitute risk factors for developing MCC [76, 77]. Mechanoreceptor cells (located in the basal layer of the epidermis) with MCC tumor cells that originated from the epidermal progenitors during embryonic development play an essential role in the sensory system of the skin [78, 80–82]. As a result of its scarcity and its resemblance with other more common neuroendocrine tumors, such as small cell lung carcinoma determining the incidence of MCC has been challenging. Across the regions of the world, the incidence rate of MCC is varied. In the USA in 2018, the incidence rate reported by SEER analysis (surveillance, epidemiology, and end results) was 0.79 per 100,000 [83]. According to the RARECARE database, reported incidence of MCC in Europe, are 0.13 per 100,000 (1995 and 2002) [84]. In the last 20 years in the USA and Europe, the incidence of this neoplasm has quadrupled, perhaps due to systemic immune suppression, increasing UV exposure, and longer lifespan [83]. It is also reported Australia has the highest incidence of 1.6 per 100,000 from 1993 to 2010 [85]. According to a recent study from 2000 to 2013, the incidence of MCC is outpacing that of other cancers with an increase of 95% [86]. The authors of that study have predicted the numbers of newly diagnosed cases would possibly increase from 2488 to 3284 in a leap of years from 2013 to 2025 [86, 87]. It is discovered that integration of polyomavirus genome in the genome of MCC tumor cells increases the tumor insidence. This created a major paradigm shift in the understanding of the etiology of MCC. MCC was chosen and subjected to digital transcriptome subtraction (DTS), a direct sequencing-based method due to its strong association with immunosuppression and because of its epidemiology [88, 89]. Polyomaviruses have also been previously connected to human disease [90]. However, unlike other polyomaviruses, MCV found to be the first polyomavirus and a causative agent, which is convincingly linked to human cancer [91]. World Health Organization (WHO) and the International Agency for Research on Cancer (IARC) classified it as a Group 2A carcinogen due to its compelling evidence of causation [92]. Type of MCC was identified by MCPyV-negative and MCPyV-positive tumor incidence, and MCPyV-negative has a higher number of chromosomal aberrations and UV-specific mutation burden [93–97]. This is reported that virus-negative tumors may be clinically more aggressive [98]. This aggressive nature of MCC tumor has been associated with higher exposure to risk factors, as well as a changed immune system. UV radiation is a risk factor for MCC. The appearance of tumors is more common in skin areas with substantial UV radiation exposure; the incidence of MCC associates with UVB radiation index and other skin cancers subsequent from sun exposure. White patients are frequently affected than other races. Patients with the underlying immunosuppressed condition, such as those with hematologic malignancies, a developed immunodeficiency syndrome (AIDS), autoimmune disease, and a history of solid organ transplant, are at higher risk for developing MCC [94–98].

1.8 Microcystic Adnexal Carcinoma

Microcystic adnexal carcinoma (MAC) is a type of skin cancer which is described in literature as aggressive trichofolliculoma, combined adnexal tumor, carcinoma with syringomatous features, malignant syringoma, sclerosing sweat duct carcinoma, sweat gland tumor. MAC was first defined as a separate subject in 1982 by Goldstein et al. [99]. The origin of MAC is from pluripotent adnexal keratinocytes and it is capable of both eccrine and follicular differentiation. MAC is not clearly observed with pathogenesis but may involve exposure to ionizing and UVR that may lead to the growth of MAC as long as 40 years [100]. MAC is very aggressive and has a high rate of local recurrence with nearby damaging cutaneous appendageal neoplasm but has a low rate of metastasis. It mainly affects White, middle-aged people, though it has been reported in children and Blacks. Comparative to further main cutaneous malignancies, MAC shows a small female prevalence. CD 10 expression is found to have 60% of infiltrative basal cell carcinoma, 31% of microcystic adnexal carcinoma, and 25% of squamous cell carcinoma. The expression of BerEP4 was reported in 38% of microcystic adnexal carcinoma, desmoplastic trichoepithelioma has 57%, infiltrative basal cell carcinoma is 100%, and 38% of squamous cell carcinoma [101].

1.9   Sebaceous Carcinoma

Sebaceous carcinoma (SC) is a type of skin cancer that has variable sites of origin it develops a malignant adnexal tumor, it observed through histologic growth patterns, and clinical presentations. Around 75% of SCs are periocular in location [102]. Periocular SC might arise from Meibomian glands and a few from the glands of Zeis. Eyelids are most frequently involved in SC development, and approximately 25% of cases of SC involve extraocular sites, which might be included in the head and neck, trunk, salivary glands, and external genitalia [103]. Globally SC affects most of the race, but Asian race is more vulnerable to the SC disease. With a noticeable ratio of 2:1, women are affected more commonly than men. SC is associated with sebaceous adenomas, radiation exposure, and Muir Torre syndrome and classically presents in the seventh to ninth decades [104]. As SC shows robust connotation with Muir Torre syndrome, colonoscopy is used to understand the colon cancer incidence. Repetitive genetic screening for Muir Torre in the absence of colon lesions is not commonly observed. Sebaceous carcinoma typically presents in older age mostly after 60 years, on the eyelid, head and neck, and trunk. Diagnosis through deep biopsy is frequently required; also, differential diagnoses that imitate the condition can be omitted with special histological stains [105]. It is quite common to detect false benign conditions, follow-on in inappropriate management. Therefore, this is of utmost importance to uphold a high index of doubt. Notwithstanding earlier reports, sebaceous carcinoma might have occurred with similar frequency in Asians and Whites. Genetic data suggest that there are numerous mutational groups of sebaceous carcinomas, help the way for specific treatment of SC.

1.10 Extramammary Paget Disease

Extramammary Paget disease (EMPD) is a rare cutaneous malignancy condition that occurs mostly on apocrine rich skin of mid-age to older individuals, frequently on the genitalia. Paget disease was described in 1874, by Sir James Paget, also known as mammary Paget disease. This disease reintroduced as extramammary Paget disease (EMPD) of the scrotum and penis in 1889. Although there is a slight female prevalence in Caucasian patients, there is a strong 4:1 male prevalence in Asians [106].

It is histologically similar to Paget disease of the breast, EMPD is another class of disease other than breast cancer with a distinct. Mostly EMPD is a malignant form of cancer from a primary intraepidermal origin which is from eccrine or apocrine glands. It is also associated with internal malignancy in 15% to 30% of cases, usually colon, bladder, or prostate cancer [107] that could lead to secondary EMPD with less prognosis than primary EMPD. Surgical operation is the treatment of choice; nevertheless, procedures tend to be extensive and associated with a high rate of recurrence. EMPD is a slowly red plaque disease that looks like an inflammatory condition and this affects diagnosis delay. Diagnosis requires histopathologic examination and is frequently supported by immunohistochemical analysis. EMPD diagnosis in the patient is evaluated further for malignancy. Data suggested that Mohs micrographic surgery might have superior clinical outcomes and lower recurrence rates. Substitutes therapy, photodynamic therapy, and topicals have been explored and may be suitable in some cases. Patients with EMPD generally have a good prognosis with a 5-year overall survival rate of 75% to 95%. Although mammary and extramammary Paget disease are both characterized by epidermal Paget cells and part a parallel clinical presentation, their exclusivity deceits in anatomical site and histogenesis. Immunohistochemical staining lets for differentiation among primary and secondary EMPD in adding to the various other disease objects that clinically look like this malignancy. Surgical removal is utilized as first-line therapy and the prognosis is frequently favorable. Current developments inside the ground have inspected the expression of chemokine receptors inside tumors, which may be appropriate in decisive prognosis [108].

1.11 Atypical Fibroxanthoma and Malignant Fibrous Histiocytoma

Atypical fibroxanthoma (AFX) is a rare cutaneous soft tissue tumor, atypical fibroxanthoma (AFX) and malignant fibrous histiocytoma were supposed to be two separate parts of the same malignancy. WHO describes AFX as soft tissue sarcomas that identifies cell line beginning in the classification of tumors. As earlier considered, maximum cases of malignant fibrous histiocytoma, were found to be simply a morphologic pattern somewhat a defined pathologic condition [109]. In most of the cases, ultrastructural and immunohistochemical inspection permitted for recognition into distinct histologic subtypes of sarcomas. On that basis updated classification of the term malignant fibrous histiocytoma is presented as a substitute for undistinguishable pleomorphic sarcoma (UPS). This cancer type is a deep-seated subcutaneous nodule infrequently comes across in the skin; it is mostly seen on the limbs of old aged individuals. UPS has a very poor prognosis that leads to aggressive tumor development. Though surgical excision is the first-line treatment (normally with adjuvant RT), up to 50% of patients may have distant metastasis at the time of initial condition, and the nearest affected organ is the lung. It affects typically the elderly on sun-exposed skin.

Atypical fibroxanthoma presents as a red nodule or plaque, and as frequently AFX effect on the head and neck of sun-exposed people and on the trunk and edges of younger patients [110]. AFX has similar histologic features to undifferentiated pleomorphic sarcoma, and it is less aggressive. Tumor development in the AFX characterized by the time point of the head and neck present during the eighth phase, while tumors connecting the boundaries often present during the fourth phase [111, 112]. The gender ratio is almost to be equal. A very small number of cases are reported with xeroderma pigmentosum. AFX pathogenesis involves UV exposure, ionizing radiation, and abnormal immune host response. The most common mutation with UVR showed TSG p53 mutation. Typically, after ionization radiation tumors might occur after 10–15 years. A high number of AFX incidences occurred in patients with renal transplant and metastatic condition and patient with chronic lymphocytic leukemia [113].

1.12 Carcinoma Metastatic to Skin

The metastatic tumors of the skin are primary tumors same as of the breast, lung, or melanoma; and skin metastases also become sporadic by other primary carcinomas. Metastasis stage of cutaneous visceral carcinomas normally occurs in patients with progressive disease and is linked with a poor prognosis. Cutaneous participation is also seen in the leukemias, with an extensive disparity in the morphology of lesions. Cutaneous metastatic disease is most common in the scalp. It may be helpful to utilize immunohistochemical stains to determine the place of the primary tumor. Management strategies such as prompt consultation with oncologists may help in the pathogenesis of tumor stage determination [114].

1.13 Conclusion

Ultraviolet (UV) light from the sun is the main cause of most skin cancers. DNA damage by UV light predominantly plays important role in skin cancer. Too much sun exposure from an early age is the primary cause of developing basal cell carcinomas (BCCs) or squamous cell carcinoma (SCCs). Sun exposure over a long time can cause both types of skin cancer but it is most common in SCC. People who work outdoors such as farmworkers, builders, and gardeners are more at risk of developing skin cancer. Normally skin cancer comes very late at an age like after

40 and commonly occurs in older age. Though the rising number of incidences is seen in younger. Using sunbeds and sunlamps rises the risk of emerging some skin cancers. Squamous cell carcinoma in situ is also called Bowen's disease. That abnormal growth of cells leads to outer layer of the skin (the epidermis), and these cells do not spread into the deeper layers of the skin. Sometime when Bowens disease left untreated may cause to develop SCC. A weak Immune system is also a prominent factor in developing SCC. Another possible rare cause for nonmelanoma skin cancer is overexposure to certain chemicals, usually at work. Most skin cancer is not genetically transferred on to other family members. Biological families are possible to have the same skin characters that may lead to their risk of developing cancer in the skin. In some cases, such as rare genetic like Gorlin syndrome, epidermolysis bullosa (EB), xeroderma pigmentosum (XP) have a higher risk of developing skin cancer. Persistent ingestion of arsenic in drinking water is associated with a higher risk of skin cancer and bladder cancer, and as it is reported occupational and medical exposure to arsenic has been clearly associated with skin cancer in epidemiological studies.

Conflict of Interest The author declares no conflict of interest.

References

1. Madan V, Lear JT, Szeimies RM (2010) Non-melanoma skin cancer. Lancet 375:673–685
2. Stern RS (2010) Prevalence of a history of skin cancer in 2007: results of an incidence-based model. Arch Dermatol 146:279–282
3. Rogers HW, Weinstock MA, Harris AR et al (2010) Incidence estimate of nonmelanoma skin cancer in the United States, 2006. Arch Dermatol 146:283–287
4. Berman B, Amini S, Valins W et al (2009) Pharmacotherapy of actinic keratosis. Expert Opin Pharmacother 10:3015–3031
5. Schwartz RA (1997) The actinic keratosis. A perspective and update. Dermatol Surg 23:1009–1019
6. Salasche SJ (2000) Epidemiology of actinic keratoses and squamous cell carcinoma. J Am Acad Dermatol 42:4–7
7. Rodriguez-Vigil T, Vazquez-Lopez F, Perez-Oliva N (2007) Recurrence rates of primary basal cell carcinoma in facial risk areas treated with curettage and electrodesiccation. J Am Acad Dermatol 56:91–95
8. Brash DE, Ziegler A, Jonason AS et al (1996) Sunlight and sunburn in human skin cancer: p53, apoptosis, and tumor promotion. J Investig Dermatol Symp Proc 1:136–142
9. Ulrich C, Bichel J, Euvrard S et al (2007) Topical immunomodulation under systemic immunosuppression: results of a multicentre, randomized, placebo-controlled safety and efficacy study of imiquimod 5% cream for the treatment of actinic keratoses in kidney, heart, and liver transplant patients. Br J Dermatol 157:25–31
10. Tanghetti E, Werschler P (2007) Comparison of 5% 5-fluorouracil cream and 5% imiquimod cream in the management of actinic keratoses on the face and scalp. J Drugs Dermatol 6:144–147
11. Cognetta AB, Howard BM, Heaton HP et al (2012) Superficial x-ray in the treatment of basal and squamous cell carcinomas: a viable option in select patients. J Am Acad Dermatol 67:1235–1241

12. Veness MJ (2008) The important role of radiotherapy in patients with non-melanoma skin cancer and other cutaneous entities. J Med Imaging Radiat Oncol 52:278–286
13. Krawtchenko N, Roewert-Huber J, Ulrich M et al (2007) A randomised study of topical 5% imiquimod vs. topical 5-fluorouracil vs. cryosurgery in immunocompetent patients with actinic keratoses: a comparison of clinical and histological outcomes including 1- year follow-up. Br J Dermatol 157:34–40
14. Piacquadio DJ, Chen DM, Farber HF et al (2004) Photodynamic therapy with aminolevulinic acid topical solution and visible blue light in the treatment of multiple actinic keratoses of the face and scalp: investigator-blinded, phase 3, multicenter trials. Arch Dermatol 140:41–46
15. Smith S, Piacquadio D, Morhenn V et al (2003) Short incubation PDT versus 5-FU in treating actinic keratoses. J Drugs Dermatol 2:629–635
16. Poojan S, Kumar S, Verma V, Dhasmana A, Lohani M, Verma MK (2015) Disruption of skin stem cell homeostasis following transplacental arsenicosis; alleviation by combined intake of selenium and curcumin. PLoS One 10(12):e0142818
17. Szeimies RM, Karrer S, Radakovic-Fijan S et al (2002) Photodynamic therapy using topical methyl 5-aminolevulinate compared with cryotherapy for actinic keratosis: a prospective, randomized study. J Am Acad Dermatol 47:258–262
18. Rivers JK, Arlette J, Shear N et al (2002) Topical treatment of actinic keratoses with 3.0% diclofenac in 2.5% hyaluronan gel. Br J Dermatol 146:94–100
19. Weiss ET, Brauer JA, Anolik R et al (2013) 1927-nm fractional resurfacing of facial actinic keratosis: a promising new therapeutic option. J Am Acad Dermatol 68:98–102
20. Lacour JP (2002) Carcinogenesis of basal cell carcinomas: genetics and molecular mechanisms. Br J Dermatol 146:17
21. Wang Y, Wells W, Waldron J (2009) Indications and outcomes of radiation therapy for skin cancer of the head and neck. Clin Plast Surg 36:335–344
22. Clarissa PHR, Renato MB (2019) Actinic keratoses: review of clinical, dermoscopic, and therapeutic aspects. An Bras Dermatol 94(6):637–657
23. Dai J, Lin K, Huang Y, Lu Y, Chen WQ, Zhang XR, He BS, Pan YQ, Wang SK, Fan WX (2018) Identification of critically carcinogenesis-related genes in basal cell carcinoma. Onco Targets Ther 11:6957–6967
24. De Giorgi V, Savarese I, Gori A, Scarfi F, Topa A, Trane L, Portelli F, Innocenti A, Covarelli P (2020) Advanced basal cell carcinoma: when a good drug is not enough. J Dermatolog Treat 31(6):552–553
25. Martens MC, Seebode C, Lehmann J, Emmert S (2018) Photocarcinogenesis and skin cancer prevention strategies: an update. Anticancer Res 38(2):1153–1158
26. Watt TC, Inskip PD, Stratton K et al (2012) Radiation-related risk of basal cell carcinoma: a report from the childhood cancer survivor study. J Natl Cancer Inst 104:1240–1250
27. Epstein EH (2008) Basal cell carcinomas: attack of the hedgehog. Nat Rev Cancer 8:743–754
28. Grossman D, Leffell DJ (1997) The molecular basis of nonmelanoma skin cancer: new understanding. Arch Dermatol 133:1263–1270
29. Situm M, Buljan M, Bulat V et al (2008) The role of UV radiation in the development of basal cell carcinoma. Coll Antropol 32(suppl 2):167–170
30. Lupi O (2007) Correlations between the sonic hedgehog pathway and basal cell carcinoma. Int J Dermatol 46:1113–1117
31. Ziegler A, Leffell DJ, Kunala S et al (1993) Mutation hotspots due to sunlight in the p53 gene of nonmelanoma skin cancers. Proc Natl Acad Sci U S A 90:4216–4220
32. Kamath P, Darwin E, Arora H, Nouri K (2018) A review on imiquimod therapy and discussion on optimal management of basal cell carcinomas. Clin Drug Investig 38(10):883–899
33. Chahal HS, Rieger KE, Sarin KY (2017) Incidence ratio of basal cell carcinoma to squamous cell carcinoma equalizes with age. J Am Acad Dermatol 76:353–354
34. Karia PS, Han J, Schmults CD (2013) Cutaneous squamous cell carcinoma: estimated incidence of disease, nodal metastasis, and deaths from disease in the United States in 2012. J Am Acad Dermatol 68:957–966

35. Venables ZC, Nijsten T, Wong KF, Autier P, Broggio J, Deas A, Harwood CA, Hollestein LM, Langan SM, Morgan E et al (2019) Epidemiology of basal and cutaneous squamous cell carcinoma in the U.K. 2013-15: a cohort study. Br J Dermatol 181:474–482

36. Que SKT, Zwald FO, Schmults CD (2018) Cutaneous squamous cell carcinoma: incidence, risk factors, diagnosis, and staging. J Am Acad Dermatol 78:237–247

37. Gloster HM Jr, Brodland DG (1996) The epidemiology of skin cancer. Dermatol Surg 22:217–226

38. Inman GJ, Wang J, Nagano A, Alexandrov LB, Purdie KJ, Taylor RG, Sherwood V, Thomson J, Hogan S, Spender LC et al (2018) The genomic landscape of cutaneous SCC reveals drivers and a novel azathioprine associated mutational signature. Nat Commun 9:3667

39. Kim YW, Kim YH, Song Y et al (2019) Monitoring circulating tumor DNA by analyzing personalized cancer-specific rearrangements to detect recurrence in gastric cancer. Exp Mol Med 51(8):1–10

40. Condorelli AG, Dellambra E, Logli E, Zambruno G, Castiglia D (2019) Epidermolysis bullosa-associated squamous cell carcinoma: from pathogenesis to therapeutic perspectives. Int J Mol Sci 20(22):5707

41. Young RJ, Brown NJ, Reed MW, Hughes D, Woll PJ (2010) Angiosarcoma. Lancet Oncol 11:983–991

42. Mark RJ, Poen JC, Tran LM, Fu YS, Juillard GF (1996) Angiosarcoma. A report of 67 patients and a review of the literature. Cancer 77:2400–2406

43. Khan JA, Maki RG, Ravi V (2018) Pathologic angiogenesis of malignant vascular sarcomas: implications for treatment. J Clin Oncol 36:194–201

44. Buehler D, Rice SR, Moody JS, Rush P, Hafez GR, Attia S, Longley BJ, Kozak KR (2014) Angiosarcoma outcomes and prognostic factors: a 25-year single institution experience. Am J Clin Oncol 37:473–479

45. Mullin C, Clifford CA (2019) Histiocytic sarcoma and hemangiosarcoma update. Vet Clin North Am Small Anim Pract 49:855–879

46. Buehler D (2014) Angiosarcoma outcomes and prognostic factors. Am J Clin Oncol 37:473–479

47. Lahat G, Dhuka AR, Hallevi H, Xiao L, Zou C, Smith KD, Phung TL, Pollock RE, Benjamin R, Hunt KK, Lazar AJ, Lev D (2010) Angiosarcoma: clinical and molecular insights. Ann Surg 251:1098–1106

48. Yin M, Wang W, Drabick JJ, Harold HA (2017) Prognosis and treatment of non-metastatic primary and secondary breast angiosarcoma: a comparative study. BMC Cancer 17:295

49. Verdura V, Di Pace B, Concilio M, Guastafierro A, Fiorillo G, Alfano L, Nicoletti GF, Savastano C, Cascone AM, Rubino C (2019) A new case of radiation-induced breast angiosarcoma. Int J Surg Case Rep 60:152–155

50. Peterson CB, Beauregard S (2016) Radiation-induced breast angiosarcoma: case report and clinical approach. J Cutan Med Surg 20:304–307

51. Virtanen A, Pukkala E, Auvinen A (2007) Angiosarcoma after radiotherapy: a cohort study of 332,163 finnish cancer patients. Br J Cancer 97:115–117

52. Disharoon M, Kozlowski KF, Kaniowski JM (2017) Case 242: radiation-induced angiosarcoma. Radiology 283:909–916

53. Amajoud Z, Vertongen AS, Weytens R, Hauspy J (2018) Radiation induced angiosarcoma of the breast: case series and review of the literature. Facts Views Vis Obgyn 10:215–220

54. Miller R, Mudambi L, Vial MR, Kalhor N, Grosu HB (2017) Radiation-induced angiosarcoma as a cause of pleural effusion. Am J Respir Crit Care Med 196:e10–e11

55. Plichta JK, Hughes K (2017) Radiation-induced angiosarcoma after breast-cancer treatment. N Engl J Med 376:367

56. Alves I, Marques JC (2018) Radiation-induced angiosarcoma of the breast: a retrospective analysis of 15 years' experience at an oncology center. Radiol Bras 51:281–286

57. Seo CJ, Lek SM, Tan GHC, Teo M (2017) Radiation-associated peritoneal angiosarcoma. BMJ Case Rep 2017:217887

58. Pereira ES, Moraes ET, Siqueira DM, Santos MA (2015) Stewart Treves syndrome. An Bras Dermatol 90(Suppl 1):229–231
59. Berebichez-Fridman R, Deutsch YE, Joyal TM, Olvera PM, Benedetto PW, Rosenberg AE, Kett DH (2016) Stewart-Treves syndrome: a case report and review of the literature. Case Rep Oncol 9:205–211
60. Cui L, Zhang J, Zhang X, Chang H, Qu C, Zhang J, Zhong D (2015) Angiosarcoma (Stewart-Treves syndrome) in postmastectomy patients: report of 10 cases and review of literature. Int J Clin Exp Pathol 8:11108–11115
61. Mesli SN, Ghouali AK, Benamara F, Taleb FA, Tahraoui H, Abi-Ayad C (2017) Stewart-Treves syndrome involving chronic lymphedema after mastectomy of breast cancer. Case Rep Surg 2017:4056459
62. Benmansour A, Laanaz S, Bougtab A (2014) Stewart-Treves syndrome: a case report. Pan Afr Med J 19:2
63. Tripke V, Heinrich S, Huber T, Mittler J, Hoppe-Lotichius M, Straub BK, Lang H (2019) Surgical therapy of primary hepatic angiosarcoma. BMC Surg 19:5
64. Chaudhary P, Bhadana U, Singh RA, Ahuja A (2015) Primary hepatic angiosarcoma. Eur J Surg Oncol 41:1137–1143
65. Choi JH, Ahn KC, Chang H, Minn KW, Jin US, Kim BJ (2015) Surgical treatment and prognosis of angiosarcoma of the scalp: a retrospective analysis of 14 patients in a single institution. Biomed Res Int 2015:321896
66. Tran Minh M, Mazzola A, Perdigao F, Charlotte F, Rousseau G, Conti F (2018) Primary hepatic angiosarcoma and liver transplantation: radiological, surgical, histological findings and clinical outcome. Clin Res Hepatol Gastroenterol 42:17–23
67. Blatt J, Finger M, Price V, Crary SE, Pandya A, Adams DM (2019) Cancer risk in Klippel-Trenaunay syndrome. Lymphat Res Biol 17(6):630–636
68. Cao J, Wang J, He C, Fang M (2019) Angiosarcoma: a review of diagnosis and current treatment. Am J Cancer Res 9(11):2303–2313
69. Kampshoff JL, Cogbill TH (2009) Unusual skin tumors: Merkel cell carcinoma, eccrine carcinoma, glomus tumors, and dermatofibrosarcoma protuberans. Surg Clin North Am 89:727–738
70. Abbott JJ, Oliveira AM, Nascimento AG (2006) The prognostic significance of fibrosarcomatous transformation in dermatofibrosarcoma protuberans. Am J Surg Pathol 30:436–443
71. Gu W, Ogose A, Kawashima H et al (2005) Congenital dermatofibrosarcoma protuberans with fibrosarcomatous and myxoid change. J Clin Pathol 58:984–986
72. Monnier D, Vidal C, Martin L, Danzon A, Pelletier F, Puzenat E, Algros MP, Blanc D, Laurent R, Humbert PH, Aubin F (2006) Dermatofibrosarcoma protuberans: a population-based cancer registry descriptive study of 66 consecutive cases diagnosed between 1982 and 2002. J Eur Acad Dermatol Venereol 20(10):1237–1242
73. Arora R, Rekhi B, Chandrani P, Krishna S, Dutt A (2019) Merkel cell polyomavirus is implicated in a subset of Merkel cell carcinomas, in the Indian subcontinent. Microb Pathog 137:103778
74. Haag ML, Glass LF, Fenske NA (1995) Merkel cell carcinoma. Diagnosis and treatment. Dermatol Surg 21:669–683
75. Rockville Merkel Cell Carcinoma Group (2009) Merkel cell carcinoma: recent progress and current priorities on etiology, pathogenesis, and clinical management. J Clin Oncol 27:4021–4026
76. Hodgson NC (2005) Merkel cell carcinoma: changing incidence trends. J Surg Oncol 89:1–4
77. Becker JC, Stang A, DeCaprio JA, Cerroni L, Lebbe C, Veness M et al (2017) Merkel cell carcinoma. Nat Rev Dis Primers 3:17077
78. Schadendorf D, Lebbe C, Zur Hausen A, Avril MF, Hariharan S, Bharmal M et al (2017) Merkel cell carcinoma: epidemiology, prognosis, therapy and unmet medical needs. Eur J Cancer 71:53–69

79. Lemos B, Nghiem P (2007) Merkel cell carcinoma: more deaths but still no pathway to blame. J Investig Dermatol 127:2100–2103
80. Haeberle H, Fujiwara M, Chuang J, Medina MM, Panditrao MV, Bechstedt S et al (2004) Molecular profiling reveals synaptic release machinery in Merkel cells. Proc Natl Acad Sci U S A 101:14503–14508
81. Lucarz A, Brand G (2007) Current considerations about Merkel cells. Eur J Cell Biol 86:243–251
82. Van Keymeulen A, Mascre G, Youseff KK, Harel I, Michaux C, De Geest N et al (2009) Epidermal progenitors give rise to Merkel cells during embryonic development and adult homeostasis. J Cell Biol 187:91–100
83. Fitzgerald TL, Dennis S, Kachare SD, Vohra NA, Wong JH, Zervos EE (2015) Dramatic increase in the incidence and mortality from Merkel cell carcinoma in the United States. Am Surg 81:802–806
84. van der Zwan JM, Trama A, Otter R, Larranaga N, Tavilla A, Marcos-Gragera R et al (2013) Rare neuroendocrine tumours: results of the surveillance of rare cancers in Europe project. Eur J Cancer 49:2565–2578
85. Youlden DR, Soyer HP, Youl PH, Fritschi L, Baade PD (2014) Incidence and survival for Merkel cell carcinoma in Queensland, Australia, 1993-2010. JAMA Dermatol 150:864–872
86. Paulson KG, Park SY, Vandeven NA, Lachance K, Thomas H, Chapuis AG et al (2018) Merkel cell carcinoma: current US incidence and projected increases based on changing demographics. J Am Acad Dermatol 78:457–463
87. Voelker R (2018) Why Merkel cell cancer is garnering more attention. JAMA 320(1):18–20
88. Feng H, Shuda M, Chang Y, Moore PS (2008) Clonal integration of a polyomavirus in human Merkel cell carcinoma. Science 319:1096–1100
89. Feng H, Taylor JL, Benos PV, Newton R, Waddell K, Lucas SB et al (2007) Human transcriptome subtraction by using short sequence tags to search for tumor viruses in conjunctival carcinoma. J Virol 81:11332–11340
90. Gjoerup O, Chang Y (2010) Update on human polyomaviruses and cancer. Adv Cancer Res 106:1–51
91. DeCaprio JA (2017) Merkel cell polyomavirus and Merkel cell carcinoma. Philos Trans R Soc Lond B Biol Sci 372:20160276
92. Bouvard V, Baan RA, Grosse Y, Lauby-Secretan B, El Ghissassi F, Benbrahim-Tallaa L et al (2012) Carcinogenicity of malaria and of some polyomaviruses. Lancet Oncol 13:339–340
93. Goh G, Walradt T, Markarov V, Blom A, Riaz N, Doumani R et al (2016) Mutational landscape of MCPyV-positive and MCPyV-negative Merkel cell carcinomas with implications for immunotherapy. Oncotarget 7:3403–3415
94. Paulson KG, Lemos BD, Feng B, Jaimes N, Penas PF, Bi X et al (2009) Array-CGH reveals recurrent genomic changes in Merkel cell carcinoma including amplification of L-Myc. J Investig Dermatol 129:1547–1555
95. Starrett GJ, Marcelus C, Cantalupo PG, Katz JP, Cheng J, Akagi K, Thakuria M, Rabinowits G, Wang LC, Symer DE, Pipas JM, Harris RS, DeCaprio JA (2017) Merkel cell polyomavirus exhibits dominant control of the tumor genome and transcriptome in virus-associated Merkel cell carcinoma. MBio 8(1):e02079–e02016
96. Harms PW, Collie AM, Hovelson DH, Cani AK, Verhaegen ME, Patel RM et al (2016) Next generation sequencing of cytokeratin 20-negative Merkel cell carcinoma reveals ultraviolet-signature mutations and recurrent TP53 and RB1 inactivation. Mod Pathol 29:240–248
97. Harms PW, Vats P, Verhaegen ME, Robinson DR, Wu YM, Dhanasekaran SM et al (2015) The distinctive mutational spectra of polyomavirus-negative Merkel cell carcinoma. Cancer Res 75:3720–3727
98. Moshiri AS, Doumani R, Yelistratova L, Blom A, Lachance K, Shinohara MM et al (2017) Polyomavirus-negative Merkel cell carcinoma: a more aggressive subtype based on analysis of 282 cases using multimodal tumor virus detection. J Investig Dermatol 137:819–827

99. Goldstein DJ, Barr RJ, Santa Cruz DJ (1982) Microcystic adnexal carcinoma: a distinct clinicopathologic entity. Cancer 50:566–572
100. Leibovitch I, Huilgol SC, Selva D et al (2005) Microcystic adnexal carcinoma: treatment with Mohs micrographic surgery. J Am Acad Dermatol 52:295–300
101. Hoang MP, Dresser KA, Kapur P, High WA, Mahalingam M (2008) Microcystic adnexal carcinoma: an immunohistochemical reappraisal. Mod Pathol 21(2):178–185
102. Eisen DB, Michael DJ (2009) Sebaceous lesions and their associated syndromes: part I. J Am Acad Dermatol 61:549–560
103. Dasgupta T, Wilson LD, Yu JB (2009) A retrospective review of 1349 cases of sebaceous carcinoma. Cancer 115:158–165
104. Tan KC, Lee ST, Cheah ST (1991) Surgical treatment of sebaceous carcinoma of eyelids with clinico-pathological correlation. Br J Plast Surg 44:117–121
105. Owen JL et al (2019) Sebaceous carcinoma: evidence-based clinical practice guidelines. Lancet Oncol 20(12):e699–e714
106. Lee K, Roh MR, Chung WG et al (2009) Comparison of Mohs micrographic surgery and wide excision for extramammary Paget's disease: Korean experience. Dematol Surg 35:34–40
107. Ito Y, Igawa S, Ohishi Y et al (2012) Prognostic indicators in 35 patients with extramammary Paget's disease. Dermatol Surg 38:1938–1944
108. St Claire K, Hoover A, Ashack K, Khachemoune A (2019) Extramammary Paget disease. Dermatol Online J 25(4):13030
109. Fletcher CD (2006) The evolving classification of soft tissue tumours: an update based on the new WHO classification. Histopathology 48:3–12
110. Tanese K (2019) Diagnosis and management of basal cell carcinoma. Curr Treat Options Oncol 20(2):13
111. Scelsi CL, Wang A, Garvin CM, Bajaj M, Forseen SE, Gilbert BC (2019) Head and neck sarcomas: a review of clinical and imaging findings based on the 2013 World Health Organization classification. Am J Roentgenol 212:644–654
112. Chaturvedi AK, Engels EA, Pfeiffer RM, Hernandez BY, Xiao W, Kim E, Jiang B, Goodman MT, Sibug-Saber M, Cozen W, Liu L, Lynch CF, Wentzensen N, Jordan RC, Altekruse S, Anderson WF, Rosenberg PS, Gillison ML (2011) Human papillomavirus and rising oropharyngeal cancer incidence in the United States. J Clin Oncol 29(32):4294–4301
113. Dei Tos AP, Maestro R, Doglioni C et al (1994) Ultraviolet-induced p53 mutations in atypical fibroxanthoma. Am J Pathol 145:11–17
114. Ruiz SJ, Al Salihi S, Prieto VG et al (2019) Unusual cutaneous metastatic carcinoma. Ann Diagn Pathol 43:151399

Therapeutic Intervention in Skin Cancer: Future Prospects

Ratika Srivastava

Abstract

There have been remarkable advancements in melanoma therapy. Melanomas treatment specifically has received maximum number of different drug moieties being approved by Food and Drug Administration, USA. Among all the different therapeutics, immunotherapy has gained maximum attention with the advent of checkpoint inhibitor based approaches, which mainly work upon retrieving back host own anti-cancer immunity through blocking of the specific molecules suppressing such responses. Besides that many other immunotherapy approaches such as vaccines development have gained attention. Among nonimmunotherapy approaches, many signaling pathway inhibitors are also delivered in form of small molecule based drugs. Most of the approaches have led the treatment approaches towards personalized therapies. Hence, biomarkers for decision-making at stage of opting therapy, patient management, toxicity profiling, are need of future.

Keywords

Immuno-oncology · Immunotherapy · Checkpoint inhibitor · Melanoma vaccine · Oncolytic viruses · Circulating cell free DNA · Microbiome · Targeted therapy

Metastatic melanoma is considered as one of the most incurable cancers with most of the patients dying within 2 years of diagnosis. Conventional treatment options like surgery, radiotherapy, and chemotherapy were the only options patients had till last decade. In recent past, potential of host own immune response to eliminate cancer cells has been realized gradually with emergence of concept of hot and cold tumors.

R. Srivastava (✉)
Department of Microbiology and Biotechnology Center, The Maharaja Sayajirao University of Baroda, Vadodara, Gujarat, India

© The Author(s), under exclusive license to Springer Nature Singapore Pte Ltd. 2021
A. Dwivedi et al. (eds.), *Skin Cancer: Pathogenesis and Diagnosis*,
https://doi.org/10.1007/978-981-16-0364-8_2

21

With better understanding of mechanisms of T cell response at tumor site has led to design and deliver immune response based therapies known as immunotherapy. Major objective of immunotherapy is to augment antitumor immunity by eliminating the hurdles which do not allow host immune response to mount to the required extent. Success of such approach can be assessed by the fact that U.S. Food and Drug Administration (FDA) approved seven novel immunotherapeutic agents in just 5 years (2011–2015).

Patients who are undergoing surgery still further need to undergo radio and/or chemotherapy for postoperative clinical management. There are multiple concerns associated with radio and chemotherapy including resistance or no responsiveness, related side effects and variability in patient to patient tolerability towards radio- and chemotherapy. To overcome these challenges as well to augment the overall antitumor efficacy, the neoadjuvant and immune response based approaches came into limelight. With the best advancements in the field in last one decade, beside the conventional therapies, following new treatment options are being offered to melanoma patients either as monotherapy or combination therapy with conventional therapies or other non-conventional therapies.

1. Immunotherapy
2. Targeted therapy
3. Oncolytic virus based therapy
4. Photodynamic therapy

In all the above mentioned class of therapy, exciting new innovations are being added up rapidly, raising a new hope for melanoma patients. In this chapter we will review these new treatment options, challenges associated with, and future challenges.

2.1   Immunotherapy

It has been well proven that the immune cells play a key role in eradication of cancer. If a person can mount sufficient anti-cancer immune response, the cancer can be cured in highly significant manner. In that case, the question arises that if we all have intact immunity (not immune-compromised), why the incidence rate of the cancer is high? Why do not we develop good anti-cancer immune response? The major reason is the cancer microenvironment, which is highly adaptive in nature and does not allow effective immune response to mount against cancerous cells by multiple ways.

2.1.1   Immune Checkpoint Inhibitors (ICIs) Therapy and Their Combinations

Antitumor T cell immunity is crucial for cancer remission. For efficient T cell signaling, three signals are essential including T cell receptor recognizing the antigens, second one of co-stimulatory nature which is crucial for achieving the desired activation threshold for overall signaling, and third one derived from cytokines which is essential for survival and proliferation of T cells. Co-stimulatory signals can be of positive and negative regulatory in nature. Positive ones enhance the overall avidity of T cell signaling allowing optimal effector responses, while the negative ones diminish the overall signal strength resulting in lack of immune response.

Expression of negative co-stimulatory molecules on the cancer cells hampers the T cell responses. These proteins bind to their corresponding receptors present on T cells and dampen the T cell signaling. Hence, the effective T cell responses are not generated against the cancer cells. Such T cell negative co-stimulatory molecules were blocked so that T cell immune response can be retained back. This strategy has shown promising results in clinic and popularly known as immune checkpoint inhibitor therapy. The very first FDA approval for checkpoint inhibitor for treatment of patients was given for advanced melanoma. The noble prize of medicine and physiology awarded for this discovery in year 2018.

FDA approval for usage of checkpoint inhibitors has revolutionized melanoma treatment in past decade with various antibody based antagonists being in place commercially. These are designed against mainly two receptor ligand combinations PD-1:PD-1 L and CD80/86:CTLA-4 being expressed on T cells and cancer cell, respectively (Table 2.1).

PD-1 (programmed death receptor-1) is a co-inhibitory molecule which is expressed late during the process of T cells activation process. Delayed expression of PD-1 makes sure that initially robust immune response is generated and then it is controlled through negative regulation. Such negative effects are generated when PD-1 binds to its ligands known as PD-L1 (programmed cell death ligand 1) and PD-L2 (programmed cell death ligand 2).

PD-L1 is the major inhibitory ligand between the two. Conventionally these ligands are expressed on the specialized cells known as APC (antigen presenting cells) which process the antigen and present them to T cells in the form of peptides. Tumor cells under conditioned tumor microenvironment express these ligands profoundly and use them to escape immune response. When the T cells reach tumor microenvironment and attack tumor cells, PD-L1 and L2 on tumor cells engage with PD-1 on T cells and reduce the overall avidity/signal strength [1]. This leads to feeble antitumor immunity and no killing of tumor cells by CD8 T cells.

CTLA-4 (cytotoxic T lymphocyte-associated protein 4) is another inhibitory receptor playing crucial role in dampening immune response in similar manner as PD-1 [2]. It competes with another positive co-stimulatory molecule on T cells

Table 2.1 FDA approved immune checkpoint inhibitors for melanoma

S. no.	Target	Name of drug	Year of approval
1.	PD-1	Nivolumab	2014
2.	PD-1	Pembrolizumab	2014
3.	CTLA-4	Ipilimumab	2011

known as CD28. CD80/86 protein is common ligand for both CD28 and CTLA-4. CTLA-4 binds with much higher affinity to CD80/86 than CD28 does. Competing with CD28, CTLA-4 dominates and successfully diminishes the T cell responses. CTLA-4 overexpression has been reported in almost all the cancer type tissues [3]. It leads to blocking of T cell responses of tumor-infiltrating T cells.

Both approaches, i.e. blocking receptor and blocking ligand of PD-1 and CTLA-4 have been tested and clinically approved by FDA as listed in Table 2.1.

There is emergence of concept of hot and cold tumors in onco-immunology. Hot tumors are those which have significant infiltration of immune cells, while tumors with few immune cells only are considered as cold tumors. It has been observed that level of CD8 T cells residing in the melanoma site positively correlates with performance of PD-1 based immunotherapy.

Checkpoint inhibitors therapy is also an approach to convert the cold tumors to hot ones so that optical local antitumor immunity can be mounted. Anti-CTLA-4 agent ipilimumab leads to increase in tumor-infiltrating lymphocytes (TILs) post-treatment [4–6].

All the forms of receptor or ligand based immune checkpoint inhibitors ipilimumab, nivolumab, and pembrolizumab have shown significant efficacy in metastatic melanoma patients, still many patients suffer from significant adverse effects and need considerable additional interventions.

2.1.1.1 Performance of ICIs

The clinical trials do not provide the right data of the real world efficacy and toxicity of the drug due to stringent inclusion and exclusion criteria. With FDA approval of ipilimumab (anti-CTLA-4) in 2011 and later availability of pembrolizumab and nivolumab (both inhibitors of the programmed death-1, PD-1, pathway) in market by 2014, their performance was reviewed in wider patient cohort. Based on the satisfactory performance of this class of blocking antibodies, checkpoint inhibitors were recommended as first-line treatment for metastatic melanoma. Not only single regimen but combinations with these inhibitors were also assessed and showed promising results. Later in 2016, monotherapy with pembrolizumab and nivolumab and combination of nivolumab/ipilimumab were considered first-line therapy, while ipilimumab as second-line regimen. By 2016, checkpoint inhibitors became the first-line therapy for almost 60% of the melanoma patients. On an average, based on various studies, the progression free survival and the overall survival of the patients increased not more than couple of months. Also, the efficacies of either single or combination of checkpoint inhibitors have not exceeded anything more than 20%.

2.1.1.2 Concerns with ICIs

Developing immune-related adverse events (irAEs) is common in many patients. As the therapy is based on basic principal of augmentation of overall immune responses, it also leads to excessive systematic inflammation leading to various complications including diarrhea, lung inflammation, rashes and itchiness, hormonal abnormalities, and renal dysfunction [7]. Beside that few patients develop infusion reaction with symptoms like allergies and autoimmunity as well. Type 1 diabetes mellitus or diabetic ketoacidosis is most common endocrine abnormality observed in patients. Abnormal pancreatic function has also been observed in patients with chronic treatment.

2.1.1.3 Reason for Lack of Efficacy of ICIs

With the advent of checkpoint inhibitor as their approval as therapy, melanoma treatment has been revolutionized. Almost 60% of the patients have them as some or other stage of the disease. Still there is a lot of scope to improve the efficacy of these inhibitors along with reduced toxicity.

In principal, two components are essential for checkpoint inhibitor therapy to work. First and foremost there should be good infiltration of T cells to the tumor site. Tumors with considerable number of immune cells present in them are known as hot tumors in contrast to cold tumors which do not have immune cell in their microenvironment. Another major lacuna in good efficacy is lack of good antigen presentation to T cells within tumor microenvironment. Based on the three signal hypothesis, the three essential signals required for T cell activation include binding of three receptor ligands on T cells and the corresponding antigen presenting cell. First and the foremost the T cell receptor should recognize the complementary peptide bound to the MHC of the APC cells. Second is positive co-stimulation to strengthen signal 1 in order to cross the threshold of activation and third are cytokine responses for the survival and proliferation of the activated T cell. The bottle neck in this whole process is that the lack of signal 1. Tumor microenvironment is highly immunosuppressive and adapts extensively in order to discourage the immune response to mount against the cancer cells. Immunosuppressive cytokines mainly TGF-β produced by the cancer cells do not allow the antigen presenting cells to become mature and express MHC for antigenic peptide upload. If signal 1 is not present, recovering positive co-stimulation with checkpoint inhibitors will have no impact (Fig. 2.1). Hence, it is very crucial that tumor antigen is processed and presented to the T cells so that T cells can mount antitumor immunity.

2.1.1.4 Future Prospects of ICI Therapy

In spite of becoming essential component of melanoma immunotherapy, there is limited efficacy as well a limited cohort of the patients respond to them. To overcome these issues, various novel approaches are being adopted, some of which are discussed in this chapter itself. Few of them include combination therapy within themselves, i.e. more than one checkpoint inhibitors or with other conventional regimens like radiotherapy or chemotherapy.

2.1.2 Melanoma Vaccine

In cancer conditions, vaccine adjuvants are aimed at producing more robust immune responses by increasing antigen uptake and presentation, recruiting other immune cells, and/or forming a depot effect for sustained release of antigen. There are many ongoing clinical trials studying the impacts of various antigen formats and adjuvants

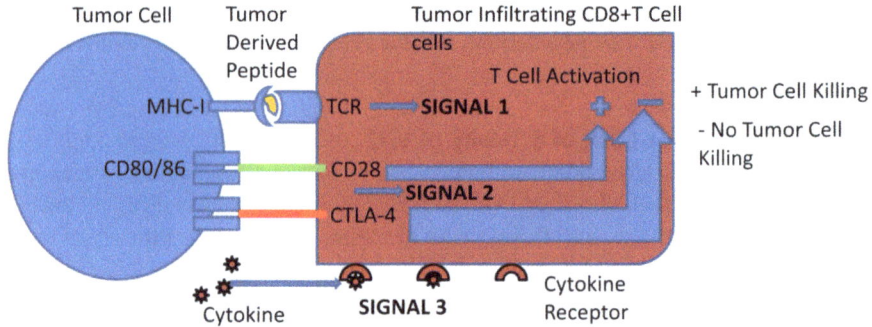

Fig. 2.1 Schematic of the three signal hypothesis for antitumor CD8 T-cell-mediated cytotoxicity

on immune responses and clinical outcomes. Among these, dendritic cells (DC) and peptide vaccines predominate. Vaccines may use antigen as whole tumor cells, RNA or DNA, single or multiple peptides, or antigen presenting cells (APCs) displaying the target antigen [8]. Both efficacy and toxicity can be related to intrinsic immunologic potency, cross-reactivity of vaccine targets to antigen on normal cells, and associated adjuvants.

Peptide vaccines use a variety of adjuvants, the most common of which is incomplete Freund's adjuvant, while the dendritic cell vaccines act as an adjuvant on their own, so do not frequently utilize additional adjuvants.

As choice of antigenic peptides, mainly 8–10 amino acid long peptides represent usually CD8 epitopes. Their effects on CD8 + T are advantageous as it activates effector cells directly, thus negating the need for further antigen processing by APCs. Another arm of long peptide vaccines refers to lengths of 20–30 amino acids and carries the potential benefit of activating both CD8 + T and CD4 + T responses [9]. RNA or DNA encoding genes for tumor antigens or immune enhancers can be introduced into APCs or myocytes through bacterial or viral vectors to synthesize peptides and mediate a vaccine effect. Some RNA vaccines involve electroporation of APCs to enable incorporation of mRNA encoding melanoma-associated antigens or immunostimulatory ligands to facilitate antigen-specific T cell responses. Whole cancer cells can be integrated into vaccines and serve as a source of antigen for APC presentation. They contain numerous mutated neoantigens that are inherent to the tumor, which does not mandate that they be identified prior to designing and manufacturing the vaccine. Whole cells can be modified to express particular tumor antigens or immune enhancers to further potentiate immune responses.

Combination therapy with vaccines provides an opportunity to target the immune system through another mechanism to augment antitumor effects and potentiate clinical benefits. The most common combination therapy for peptide vaccines is checkpoint blockade, while IL-2 is most common among combination therapies used with DC vaccines, though DC vaccines utilize more combination therapies overall.

2.1.3 Interleukin-2 Therapy

Based on the concept of three signal hypothesis, the third signal of cytokine response is crucial for maintenance as well as amplification of overall T cell responses. IL-2 is one of the cytokine not only crucial for T cell survival but also for their proliferation. Administration of IL-2 in higher dose has shown promising effects in melanoma patients. It is one of the earliest immunotherapy approved for melanoma.

2.2 Targeted Therapies

With advances in techniques involved in mutation detection and reduction in cost of sequencing, it has become quite affordable to precisely know the nature of somatic mutation a cancer patient has. Also, it is possible to calculate the mutation burden of a particular tumor precisely. Such information will not only provide the better understanding of the pathogenesis at molecular level but may also suggest targeted cancer therapies as listed below.

2.2.1 BRAF Inhibitors

BRAF is a human gene that encodes a protein called B-Raf. B-Raf is a serine/threonine protein kinase enzyme which triggers the MAP kinase/ERK-signaling pathway. MAP kinase/ERK-signaling pathway is essential for various physiological functions of cell including proliferation as well. Tumor cells exploit this pathway for aggressive cell proliferation. About 50% of melanomas harbor activating BRAF mutations to attain gain of function [10]. The most commonly reported mutation of BRAF, with BRAFV600E change has been implicated in different mechanisms leading to rapidly progressive melanoma. Blocking the activity of the kinase and its mutated forms have shown promising efficacy towards reducing tumor growth. FDA in 2011 approved vemurafenib, an inhibitor of the BRAF kinase with V600 form of protein. Later other BRAF inhibitors were approved including dabrafenib (2013), encorafenib, or LGX818 (2018). Encorafenib has shown to be better option over dabrafenib or encorafenib with greater half-life and prolonged inhibition of kinase activity. Although BFAF inhibitors show considerable efficacy but beyond a time patients do develop resistance to particular therapy within 1 year of start of therapy which is a major concern [11].

2.2.2 MEK Inhibitors

The mitogen-activated protein kinases (MAPKs) cell signaling pathway is essential for cellular development, differentiation, and proliferation. Cancer cells utilize this pathway for their own differentiation and proliferation. Mitogen-activated protein kinase kinase enzymes MEK1 and/or MEK2 are essential component of the signaling cascade. They have 80% amino acid sequence homology. Antagonists against MEK1 and MEK2 have shown promising effects in cessation of tumor growth in melanoma when used along with BRAF inhibitors. Various MEK and BRAF inhibitors combinations were approved by FDA for melanomas from 2015 onwards. The list includes cobimetinib or XL518 in combination with vemurafenib, binimetinib in combination with encorafenib for the treatment of patients with unresectable or metastatic BRAF V600E or V600K mutation-positive melanoma [12].

2.2.3 C-Kit Inhibitors

c-Kit is a receptor tyrosine kinase involved in cell survival, migration, and proliferation of various cell types. It acts as a receptor for stem cell factor mainly for hemopoiesis under normal physiology. Mutated form of c-Kit has been reported in various cancers providing survival, proliferation advantages to cancer cells. Hence, inhibiting c-Kit kinase activity stands as potential drug target for cancer therapy [13]. Inhibitor against mutated forms c-Kit (SCFR) known as PLX9486 is an orally bio-available small molecule with significant anti-proliferative activity.

2.3   Oncolytic Virus Based Therapy

Using virus to kill cancer cells is a novel concept in immune-oncology. These viruses are specific to infect only the cancer cells. Once they infect the cancer cells, they hijack their central dogma of the cancer cells. Virus divide and lyse the cancer cells turning viral infection towards specific cancer cell therapy by lysis. Adenovirus or herpes simplex virus are best choices for designing these therapies. Talimogene laherparepvec (Imlygic®) or T-VEC is first oncolytic virus to receive FDA approval in 2015 for melanoma. Another advantage of OV based therapies is that they can augment the local (intratumoral) immune response by maturing many antigen presenting cells and causing local inflammation due to dead cancer cells at local site. Such combined effect of specific cancer cell killing and augmentation of immune response leads to better efficacy in patients with melanoma [14]. In terms or side effects or toxicity, OV based therapies are quite safe with targeted killing of cancer cells only. In certain patients mild symptoms including fever, chills, diarrhea, and stomach pains are observed which is mainly due to systemic inflammation caused by anti-viral immunity itself.

OV has immense potential to be used as combination therapy with various other regimens. In particular combination of OV and checkpoint inhibitors is in various phases of clinical trials. OV with minimal toxicity and high specificity is an emerging tool for cancer therapy.

2.4   Photodynamic Therapy (PDT)

PDT is a specific therapy only for melanoma being a local therapeutic modality. It is a noninvasive local tissue exposure based therapy recently evolved for melanoma patients. Specific devices known as photosensitizers (PSs) are used to selectively target diseased tissues. PSs allow sensitization of local tissue towards the particular wavelength of laser emissions. As the particular wavelength exposure achieved, it leads to photoactivation induced cell death in tumor and not the surrounding healthy tissue. Major cytotoxic agent generated during such photo-exposures are reactive oxygen species (ROS) [15]. It leads to oxidation of various key physiologically important key enzymes, substrate essential for normal cell survival, and physiology. ROS can act on lipids, proteins making them dysfunctional and hence triggering apoptosis in the cancer cells exposed to PDT. Various additional advantages of PDT based therapy are that it can be used for particular metastatic site as well, also ROS generated in the process lead to augment local immune response which aids in overall tumor regression further [16].

2.5   Challenges and Emerging Approaches Associated with Non-Conventional Therapies

The last few decades have resulted in a period of learning, clinical experience, and research knowledge gained in tumor biology, molecular and cellular immunology, genomics, immunology, and immunotherapy of cancer, especially for melanoma. Checkpoint inhibitor emerged as landmark discovery for cancer therapy. Still, overall cumulative efficacy of these emerging immune therapies is lower [17]. On top of that around two-third of the melanoma patients become nonresponsive to ongoing therapy at some stage. Hence, drug targeting strategies must keep on evolving and back up with biomarkers with robust predictability of expected resistance.

Efforts to improvise on performance of approved therapies are focused mainly in two directions. First and foremost recognize the right therapy for the right patient, i.e. providing personalized therapy to patients based on their detailed individual cancer profile. In this direction, efforts are being made to identify the appropriate biomarkers for identification of stage, type of the disease, choosing right targeted therapy, timely/early prediction of treatment responsiveness/resistance. Second, is to try and test the combinations of the preapproved therapies (mainly immunotherapies and targeted therapies) in addition to exploring the novel drug targets related to metabolomics, gut microbiome based approaches, and many other options.

2.5.1 Biomarkers: Transition from Generalized to Personalized Therapy

Biomarkers are the molecular signatures representing particular phenotypes or trait or condition in biological system. They help in defining or predicting a particular condition. In the last decade we moved towards patients based specific therapies as compared to the generalized therapies. Discovery of various biomarkers has offered great help in this direction. One such biomarker is to evaluate the tumor mutational burden (TMB) of the patients which not only reflects the tumor adaptability inside the host but indirectly also offers new patient specific targeted therapy [18].

2.5.1.1 Clinical Endpoints

In case of conventional therapies like radiotherapy and chemotherapy some standard classical endpoints including median progression free survival, response rates, or hazard ratio (HR) are used as biomarkers. Although such markers are robust clinical stage reflectors still they have not found to be of best use in case of ICI. One of the major reasons for it delayed effects of ICI and higher patient to patient diversity in response. Approaches like assessing mortality within stipulated time period or data collection at late time points found more valuable in case of ICI [19].

2.5.1.2 Blood Counts and Derived Values

Various hematological parameters and values derived out of them have served as biomarkers in predicting disease state, treatment responsiveness, etc., ratio of peripheral blood absolute neutrophil count to the lymphocyte is known as NLR. It has been found to be altered in almost all cancers with association of systemic inflammation. Higher proportion of neutrophils as compared to other lymphocytes (i.e. high NLRs) was related to worse overall survival (OS) for melanoma patients treated with ipilimumab, nivolumab, and the combination of nivolumab and ipilimumab [20–22].

NLR has also served as marker of post-therapy outcomes. Patients with more than 30% increase in NLR, i.e. higher expansion of neutrophils but not other lymphocytes after two cycles of anti-PD-1 treatment are shown to be associated strongly with poor overall survival in melanoma patients [23].

Beside the derived ratio values even peripheral blood based absolute neutrophil count (ANC) and absolute lymphocyte count (ALC) have also served as early biomarkers related to OS in melanoma patients during nivolumab therapy [24]. More than 30% expansion of lymphocytes (high ALC) after two cycles of ipilimumab was related to a longer OS [25]. Peripheral blood counts based markers are cost-effective and easy to conduct in a follow-up manner. It is one of the most robustly clinically used biomarker.

2.5.1.3 Tumor Mutation Burden (TMB)

Somatic mutations are key for adaptability of cancer cells inside host. Many acquired somatic mutation can allow cancer cells to develop resistance to therapies as well as develop immune evasion strategies. Hence, the quantitation of mutations harbored by a cancer is also a reflection of their adaptable and aggressive form. TMB is a quantitative measure of the same. It represents the somatic mutations per tumor DNA megabase. TMB has served as prognostic marker of resistance to cytotoxic or targeted therapy.

In terms of immunological advantages, more the mutations the tumor contains, higher likelihood it has to generate new antigens which in turn increase immunogenicity of tumor [26]. Hence, TMB also predicts the efficacy of immune therapies like checkpoint inhibitors including melanoma as well. With accumulating patient data, TMB has gradually established as a clinically validated biomarker.

2.5.1.4 Lactate Dehydrogenase (LDH)

Lactate dehydrogenase is an enzyme found in nearly all living cells responsible for conversion of lactate to pyruvate and back. High LDH indicates tissue injury. It is the only soluble protein based biomarker with significant prognostic value for melanoma staging approved in clinical settings. Level of LDH significantly associates with poor survival in advanced stage IV melanoma [27]. Further, it is also a good predictor of poor outcome in patients treated with combination of dabrafenib and trametinib [28].

Reduction in LDH levels post-therapy is helpful in predicting treatment responsiveness of immunotherapy as well [29]. As an exploratory approach, many soluble proteins including S100B, C reactive protein (CRP), and melanoma-inhibiting activity (MIA) protein have been explored but not clinically approved [30].

2.5.1.5 Cytokines

Cytokines are generated by immune cells as effector molecules to mount antitumor immunity. Various pro-inflammatory cytokines have been shown to be pro-tumerogenic in nature. Various cytokines have been explored as biomarker in oncology especially in case of ICIs [31]. Increase in pro-inflammatory cytokines has been associated with adverse events during ICI treatment. Increase in IL-6 level from base line has been shown to predict occurrence of irAE in a small group of melanoma patients treated with nivolumab [32]. Various studies suggest alterations in level of cohort or combinations of particular cytokines as biomarkers such as including: granulocyte colony-stimulating factor (G-CSF), granulocyte-macrophage colony-stimulating factor (GM-CSF), Fractalkine, fibroblast growth factor 2 (FGF-2), IFN-α2, IL-12p70, IL-1a, IL-1B, IL-1RA, IL-2, and IL-13 to predict adverse events post ICI therapies [33].

2.5.1.6 Soluble Checkpoint Molecules

Beside the membrane bound form of the checkpoint inhibitor proteins, soluble forms of the same proteins are readily detected in peripheral blood of the patients. These soluble forms are generated either by splice variant of the mRNA or by shedding/cleavage of the membrane bound protein form. It has been shown to work similar to membrane bound form, i.e. they can bind the respective ligand and generate inhibitory or negative co-stimulatory effects for PD-1 [34]. Melanoma patients with a high sPD-L1 level had a worse prognosis in treatment groups receiving ipilimumab or pembrolizumab monotherapies [35].

Similar to PD-1, soluble CTLA-4 (sCTLA4) protein does exist being generated due to existence of splice variant. sCTLA-4 is capable of binding to CD80/86 and thus can do inhibitory regulation of T-cell-mediated immune response [36, 37]. Elevated basal level of sCTLA-4 concentration was associated with a lower death rate and serves as a biomarker of efficacy of ipilimumab treatment in melanoma [38, 39].

2.5.1.7 Circulating Tumor Cells

Growing tumors do release certain number of their progenies in the peripheral blood known as circulating tumor cells (CTCs). They have been explored extensively as prognostic biomarkers [40, 41]. Their presence is reported in almost all stages of the disease progression. As they are free flowing in blood the process of sampling for CTC studies is also known as "liquid biopsy." It serves as very useful non-tumor invasive marker as no tumor tissue biopsy is required for its assessment. CTC is very useful biomarker in cases where there is inaccessibility of the tumor, or multiple metastases are present in a patient.

Unit to quantify the CTC is proportion per million leukocytes [42]. Basis of the discrimination of CTC from host blood cells is based on the presence of certain tumor specific genes. Circulating melanoma cells (CMCs) have been detected in blood by qPCR of melanocyte specific genes or by enrichment using melanocyte surface markers.

Liquid biopsy based CTC analysis also has additional advantages. They can provide information about the tumor itself being its origin.

2.5.1.8 Circulating Tumor DNA (ctDNA)

Beside the whole CTCs, the DNA released by the tumor cells (ctDNA) themself can also be detected in blood and has potential to serve as biomarker. Highly fragmented DNA released by tumor cells in circulation ranges between 130 and 170n base pairs in size [43]. In advanced cancers, ctDNA has shown promising results in order to be considered as biomarker. CtDNA also provides genetics based information related to aggressiveness of the disease and pro-oncogenic characteristics. In melanoma, ctDNA has been used for the detection of mutations and suggesting targeted therapies as well as assessment of response to therapy. Cheaper next generation sequencing (NGS)-based panels with high sensitivity have increased the fields of application of ctDNA testing.

One of the major limitations of ctDNA based approach is the window period to detect these DNAs as the half-life for them is shorter ranging between minutes and 13 h [43, 44]. It can be easily cleared from circulation, hence missing the best window period for sample collection can mislead the findings [45]. ctDNA is often undetectable in the majority of early stage melanoma patients [46]. In late stage melanomas, longitudinal assessment of ctDNA levels was predictive of response [47]. Epigenetic modifications of ctDNA, such as methylation signature, are a promising avenue for biomarker discovery [48].

2.5.1.9 Exosomes

In order to establish cell to cell and cells at distant metastatic sites, tumor secretes certain molecules especially for cellular communication and cargo activity. Exosomes are one such kind of cell communication and cargo carrying moieties with 30–150 nm size equivalent to viruses. They are membrane bound vesicles, produced by all cells and capable of transporting almost all biomolecules including DNA, RNA, and proteins between cells. Using defined biochemical methods and exploiting physical properties, such as size, sedimentation rate, exosomes can be purified and further characterized to serve as biomarker.

Tumors extensively secrete exosomes which can impact the tumor survival, proliferation, and treatment response [49].

Further the content of exosome cargo also serves as cancer biomarkers. Exosome-derived micro-RNAs have shown promising results in metastatic melanoma cases [50, 51]. Still their wider clinical use needs more validation and hunt of reliable fixed set of analytes.

2.5.1.10 Gut Microbiome

Composition of the microbes residing in the gut has immense impact on host immune status, disease susceptibility, etc. Various metabolites produced by them affect immune state of the host. Short-chain fatty acids (SCFAs) produced as byproduct of microbes metabolic activity have shown to affect the efficacy of immunotherapy. Various bacterial species have been indicated as potential biomarkers for predicting efficacy of anti-PD-1 or anti-CTLA-4 therapy in melanoma.

Gopalakrishnan et al. [52] published clear discrimination in gut microbe composition between responders and non-responders melanoma patients treated with anti-PD-1 therapy. Responding patients were more diversified and were enriched with bacteria belonging to the *Ruminococcaceae* family and the *Clostridiales* order, such as *Faecalibacterium* species, whereas non-responders represented low diversity and dominance of *Bacteroidales* in composition of their gut microbiota.

Besides characterizing the gut bacteria by sequencing based method of fecal material, additional approach of estimating the related metabolites has also shown promising potential as biomarker, mainly the concentration of fecal SCFAs. It is positively correlated with clinical outcomes to treatment with anti-PD-1 therapy. SCFAs modulate immune responses regulatory T cell differentiation which can downregulate antitumor immunity. Gut microbiota enriched with *Faecalibacterium* spp. was linked with positive clinical responses to CTLA-4.

2.5.2   New Treatment Approaches

With better understanding of tumor microenvironment, its components, biochemical composition, metabolic profile of constituent cells, new treatment strategies are being evaluated. Enormous numbers of active clinical trials are ongoing at various phases with promising future prospects. Some of such approaches are discussed in the below mentioned section under immune therapeutics and nonimmune based drug target categories.

2.5.2.1 Emerging Immunotherapies

Lymphocyte-Activation Gene 3 (LAG-3)

Lymphocyte-activation gene 3 (LAG-3) is a cell surface molecule expressed on T effectors and T regulatory cells. It has suppressive function and serves as marker of T cell exhaustion. LAG-3 binds to MHC class II, hence can downregulate all the CD4 based helper responses. Such signaling also enhances regulatory T cell differentiation. These tumor residing regulatory T cells make the overall tumor microenvironment very immune suppressive and tolerizing [53]. Targeting the LAG-3 protein, results in robust T cell responses [54, 55]. More than 50 clinical trials are currently ongoing targeting LAG-3 both alone and in combination with other immune checkpoints, indicating promising therapeutic potential in future.

T Cell Immunoglobulin and Mucin-Domain-Containing Molecule 3 (TIM-3)

T-cell immunoglobulin and mucin-domain-containing molecule 3 (TIM-3) are expressed on numerous types of immune cells under exhaustion [56]. Under the influence of the various secretary as well as suppressive factors, tumor-infiltrating cells show TIM-3 expression which correlates with poor outcomes in multiple different types of cancer [57–59].

Various antagonizing approaches against TIM-3 augment CD8$^+$ T cell effectors responses including cytotoxic activity [60]. Such TIM-3 antagonists, however, also increase the autoimmunity and many adverse events related to high cytokine levels including pneumonitis [61].

Toll Like Receptors (TLRs)

Toll like receptors are innate immune cell receptors and are major components for first line of defense system of the host immunity. Tumor cells also express various TLRs. They provide pro-oncogenic help to tumors. In case of TLR both therapies using TLR agonists are currently in early phase trials.

Rationale for testing TLR agonists is based on their potential to work as adjutants. For example, the TLR9 agonists CMP-001, SD-101 are being tested as monotherapy and in combination with checkpoint inhibitors for a melanoma (https://clinicaltrials.gov/ct2/show/NCT02680184, https://clinicaltrials.gov/ct2/show/NCT03618641, https://clinicaltrials.gov/ct2/show/NCT02521870). TLR7 is also being targeted in combination with chemo-radiotherapy as well as with ICI (https://clinicaltrials.gov/ct2/show/NCT03276832).

Myeloid Derived Suppressor Cells (MDSCs)

MDSCs are specialized differentiated cell lineage profoundly existing in tumor microenvironment. They are by origin mononuclear myeloid lineage which under chronic inflammatory condition becomes highly immunosuppressive in nature.

Major mechanism of MDSCs immunosuppressive effect is through production of nitric oxide, anti-inflammatory cytokines, and reactive oxygen species. These effector molecules can lead to inhibit T cells through antigen-specific and nonspecific mechanisms. Effector molecules secreted by the MDSCs promote angiogenesis, metastasis, and resistance to chemotherapy, targeted therapy, and immunotherapy [62]. Most of the studies regarding MDSC depletion are conducted in animal models at preclinical stages except few which entered in clinical trial.

Tumor-Infiltrating Lymphocytes (TIL) Infusions

In order to mount efficient antitumor immunity, the tumor should have sufficient presence of immune cells, known as being hot tumor. Cold tumor where there is very few immune cells reach can never mount sufficient response to eradicate tumor. Converting cold to hot tumors and then enhancing antitumor immunity by additional approaches can be an effective treatment strategy.

For therapeutic purpose, tumor tissue derived lymphocytes are harvested and expanded in vitro first, followed by testing for responsiveness to specific neoepitopes. Lymphocytes predicted to recognize tumor antigens with high affinity are expanded ex vivo and reinfused into the patient. Cytokine based supplementation therapy is also provided in form of cytokine IL-2 which is given post-TIL infusion [63, 64].

2.5.2.2 Gut Microbiome Alteration

Many studies have shown association of diversity and composition of gut microbiota and treatment responsiveness and immune state of host. Although the exact mechanism of such observation is not well elucidated still strong observational data prompted scientists to test the approach of manipulating the gut microbiota in favorable way. In a single-center study of patients treated for melanoma, those with higher fiber intake had better ICI responses, but those who used probiotics had lower alpha diversity and were less likely to respond to ICI [65].

Approaches like altering the gut microbiota by using the method of fecal transplant is becoming popular but still needs to be validated for efficacy and expected side effects in any cancer including melanoma.

2.5.2.3 Metabolomics Based Approaches

In order to survive and extensively proliferate, tumor cells need considerably high level of energy and thus have different metabolic profile as compared to normal noncancerous cells. They have signature Warburg effect, with excretion of lactate into the microenvironment. This leads to quicker consumption of glucose in competition to immune cells and creating an acidic microenvironment. Such condition lead to TIL dysfunction along which tumor growth. Metabolomics based treatment approaches are emerging ones with certain adopted approaches discussed below.

Glucose Metabolism Based Targets

A number of therapeutic strategies have shown preclinical efficacy by modulating glucose metabolism. In melanoma models, phenformin and metformin have shown to reduce the differentiation of MDSCs in the tumor microenvironment. Such drugs like metformin have also shown to enhance efficacy of ICIs [66].

Such glucose emetabolism modulatory drugs have many bystander effects as well such as impact on angiogenesis, cell survival, and differentiation [67, 68]. Phenformin is currently being studied in the phase I setting together with the BRAF and MEK inhibitors dabrafenib and trametinib in patients with BRAF V600E mutant melanomas (https://clinicaltrials.gov/ct2/show/NCT03026517).

Amino Acids Based Targets
Amino acids based approaches mainly involve tryptophan and arginine.

Tryptophan
Tryptophan is an essential amino acid involvement in various physiological process except being protein based building base. Tryptophan is broken down by indoleamine 2,3-dioxygenase (IDO) enzyme and this reaction allows enhanced Treg activity and MDSC recruitment. Blocking the enzyme IDO has been proven to be effective strategy to cut down immune suppressive tumor microenvironment. Many small molecules based DO inhibitors are currently in phase I–III clinical trials either alone or in combination with other checkpoint inhibitor therapies.

Arginine
Melanoma cannot synthesize arginine due to lack of argininosuccinate synthetase, an essential enzyme for arginine synthesis. Hence they need exogenous source of arginine. Depleting the exogenous arginine affects the melanoma progression, hence approaches to diminish it have been adopted as therapy. ADI-PEG 20 monotherapy, which depletes arginine, has shown safety but limited efficacy to date [69]. On the contrary inhibition of arginine degradation is also being studied in combination with ICI in an early phase trial for patients with melanoma [70] (https://clinicaltrials.gov/ct2/show/NCT02903914).

Lipid Based Targets
Lipid content in tumor microenvironment shapes the local antitumor immunity. MDSCs with high lipid content are shown to be more tolerogeneic [71]. Preclinical studies evidence that inhibition of cholesterol esterification leads to CD8 cells which are the major tumor killer cells are impacted by the cholesterol esterification. Reducing cholesterol esterification allows better CD8 T cell proliferation. To establish the proof of concept, using preclinical animal model, anti-melanoma effects using the anti-atherosclerotic drug "Avasimibe" have been demonstrated but not yet clinically validated [72]. Another metabolomics based therapeutic approach involves modulation of fatty acid oxidation, creating potential novel avenues for future combination therapies [73].

Past decade has revolutionized the melanoma therapy which eventually has resulted in better clinical management of the patients and better overall outcomes. All this has been possible due to use of advanced techniques and novel approaches to study the components of tumor microenvironment other than cancer cells themselves. One of such components is immune cells. Understanding why they do not work up to their full potential after entering into tumor microenvironment has given us many potential drug targets. Recovering immune cells back to their best antitumor potential has given enormous hope to test newer strategies. At present most of the strategies are exploring the possibility of converting the cold tumors to hot ones and hitting them with immune cells. Such strategies have also shown us many challenges like low responsiveness, resistance, adverse effects. As cancer cells are highly adaptive and cope with the adverse conditions quickly, we need to design combination therapies with mix of different class of targets to overcome these issues. Also, we are gradually progressing towards personalized therapy. Such one-on-one approach for patients needs availability of robust and well-validated biomarkers to not only provide best clinical care to patients, but also predict expected drug nonresponsiveness earlier in course. On one hand all current and emerging approaches sound very promising but simultaneously they are quite resource intensive also. We also need to evolve in terms of making personalized therapy approaches cheaper so that majority of patient population can take benefit of all the scientific advancements in this field.

References

1. Gun SY, Lee SWL, Sieow JL, Wong SC (2019) Targeting immune cells for cancer therapy. Redox Biol 25:101174
2. Sharpe AH, Freeman GJ (2002) The B7–CD28 superfamily. Nat Rev Immunol 2:116–126
3. Seidel JA, Otsuka A, Kabashima K (2018) Anti-PD-1 and anti-CTLA-4 therapies in cancer: mechanisms of action, efficacy, and limitations. Front Oncol 8:86
4. Gibney GT, Weiner LM, Atkins MB (2016) Predictive biomarkers for checkpoint inhibitor-based immunotherapy. Lancet Oncol 17:e542–e551
5. Hamid O et al (2011) A prospective phase II trial exploring the association between tumor microenvironment biomarkers and clinical activity of ipilimumab in advanced melanoma. J Transl Med 9:204
6. Tumeh PC et al (2014) PD-1 blockade induces responses by inhibiting adaptive immune resistance. Nature 515:568–571
7. Bajwa R et al (2019) Adverse effects of immune checkpoint inhibitors (programmed death-1 inhibitors and cytotoxic T-lymphocyte-associated protein-4 inhibitors): results of a retrospective study. J Clin Med Res 11(4):225–236
8. Pan RY et al (2018) Recent development and clinical application of cancer vaccine: targeting neoantigens. J Immunol Res 2018:4325874
9. Yang H, Kim DS (2015) Peptide immunotherapy in vaccine development: from epitope to adjuvant. Adv Protein Chem Struct Biol 99:1–14
10. Haugh AM, Johnson DB (2019) Management of V600E and V600K BRAF-mutant melanoma. Curr Treat Options Oncol 20:81
11. Frederick DT et al (2013) BRAF inhibition is associated with enhanced melanoma antigen expression and a more favorable tumor microenvironment in patients with metastatic melanoma. Clin Cancer Res 19:1225–1231
12. Guo J, Si L, Kong Y et al (2011) Phase II, open-label, single-arm trial of imatinib mesylate in patients with metastatic melanoma harboring c-Kit mutation or amplification. J Clin Oncol 29 (21):2904–2909

13. Bayan C-AY et al (2018) The role of oncolytic viruses in the treatment of melanoma. Curr Oncol Rep 20(10):80. https://doi.org/10.1007/s11912-018-0729-3

14. Li X-Y et al (2020) Susceptibility and resistance mechanisms during photodynamic therapy of melanoma. Front Oncol 10:597. https://doi.org/10.3389/fonc.2020.00597

15. Anzengruber F, Avci P, de Freitas LF, Hamblin MR (2015) T-cell mediated anti-tumor immunity after photodynamic therapy: why does it not always work and how can we improve it? Photochem Photobiol Sci 14:1492–1509

16. Luke JJ, Flaherty KT, Ribas A, Long GV (2017) Targeted agents and immunotherapies: optimizing outcomes in melanoma. Nat Rev Clin Oncol 14:463–482

17. Blank CU, Haanen JB, Ribas A, Schumacher TN (2016) Cancer immunology. The 'cancer immunogram'. Science 352:658–660

18. Liang F, Zhang S, Wang Q, Li W (2018) Treatment effects measured by restricted mean survival time in trials of immune checkpoint inhibitors for cancer. Ann Oncol 29:1320–1324

19. Ferrucci PF, Gandini S, Battaglia A, Alfieri S, Di Giacomo AM, Giannarelli D, Cappellini GCA, De Galitiis F, Marchetti P, Amato G et al (2015) Baseline neutrophil-to-lymphocyte ratio is associated with outcome of ipilimumab-treated metastatic melanoma patients. Br J Cancer 112:1904–1910

20. Zaragoza J, Caille A, Beneton N, Bens G, Christiann F, Maillard H, Machet L (2016) High neutrophil to lymphocyte ratio measured before starting ipilimumab treatment is associated with reduced overall survival in patients with melanoma. Br J Dermatol 174:146–151

21. Xie X, Liu J, Yang H, Chen H, Zhou S, Lin H, Liao Z, Ding Y, Ling L, Wang X (2019) Prognostic value of baseline neutrophil-to-lymphocyte ratio in outcome of immune checkpoint inhibitors. Cancer Invest 37:265–274

22. Bartlett EK, Flynn JR, Panageas KS, Ferraro RA, Jessica JM, Postow MA, Coit DG, Ariyan CE (2020) High neutrophil-to-lymphocyte ratio (NLR) is associated with treatment failure and death in patients who have melanoma treated with PD-1 inhibitor monotherapy. Cancer 126:76–85

23. Nakamura Y, Kitano S, Takahashi A, Tsutsumida A, Namikawa K, Tanese K, Abe T, Funakoshi T, Yamamoto N, Amagai M et al (2016) Nivolumab for advanced melanoma: pretreatment prognostic factors and early outcome markers during therapy. Oncotarget 7:77404–77415

24. Kelderman S, Heemskerk B, van Tinteren H, van den Brom RRH, Hospers GAP, van den Eertwegh AJM, Kapiteijn EW, de Groot JWB, Soetekouw P, Jansen RL et al (2014) Lactate dehydrogenase as a selection criterion for ipilimumab treatment in metastatic melanoma. Cancer Immunol Immunother 63:449–458

25. Schumacher TN, Scheper W, Kvistborg P (2019) Cancer neoantigens. Annu Rev Immunol 37:173–200

26. Agarwala SS, Keilholz U, Gilles E, Bedikian AY, Wu J, Kay R, Stein CA et al (2009) LDH correlation with survival in advanced melanoma from two large, randomised trials (Oblimersen GM301 and EORTC 18951). European J Cancer 45:1807–1814

27. Long GV, Grob JJ, Nathan P, Ribas A, Robert C, Schadendorf D, Lane SR et al (2016) Factors predictive of response, disease progression, and overall survival after dabrafenib and trametinib combination treatment: a pooled analysis of individual patient data from randomised trials. Lancet Oncol 17:1743–1754

28. Diem S, Kasenda B, Martin-Liberal J, Lee A, Chauhan D, Gore M, Larkin J (2015) Prognostic score for patients with advanced melanoma treated with ipilimumab. Eur J Cancer 51:2785–2791

29. Vereecken P, Cornelis F, Van Baren N, Vandersleyen V, Baurain JFA (2012) Synopsis of serum biomarkers in cutaneous melanoma patients. Dermatol Res Pract 2012:260643

30. Dranoff G (2004) Cytokines in cancer pathogenesis and cancer therapy. Nat Rev Cancer 4:11–22. https://doi.org/10.1038/nrc1252

31. Tanaka R, Okiyama N, Okune M, Ishitsuka Y, Watanabe R, Furuta J, Ohtsuka M, Otsuka A, Maruyama H, Fujisawa Y et al (2017) Serum level of interleukin-6 is increased in

nivolumab-associated psoriasiform dermatitis and tumor necrosis factor-α is a biomarker of nivolumab reactivity. J Dermatol Sci 86:71–73

32. Lim SY, Lee JH, Gide TN, Menzies AM, Guminski A, Carlino MS, Breen EJ, Yang JYH, Ghazanfar S, Kefford RF et al (2019) Circulating cytokines predict immune-related toxicity in melanoma patients receiving anti-PD-1–based immunotherapy. Clin Cancer Res 25:1557–1563

33. Chen Y, Wang Q, Shi B, Xu P, Hu Z, Bai L, Zhang X (2011) Development of a sandwich ELISA for evaluating soluble PD-L1 (CD274) in human sera of different ages as well as supernatants of PD-L1+ cell lines. Cytokine 56:231–238

34. Zhou J, Mahoney KM, Giobbie-Hurder A, Zhao F, Lee S, Liao X, Rodig S, Li J, Wu X, Butterfield LH et al (2017) Soluble PD-L1 as a biomarker in malignant melanoma treated with checkpoint blockade. Cancer Immunol Res 5:480–492

35. Magistrelli G, Jeannin P, Herbault N, Benoit De Coignac A, Gauchat JF, Bonnefoy JY, Delneste Y (1999) A soluble form of CTLA-4 generated by alternative splicing is expressed by nonstimulated human T cells. Eur J Immunol 29:3596–3602

36. Ward FJ, Dahal LN, Wijesekera SK, Abdul-Jawad SK, Kaewarpai T, Xu H, Vickers MA, Barker RN (2013) The soluble isoform of CTLA-4 as a regulator of T-cell responses. Eur J Immunol 43:1274–1285

37. Pistillo MP, Fontana V, Morabito A, Dozin B, Laurent S, Carosio R, Banelli B, Ferrero F, Spano L, Tanda E et al (2019) Soluble CTLA-4 as a favorable predictive biomarker in metastatic melanoma patients treated with ipilimumab: an Italian melanoma intergroup study. Cancer Immunol Immunother 68:97–107

38. Leung AM, Lee AF, Ozao-Choy J, Ramos RI, Hamid O, Shin-Sim M, Morton DL, Faries MB, Sieling PA et al (2014) Clinical benefit from Ipilimumab therapy in melanoma patients may be associated with serum CTLA4 levels. Front Oncol 4:110

39. Alix-Panabieres C, Pantel K (2016) Clinical applications of circulating tumor cells and circulating tumor DNA as liquid biopsy. Cancer Discov 6:479–491

40. Marsavela G, Aya-Bonilla CA, Warkiani ME, Gray ES, Ziman M (2018) Melanoma circulating tumor cells: benefits and challenges required for clinical application. Cancer Lett 424:1–8

41. Diaz LA Jr, Bardelli A (2014) Liquid biopsies: genotyping circulating tumor DNA. J Clin Oncol 32:579–586

42. Cheng F, Su L, Qian C (2016) Circulating tumor DNA: a promising biomarker in the liquid biopsy of cancer. Oncotarget 7:48832–48841

43. Lo YM, Zhang J, Leung TN, Lau TK, Chang AM, Hjelm NM (1999) Rapid clearance of fetal DNA from maternal plasma. Am J Hum Genet 64:218–224

44. Yu SC, Lee SW, Jiang P, Leung TY, Chan KC, Chiu RW, Lo YM (2013) High-resolution profiling of fetal DNA clearance from maternal plasma by massively parallel sequencing. Clin Chem 59:1228–1237

45. Underhill HR, Kitzman JO, Hellwig S, Welker NC, Daza R, Baker DN, Gligorich KM et al (2016) Fragment length of circulating tumor DNA. PLoS Genet 12:e1006162

46. Daniotti M, Vallacchi V, Rivoltini L, Patuzzo R, Santinami M, Arienti F, Cutolo G et al (2007) Detection of mutated BRAFV600E variant in circulating DNA of stage III-IV melanoma patients. Int J Cancer 120:2439–2444

47. Lee JH, Long GV, Boyd S, Lo S, Menzies AM, Tembe V, Guminski A et al (2017) Circulating tumour DNA predicts response to anti-PD1 antibodies in metastatic melanoma. Ann Oncol 28:1130

48. Warton K, Mahon KL, Samimi G (2016) Methylated circulating tumor DNA in blood: power in cancer prognosis and response. Endocr Relat Cancer 23:R157–R171

49. Felicetti F, De Feo A, Coscia C, Puglisi R, Pedini F, Pasquini L, Bellenghi M et al (2016) Exosome-mediated transfer of miR-222 is sufficient to increase tumor malignancy in melanoma. J Transl Med 14:56

50. Pfeffer SR, Grossmann KF, Cassidy PB, Yang CH, Fan M, Kopelovich L, Leachman SA et al (2015) Detection of Exosomal miRNAs in the plasma of melanoma patients. J Clin Med 4:2012–2027

51. Lunavat TR, Cheng L, Einarsdottir BO, Olofsson Bagge R, Veppil Muralidharan S, Sharples RA, Lasser C et al (2017) BRAFV600 inhibition alters the microRNA cargo in the vesicular secretome of malignant melanoma cells. Proc Natl Acad Sci USA 114:E5930–E5939
52. Gopalakrishnan V, Spencer CN, Nezi L, Reuben A, Andrews MC, Karpinets TV, Prieto PA, Vicente D, Hoffman K, Wei SC et al (2018) Gut microbiome modulates response to anti-PD-1 immunotherapy in melanoma patients. Science 359:97–103
53. Huard B, Tournier M, Hercend T, Triebel F, Faure F (1994) Lymphocyte-activation gene 3/major histocompatibility complex class II interaction modulates the antigenic response of CD4+ T lymphocytes. Eur J Immunol 24:3216–3221
54. Woo SR et al (2012) Immune inhibitory molecules LAG-3 and PD-1 synergistically regulate T-cell function to promote tumoral immune escape. Cancer Res 72:917–927
55. Lichtenegger FS et al (2018) Targeting LAG-3 and PD-1 to enhance T cell activation by antigen-presenting cells. Front Immunol 9:385
56. Wolf Y, Anderson AC, Kuchroo VK (2019) TIM3 comes of age as an inhibitory receptor. Nat Rev Immunol 20:173–185. https://doi.org/10.1038/s41577-41019-40224-41576
57. Lu X et al (2017) Tumor antigen-specific CD8(+) T cells are negatively regulated by PD-1 and Tim-3 in human gastric cancer. Cell Immunol 313:43–51
58. Shayan G et al (2017) Adaptive resistance to anti-PD1 therapy by Tim-3 upregulation is mediated by the PI3K-Akt pathway in head and neck cancer. Onco Targets Ther 6:e1261779
59. Fourcade J et al (2010) Upregulation of Tim-3 and PD-1 expression is associated with tumor antigen-specific CD8+ T cell dysfunction in melanoma patients. J Exp Med 207:2175–2186
60. Ngiow SF et al (2011) Anti-TIM3 antibody promotes T cell IFN-gamma-mediated antitumor immunity and suppresses established tumors. Cancer Res 71:3540–3551
61. Isshiki T et al (2017) Cutting edge: anti-TIM-3 treatment exacerbates pulmonary inflammation and fibrosis in mice. J Immunol 199:3733–3737
62. Gabrilovich DI (2017) Myeloid-derived suppressor cells. Cancer Immunol Res 5:3–8
63. Rohaan MW, van den Berg JH, Kvistborg P, Haanen J (2018) Adoptive transfer of tumor-infiltrating lymphocytes in melanoma: a viable treatment option. J Immunother Cancer 6:102
64. Rosenberg SA et al (2011) Durable complete responses in heavily pretreated patients with metastatic melanoma using T-cell transfer immunotherapy. Clin Cancer Res 17:4550–4557
65. Spencer CN et al (2019) The gut microbiome (GM) and immunotherapy response are influenced by host lifestyle factors. Cancer Res 79:2838
66. Kim SH et al (2017) Phenformin inhibits myeloid-derived suppressor cells and enhances the anti-tumor activity of PD-1 blockade in melanoma. J Investig Dermatol 137:1740–1748
67. Orecchioni S et al (2015) The biguanides metformin and phenformin inhibit angiogenesis, local and metastatic growth of breast cancer by targeting both neoplastic and microenvironment cells. Int J Cancer 136:E534–E544
68. Vara-Ciruelos D et al (2019) Phenformin, but not metformin, delays development of T cell acute lymphoblastic leukemia/lymphoma via cell-autonomous AMPK activation. Cell Rep 27:690–698
69. Ott PA et al (2013) Phase I/II study of pegylated arginine deiminase (ADI-PEG 20) in patients with advanced melanoma. Investig N Drugs 31:425–434
70. Speiser DE, Ho PC, Verdeil G (2016) Regulatory circuits of T cell function in cancer. Nat Rev Immunol 16:599–611
71. Yan D et al (2019) Lipid metabolic pathways confer the immunosuppressive function of myeloid-derived suppressor cells in tumor. Front Immunol 10:1399
72. Yang W et al (2016) Potentiating the antitumour response of CD8(+) T cells by modulating cholesterol metabolism. Nature 531:651–655
73. Zhang Y et al (2017) Enhancing CD8(+) T cell fatty acid catabolism within a metabolically challenging tumor microenvironment increases the efficacy of melanoma immunotherapy. Cancer Cell 32:377–391

Melanin Based Classification of Skin Types and Their Susceptibility to UV-Induced Cancer

3

Bidisha Bhattacharya, Disha Chauhan, Abhishek Kumar Singh, and Mallika Chatterjee

Abstract

One of the characteristics that easily distinguish every human being is their skin complexion. The primary pigment that brings about this distinction is melanin. And just like most other physical characteristics, the degree of pigmentation is a genetically inherited factor. As is explained by the gradation of colours from very light to dark brown, it is understood that skin colour is not governed by one specific gene, rather it is a polygenic trait. Skin colour is also influenced to some extent by the environment as well, for example, sun exposure. That is to say, while genetic expression decides the basal level of melanin synthesis, exposure to ultraviolet radiation acts as a fine tuner and upregulates or downregulates this synthesis and distribution. It is known with some clarity that apart from imparting pigment to the skin, melanin also plays a photoprotective role by preventing the cellular and molecular damage caused due to UV radiations. However, lately it has been observed that melanin also has deleterious effects that arise due to its photolabile nature. This chapter focuses on the ethnic classifications of skin types based on the melanin synthesis and susceptibility of these skin types to UV-induced cancer. Further it elaborates on the genetic correlates of melanin synthesis and distribution. The chapter concludes with the molecular mechanisms that underlie both the protective and the deleterious effects of melanin.

Keywords

Melanocyte · Melanosomes · Eumelanin · Pheomelanin · Neuromelanin · Photoprotection · Photodegradation

B. Bhattacharya · D. Chauhan · A. K. Singh · M. Chatterjee (✉)
Amity Institute of Neuropsychology & Neurosciences, Amity University, Noida, Uttar Pradesh, India
e-mail: mchatterjee@amity.edu

3.1   Skin and Its Biological Functions

The skin, together with its appendages like various glands, nails, and hair follicles together constitute the integumentary system. It covers the entire exposed surface area of our body because of which it the largest organ in the human body. The skin, throughout the body serves multiple functions like [1]:

1. Barrier function: It protects the internal organs from environmental exposure of harmful substances like pathogenic microorganisms, toxic and corrosive chemicals, irritants and allergens, sharp objects, and ultraviolet radiations. Likewise, it also prevents the loss of fluids, electrolytes, proteins, and nutrients from within the body.
2. Immunological functions: Skin is the first line of defence for any external environmental hazard like bacterial or viral infections or toxicants that gain entry through contact.
3. Integrity: Skin is a lining that bounds all the internal organs and tissues together and ensures that they remain in contact with each other in their proper place.
4. Wound healing and repair of injury: The healing capacity of the skin allows the repair of all minor to major cuts and burns. This is essential because considering the barrier function of skin; no area can be left cut open for long.
5. Sensory organ: Sensations like touch, itch, pain, heat, and cold are all extremely important for survival of the body and are perceived from skin.

3.2   Histological Structure of Skin

The longitudinal cross-section of skin reveals two main layers—epidermis and dermis with a subcutaneous loose connective tissue called hypodermis deep within, that blends with dermis by an unclear boundary (Fig. 3.1). The uppermost epidermis is a stratified, keratinised, squamous epithelium. Dermis is the adjacent fibrous collagenous-elastic tissue containing blood vessels, nerves, and sensory receptors to support epidermis. The epidermis is further divided into five layers based on its constituent cell type, namely *stratum basale* (or *stratum germinativum*), *stratum spinosum, stratum granulosum, stratum lucidum,* and *stratum corneum*, in sequence from the innermost to the topmost layer (Fig. 3.2) [1].

There are four different cell types that make up these different layers of the epidermis – keratinocytes being the most abundant ones and the other three are specialized non-epithelial cells interspersed at specific locations namely: melanin-producing melanocytes, tactile Merkel cells, and antigen-presenting Langerhans cells.

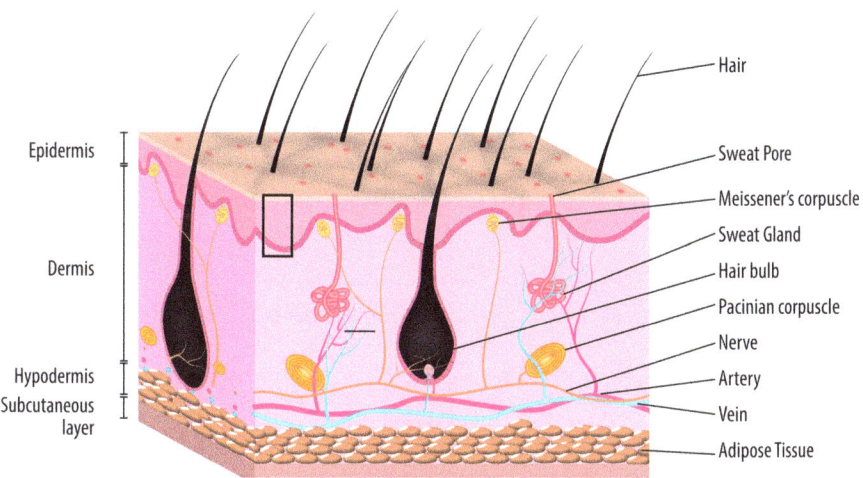

Fig. 3.1 Longitudinal section of skin

3.3   Melanocyte and Skin Pigmentation

Neural crest cells-derived melanocytes constitute the pigment system of skin and are the second most populous cell type in the epithelium (Fig. 3.2). Hair bulbs have follicular melanocytes for transference of melanin to the hair. Typically, human skin has between 1000 and 2000 melanocytes per mm^2 that comprise around 2–3% of the total epidermal cells. There are primarily four functions that characterize a melanocyte - the synthesis of melanin granules; the growth and maintenance of dendrites; the translocation of melanin granules within the cytoplasm in response to hormones or neurotransmitters; the transfer of melanin granules to adjacent cells that have phagocytic capacities. They have a round cell body with a clear cytoplasm since they continuously transfer the secreted melanin pigment to their satellite epidermal keratinocytes through the thin dendritic cytoplasmic extensions. Phagosomes release their melanin granules into the cytoplasm of keratinocytes which accumulate in supranuclear areas like an umbrella. Melanin protects the DNA of the cells by absorbing and scattering the harmful destructive ultraviolet (UV) rays. The exposed amount of UV radiation proportionally stimulates the production of melanin and accelerates its transfer to keratinocytes. This also darkens the existing ones. Along with this, melanin also plays an important role in determining the colour of skin (shades in gradation from brown to black). A darker skin colour depends on the amount of melanin production in melanocytes and their transfer rate to keratinocytes [1].

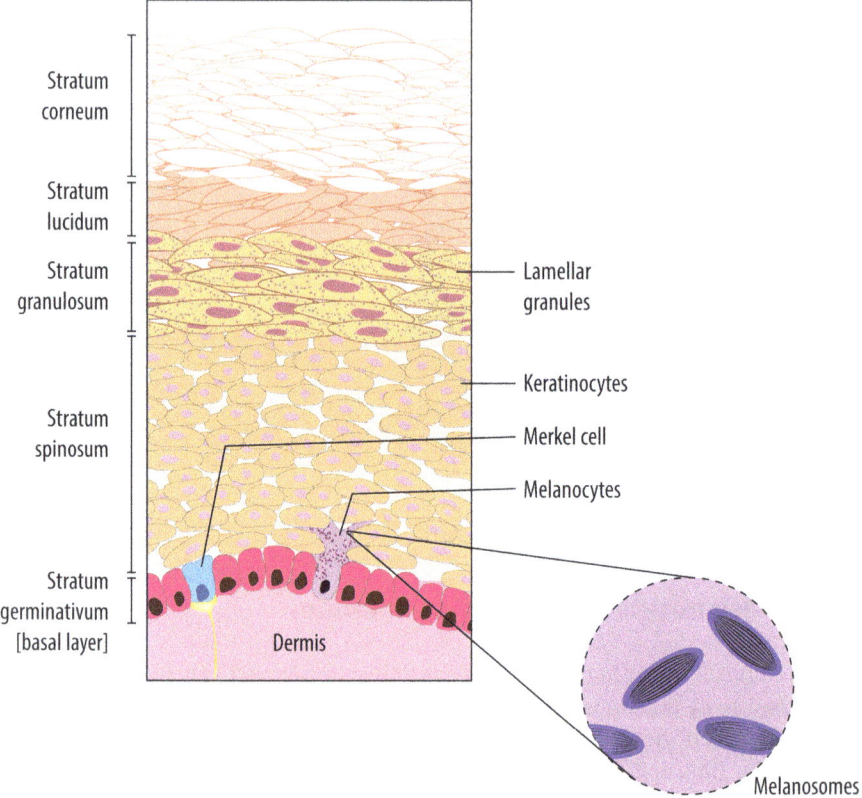

Fig. 3.2 Magnified cartoon of skin (boxed area in Fig. 3.1) showing layers containing melanocytes and melanosomes

3.4 Melanocyte Ultrastructure and Intracellular Dynamics

Melanocytes are highly functionally active cells that undergo dynamic changes in internal cellular composition and the overall cellular structure as is seen in studies that focus on each step of their functionality (Fig. 3.3) [2, 3]:

1. Synthesis of Melanin Granules

   Melanin granules are the secretions of the single membrane-bound organelles called melanosomes present specifically within melanocytes. Like any other secretory organelle, they are bound by a single membrane and have an organized matrix structure of melanin pigment. Melanisation takes place on the surface of thin melanofilaments which are present within the melanosome. These gradually thickening filaments due to melanin deposition fuse together laterally and form

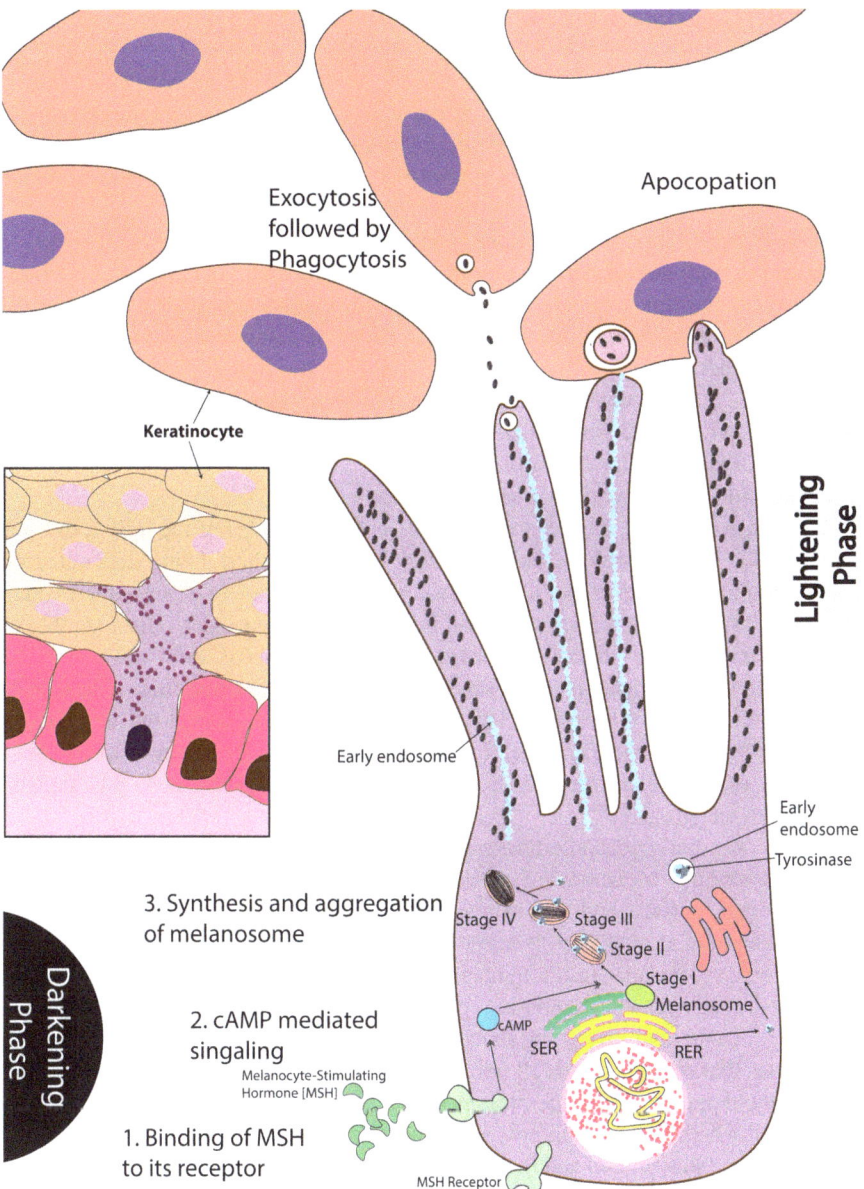

Fig. 3.3 Schematic representation of synthesis and distribution of melanin (based on data from Moellmann et al. [2])

intricate lattice like arrangement with the thickness of a single filament within the melanosome.

These melanosomes develop as a focal dilation of the smooth endoplasmic reticulum (SER) that is in continuation with the rough endoplasmic reticulum (RER). After pinching off from the endoplasmic reticulum, the melanosomal membrane distally fuses with tyrosinase-rich coated vesicles originating from the Golgi apparatus, forming the mature functional melanosome.

2. Growth and Maintenance of Melanocytic Dendrites

Several functional similarities exist between melanocytic dendrites and neurites. These are the thin processes that project from the melanocyte cell body to the nearby keratinocytes and structurally resemble neuronal dendrites. Many microtubules and microfilaments run parallel to the longitudinal axes of these processes. Apart from these cytoskeletal proteins, these processes also contain axially oriented mitochondria, membrane-bound vesicles, and rough endoplasmic reticulum along with melanosomes.

3. Intracellular Translocation of Melanin Granules

The translocation of the melanin granules in the dendrites of the melanocytes is somewhat similar to the axoplasmic flow in neurons, both being dependent on microtubules. However, the difference lies in the direction of translocation which is centrifugal in axons and centripetal in melanocytic processes. The assembly of subsequent tubulin subunits to form the microtubules is only needed in the direction of centripetal aggregation of melanin granules while their disassembly aids in dispersion of the melanin granules in all directions within the melanocyte. This dispersion is also facilitated by many intradendritic melanocytic filaments in such a manner that when these filaments disappear in the cell, the melanin granules reaggregate.

The skin undergoes alternate periods of darkening and lightening depending on interaction of Melanocyte Stimulating Hormone(MSH) with its receptor on the melanocyte surface and downstream cAMP signaling that stimulates melanin synthesis and aggregation corresponding to the darkening phase followed by dispersion of granules in the lightening phase.

In the subsequent lightening phase, the melanin granules get dispersed throughout the cytoplasm and the nucleus shifts to a more central location. The granules that remain in the cell body remain dispersed randomly while those that enter the dendrites orient themselves along the longitudinal axes. The cytoplasm of dendrites shows that the processes are packed with microfilaments of 10-nm type (neurofilamentous) and few or no microtubules are present. At the molecular level, cAMP is the switch between darkening and lightening phase as it induces the formation of 10-nm filaments and simultaneously reduces the number of microtubules.

4. Transfer of Melanin Granules to Keratinocytes

Each melanocyte transfers melanosomes to around 30 surrounding keratinocytes, forming the melano-epidermic unit. The ratio of keratinocytes to melanocytes in the melano-epidermic unit changes in different skin patches and animals, and is attributed to a genetic control. There are two proposed mechanisms that explain the transfer of melanin granules from melanocytes to adjacent keratinocytes. According to one of these, the melanin granules escape from the tip of the melanocyte dendrite by exocytosis into the extracellular matrix followed by its phagocytosis by the nearest keratinocyte. Yet another mechanism suggests that the entire distal end of the melanocyte dendrite is engulfed by the keratinocyte, termed as 'apocopation' such that melanin granule exchange takes place.

3.5   Melanin Pigment and Its Synthesis

Melanin is the generic name given to the most ubiquitous, resistant, heterogeneous, and ancient natural pigment. It is more commonly known as an animal cutaneous pigment, however, it is also found in plant, fungi, and bacterial kingdoms. From a structural point of view, melanin is a heterogeneous polymer derived by the oxidation of phenols and subsequent polymerization of intermediate phenols and their resulting quinones. It is defined with the molecular formula $C_{18}H_{10}O_4N_2$, an average mass of 318.3 for the minimal unit, and the systematic name *3,8-dimethyl-2,7-dihydrobenzo[1,7]isoindolo[6,5,4   cd]indole-4,5,9,10-tetrone*. Although most melanins are dark in colour, there exists a wide gradient in shades of black, brown, reddish, and yellowish. On this basis, different terms have emerged that represent a particular type and shade of melanin.

Accordingly, animal melanin is categorized into two broad categories – eumelanin (eu; good) and pheomelanin (pheo; cloudy or dusky). Eumelanin provides mainly dark colours, from brown to black. Small amounts can give place to sepia or grey colours, as in human hair at mature age. The other pigment pheomelanin provides fair colour, from reddish to yellowish. It is predominant in higher animals: mammals, birds, and reptiles but is still very rare in lower organisms [4].

L-Tyr and L-Dopa act as the precursors for the synthesis of eumelanin by activity of tyrosinase, the key enzyme of melanogenesis in animals and many microorganisms (Fig. 3.4). The tetrone simplified model of melanin has the empirical composition $C_{18}H_{10}O_4N_2$. On the other hand, the precursor for pheomelanin is 5-Cys-dopa monomer which consists of two main units—benzothiazines and benzothiazoles (Fig. 3.5).

However, melanin is not restricted to skin and hair. The extra-cutaneous melanogenic system imparts colour to the tissue underlying the iris of the eye, eyespots, retinal epithelial pigment (REP), and the *stria vascularis* of the inner ear. It is also found in adrenal glands of some mammals, adipose tissue, and certain brain regions like the catecholaminergic neurons in substantia nigra where it is called neuromelanin. Neuromelanin is a mixture of pheomelanin and eumelanin with pheomelanin at the core and eumelanin covering it to form the surface. Neuromelanin is the only type of mammalian melanins that is not formed in melanocytes, but in catecholaminergic neurons. This location is related to the double-edged sword properties sometimes attributed to neuromelanin, as melanin formation in the cytosol of neurons could have cytotoxic properties. While the

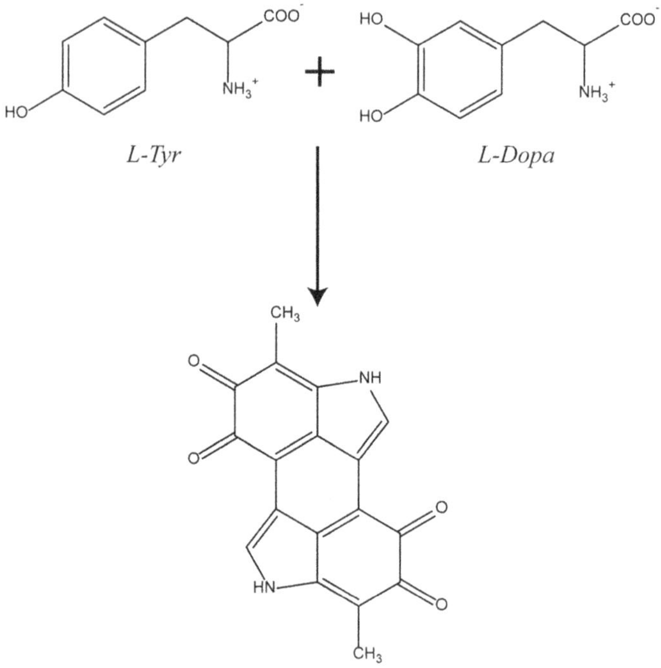

Fig. 3.4 Synthesis of eumelanin

process of melanin formation can be damaging for the cell, once the polymer is formed, it can act as a cytosolic scavenger for potentially neurotoxic sub-products, as Fe (III) or reactive oxygen species (ROS) due to oxidation of catecholamine neurotransmitters. Although it is produced as a waste product of catecholamine metabolism, its specific functions in dopaminergic neurons of the substantia nigra are critical factors to explain the vulnerability of this brain region to early and massive degeneration in Parkinson's disease (PD) [4].

Keeping in mind the variety of structures and occurrences of melanin, its biogenesis is not a single and universal biochemical pathway. However, the entire process can be generalized as an initial phase with the enzyme-catalysed oxidation of phenolic precursors to quinones followed by a final phase consisting of the mostly unregulated polymerization of quinones. The universal and well-known route for eumelanin and pheomelanin is the Raper–Mason pathway (Fig. 3.6) [4].

The initial phase up to L-dopaquinone production is common to both pheomelanin and eumelanin. It is formed by oxidation of L-tyrosine by the two enzymatic activities of tyrosinase—that of tyrosine hydroxylase and of dopa oxidase. L-Dopaquinone is thus the pivotal intermediate. Addition of L-cysteine gives place to benzothiazine units and then to pheomelanins (Fig. 3.6, right). In the absence of L-cysteine, eumelanogenesis takes place since L-dopaquinone is spontaneously cycled to L-leukodopachrome. The reaction between indoline and L-dopaquinone is very spontaneous that yields L-dopachrome. L-Dopachrome is

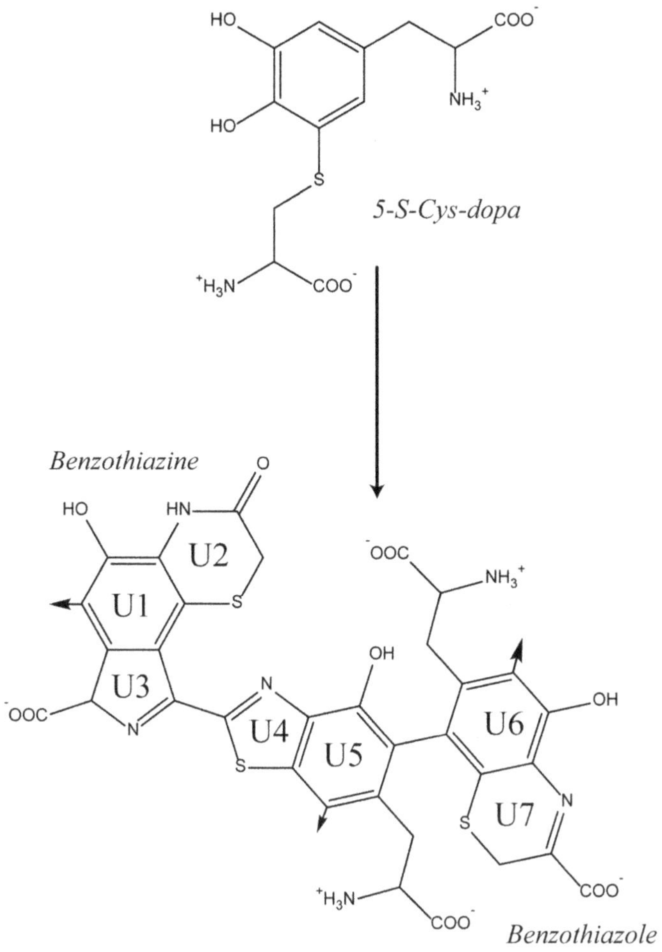

Fig. 3.5 Synthesis of pheomelanin

then converted to 5,6-dihydroxyindole (DHI) and 5,6-dihydroxyindole-2-carboxylic acid (DHICA) mixtures, depending on the Trp2 activity and decarboxylation rate. Further oxidation of these dihydroxyindoles by tyrosinase or Trp1 gives rise to indolequinones while subsequent crosslink reactions between hydroxyl and quinone forms lead to formation of the polymer. In the final phase of polymerization, the Pmel17 protein located in the melanosome seems to have a role in the regulation and deposition of the polymer on that organelle [4].

Neuromelanin formation is yet another pathway and is not a random mixture of eumelanin and pheomelanin generated from the Raper–Mason pathway. The initial precursor in this case is L-tyrosine, which is hydroxylated to L-dopa by neuronal tyrosine hydroxylase (Fig. 3.7). Catecholaminergic neurons show high amino acid decarboxylase activity. This yields dopamine and which is later oxidized to

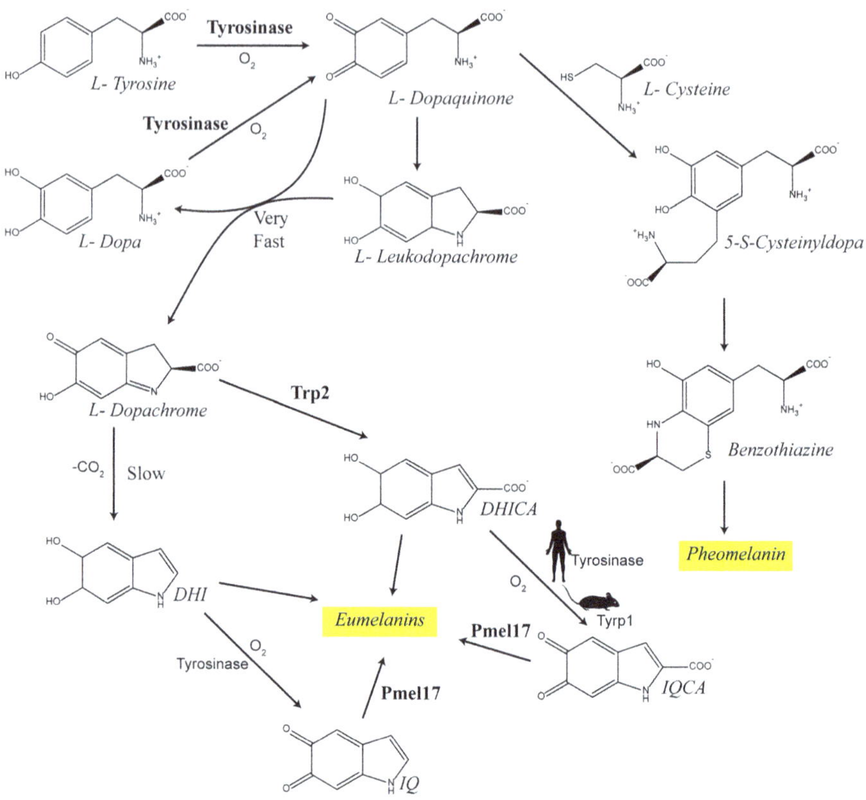

Fig. 3.6 Raper–Mason pathway for synthesis of eumelanin and pheomelanin

dopamine quinone. This is either catalysed by a peroxidase or it occurs spontaneously by the action of ROS. Similar to L-dopaquinone in the Raper–Mason pathway, this quinone is also pivotal in the route, giving place to 5-S-cysdopamine or DHI depending on the presence or the absence of L-cys during the dopamine quinone formation. Since both indole and benzothiazine units are incorporated into the structure, hence neuromelanin is usually a mixed melanin.

Since melanin synthesis involves quinone formation and the latter species are potentially cytotoxic, due to the ROS generated during its formation and polymerization, melanin formation should be restricted to specific cellular and subcellular compartments. This explains the presence of the specialized cells, melanocytes and the function specific organelles, the melanosomes. Based on the type of melanin synthesized, there are two main types of melanosomes, spherical pheomelanosomes and ovoid eumelanosomes. Apart from the difference in the type of melanin pigment formed, differences in the amino acid transport systems to these organelles to control the availability of L-tyrosine and also of L-cysteine or glutathione inside the organelle also regulates the formation of pheo-oreumelanin [4].

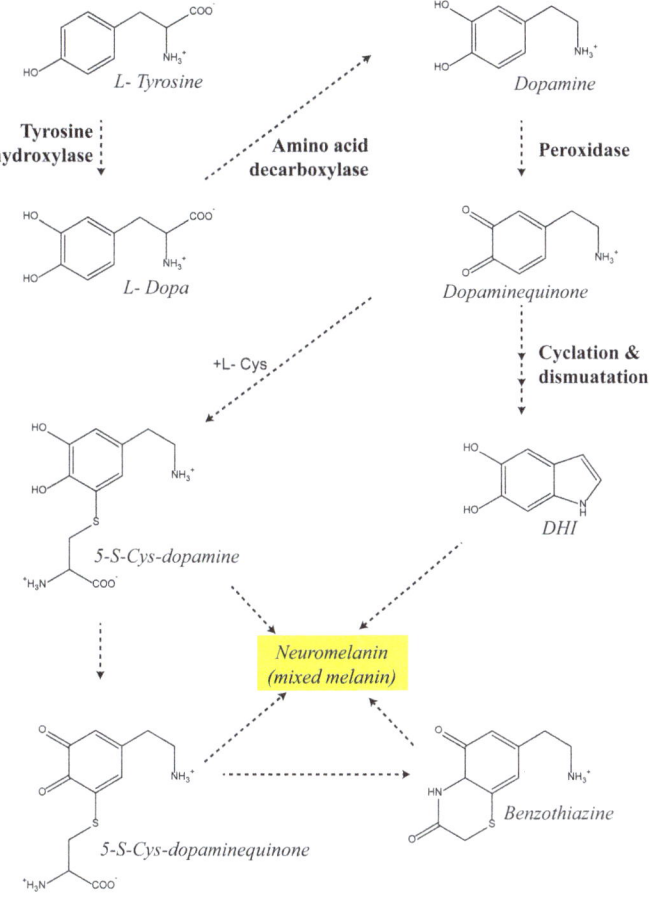

Fig. 3.7 Synthesis of neuromelanin

3.6 Regulation of Melanin Synthesis by Sun Exposure

Based on an individual's melanogenic potential, the ability to adjust melanin concentration in the melanocytes with respect to solar exposure has given rise to two types of skin pigmentation, namely – Constitutive and Facultative. Constitutive skin colour results from the genetically determined levels of melanin in the skin that is not influenced by any internal or external factors. On the other hand, facultative pigmentation is due to induced increase in epidermal melanin content as a defence mechanism to guard against the damaging effects of UV radiation. This UV-induced pigmentation proceeds in certain distinct steps [5–7]:

Table 3.1 Classification of skin phototypes based on skin pigmentation upon UV exposure

Skin phototype	Characteristics
I	Very fair skin who always burn and never tan when exposed to the sun
II	Tan minimally with difficulty and burn easily
III	Tan moderately and uniformly and burn moderately
IV	Burn minimally and tan moderately and easily
V	Very dark skin who rarely burn and tan profusely
VI	Never burn and tan profusely upon sun exposure

1. Immediate pigment darkening (IPD): Within minutes of UV exposure, it appears as a greyish-brown colouration, not due to synthesis of new melanin pigment, but, rather due to photo-oxidation of pre-existing melanin and the redistribution of existing melanosomes from a perinuclear to a peripheral dendritic location.
2. Persistent pigment darkening (PPD): Prolonged second phase of tan brown colouration due to melanin oxidation that occurs within hours after UV exposure and persists at least 3–5 days. It is elicited more strongly by UVA than by UVB exposure.
3. Delayed tanning (DT): This step occurs after 2–3 days of UV exposure and as a result of stimulation of melanin synthesis. It involves increase in the number and activity of functional melanocytes, increased dendricity, increased synthesis and transfer as well as altered packaging of melanosomes. Simultaneously, there is an increase in the activity of tyrosinase, the rate-limiting enzyme in the melanogenic pathway. UVB-induced DT is photoprotective while UVA-induced DT is not considered to be so.

Individuals with different constitutive pigmentation have varying degrees of burning or tanning in response to UV exposure which forms the basis of classification of skin phototypes as listed in Table 3.1 [8].

3.7   Skin Pigmentation Diversity and Classification of Skin Types

Skin pigmentation is a highly variable phenotype in humans and available evidence indicates that this observed variation in the trait, both inter-population and intra-population, is due to natural selection. The current evolutionary hypothesis in support of natural selection is the Vitamin D/Folate hypothesis which states that a compromise exists between the requirements for photoprotection on the one hand and vitamin D3 synthesis on the other hand. The geographic distribution of skin pigmentation is strongly correlated with latitude and UV radiation intensity. World map of skin colour shows that darker skin types can be found mostly in tropical regions and is strongly correlated to the world map of yearly mean of daily irradiation in UV (280–400 nm) (Figs. 3.8 and 3.9).

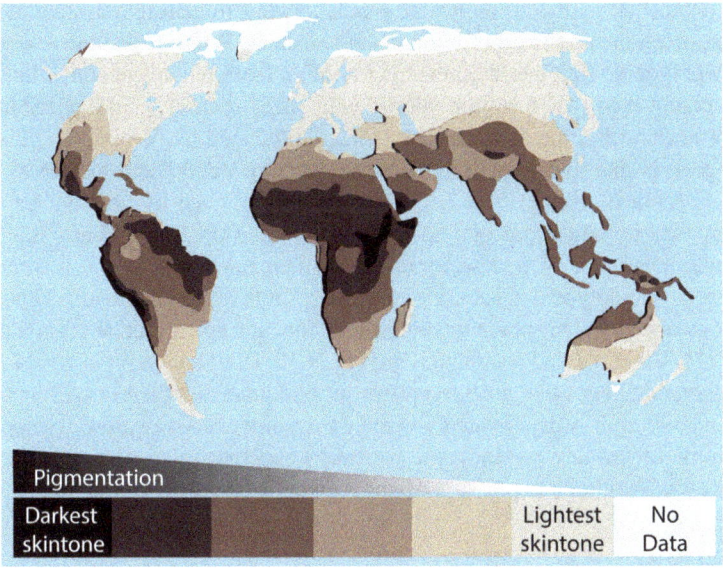

Fig. 3.8 World map of skin tone distribution (adapted from Del Bino et al. [9])

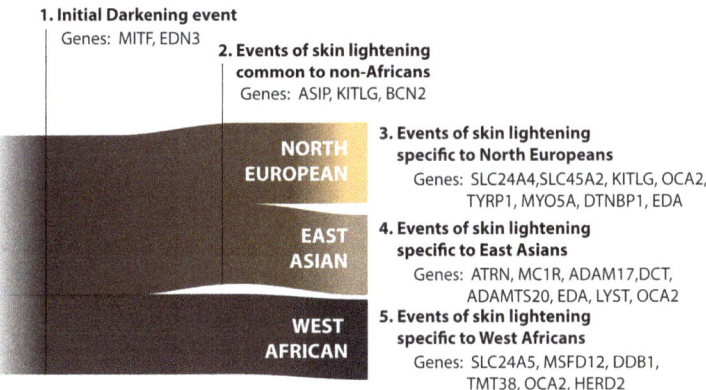

Fig. 3.9 Speculative Sankey chart representation for human skin pigmentation (adapted from McEvoy et al. [10]). Shading in the chart shows deduced pigmentation levels of populations. Genes hypothesized to have been subject to positive selection are listed

Although all races of human beings possess a similar concentration of melanocytes in their skin, melanocytes in different ethnic groups and among some individuals differ in the level of expression of the genes related in melanin production, which can alter significantly due to the presence of small nucleotide polymorphisms (SNPs) affecting various steps of the melanogenesis process, thereby conferring a greater or lesser melanin amounts in the skin and hair, and in the relative amounts of eumelanin and pheomelanin produced. This process is mostly controlled by the hormonealpha-melanocyte stimulating hormone (α-MSH), produced from the precursor proopiomelanocortin (POMC). Constitutive pigmentation is a polygenic trait based on the quality of melanin with respect to relative ratio of eumelanin and pheomelanin along with size, quantity, and distribution of melanosomes within the epidermis. It is also influenced by paracrine regulation of melanogenesis due to cross-talk between melanocytes and keratinocytes as well as dermal fibroblasts. However, it is not particularly affected by varying melanocyte densities that remain more or less constant in all skin types. Since this trait is polygenic, a number of genes controlling melanogenesis give rise to four major ethnic skin phenotypes- Caucasian, Oriental, Indian, and African. The genetic alterations and resultant phenotypes in these four groups are detailed in Table 3.2 [9, 10, 21]. Table 3.3 and accompanying Fig. 3.10 detail the chromosomal locations of melanogenic genes that are susceptible to mutations and therefore of importance in understanding disorders related to melanin dysbiogenesis. Figure 3.11 depicts the interactome of the key melanogenic pathways and the principal genes within this network, whose altered expression affect pigmentation in the ethnic groups.

3.8 Skin Cancer and UV-Induced Damage

According to the World Health Organisation (WHO), skin cancer is the most common malignancy in the white population that inhabit the Western world, particularly the Caucasians. Skin cancer is an umbrella term under which reside many categories based on the cells they originate from and their clinical behaviour. These categories are depicted below (Fig. 3.12) [22].

1. Non-melanocytic skin cancer (NMSC): As is understood from the term 'non-melanocytic', the skin cell types affected in this type of cancer are those other than the melanocytes. It is in general the most common malignancy found in humans. The most important etiological factors include certain chemical carcinogens, UV light, and ionizing radiations. Further specific to the cell type, there are two sub-categories namely –.
   (a) Basal cell carcinoma (BCC): It represents 80–85% of all NMSCs, which makes it the most common skin cancer type. Moreover, its worldwide incidence has a trend of 10% increase annually and mostly affects older men but is also seen to occur in younger women.
   (b) Squamous cell carcinoma (SCC): It represents the remaining 15–20% of the NMSCs. It is benign in terms of its growth pattern and localized tissue distribution. However, it is fatal more often than not when compared to BCC. Its incidence rate is also increasing but the rate of increase varies with the geographical location.
2. Malignant melanoma (MM): This marks the cancerous progression specifically in the melanocytes. Its incidence is still on the rise in areas with fair complexion population that is overly exposed to sun radiation. The incidence in the Caucasian population is 16 times greater than in Afro-Americans and 10 times greater than in Latin-Americans. The incidence rate, however, is higher in males, making it

Table 3.2 Single nucleotide polymorphism (SNP) in melanogenic genes and resultant different skin types

Gene	Function	Ethnic group	Genetic alterations and phenotype	Ref.
Melanin synthesis				
MC1R	Melanocortin-1-receptor (switch between eumelanin and pheomelanin synthesis within the melanocytes)	Caucasian	SNP (rs1805005 G > T, rs1805006 C > A, rs1805007 C > T), sun sensitivity and freckles	[11, 12]
		Oriental	SNP, lighter skin reflectance and freckles	
IRF4	Interferon regulatory factor 4 (strongly associated with skin colour, skin tanning response, freckling, and nevus count)	Caucasian	SNP (rs12203592 C > T), reduced skin tanning response, freckling, and sun sensitivity	[11, 13]
ASIP	Agouti signaling protein (antagonist of MC1R and upon binding to its receptor, ASIP promotes the synthesis of pheomelanin)	Caucasian	Polymorphism associated with sensitivity to sun and freckling	
		Oriental	SNP (rs 6,058,017 G)	[14]
TYR	Tyrosinase (encodes a key enzyme in melanogenesis)	Caucasian	Involved in normal variation of pigmentation. Polymorphism correlated with the levels of serum 25[OH]D, impact on vitamin D status and deficiency	
		Indian	Accounts for the differences between darkest and lightest skin reflectance	
TYRP1	Tyrosinase related protein 1 (aids TYR in melanogenesis)	Caucasian	Polymorphism correlated with the levels of serum 25[OH]D, impact on vitamin D status and deficiency	
		Oriental	SNP (rs1393350 A, rs1408799 C > T, rs2733832 C > T)	[11, 12]
		Indian	SNP, frequently associated with red-bronze skin	
		African	SNP (rs34803545), frequently associated with red-bronze skin	[15]

(continued)

Table 3.2 (continued)

Gene	Function	Ethnic group	Genetic alterations and phenotype	Ref.
Melanocyte biogenesis and survival				
KITLG	Hyper-pigmentation c-KIT receptor	Caucasian	SNP (rs12821256 T > C)	[11, 12]
		Oriental	SNP (rs642742 A > G)	[11]
DDB1	Damage specific DNA binding protein 1	Caucasian	SNP (rs11230664 C > T)	[16]
		Oriental	SNP (rs11230664 C > T)	[16]
		Indian	SNP (rs11230664 C > T, rs7120594 T, rs11230664 C)	[16]
		African	SNP (rs7120594 T, rs11230664 C)	[16]
HERC2	HECT and RLD domain containing E3 ubiquitin protein ligase 2	Caucasian	SNP (rs 6,497,271 A > G)	[16]
		Indian	SNP (rs 6,497,271 A)	[16]
		African	SNP (rs4932620 C > T)	[16]
SMARCA2	SWI/SNF related, matrix associated, actin dependent regulator of chromatin, subfamily A, member 2	African	SNP (rs7866411)	[15]
VLDLR	Very low density lipoprotein receptor	African	SNP (rs2093385)	[15]
Melanosome biogenesis and trafficking				
SLC24A5	Solute carrier family 24 member 5 (cation exchanger that has a key role in melanosome morphogenesis and melanogenesis)	Caucasian	SNP, mutations disrupt melanosomal maturation and melanin biosynthesis	
		Oriental	SNP (rs1426654 G > A)	[11,17,18]
		Indian	SNP at very high frequencies (rs1426654 G > A, rs1426654)	[11,15, 17, 18]
		African	SNP at very high frequencies (rs1426654 G, rs2470102)	[15,17, 18]
SLC45A2/ MATP	Solute carrier family 45 member 2/membrane associated transporter protein	Caucasian	Polymorphism associated with olive skin and immature melanosomes	
		Oriental	SNP (rs16891982 C > G)	[11, 17]
		Indian	SNP (rs16891982 C, rs26722 G > A)	[11, 17]
		African	SNP (rs16891982 C)	[17]

(continued)

Table 3.2 (continued)

Gene	Function	Ethnic group	Genetic alterations and phenotype	Ref.
OCA2	Chloride anion channel identified as effectors of melanosomal pH	Caucasian	SNP (rs1800407 G > A, rs1667394 A, rs7495174 A)	[11, 12]
		Oriental	SNP, major gene contributing to skin lightening	
		Indian	SNP (rs26722 G > A, rs1800414 A > G)	[11, 19, 20]
		African	SNP (rs1800404 C)	[11, 16]
MFSD12	Major facilitator superfamily domain containing 12 (transmembrane solute transporter that locates to late endosomes and/or lysosomes in melanocytes and not to eumelanosomes)	African	SNP (rs56203814 C > T, rs10424065 C > T, rs6510760 G, rs6510760 G > A)	[16]
SNX13	Regulates lysosomal degradation and G protein signaling associated with skin pigmentation	African	SNP (rs2110015 > T)	[15]
TMEM38	Transmembrane protein 38 (DNA repair)	African	SNP (rs7948623 A, rs7948623 A > T)	[16]

more common in males than in females worldwide. Once it becomes metastatic, the prognosis is very poor. Therefore, early identification of this cancer is crucial for the success of patient treatment [23]. There are multiple risk factors for MM namely:

(a) Skin type: Highest risk is in light skin population (1 in 40) while it is considerably lower in dark skinned people (1 in 1000) or Latin-American (1 in 200).

(b) Sun radiation: Both UVA and UVB of natural or artificial origin are carcinogenic. It is true that UV rays exert a positive effect by inducing desired tanning and Vitamin D synthesis; however, they also have a mutagenic effect and depress the immune system. The most important risk factor is the so-called intermittent sun exposure as against the much weaker risk factor of chronic or professional exposure.

(c) Age: Incidence of MM increases with age. The average age of a patient is 62 years. Nevertheless, MM is still one of the most common cancers in young adults as well.

Table 3.3 Chromosomal locations of melanogenic genes susceptible to mutations (chromosome length details from https://www.ncbi.nlm.nih.gov/grc/human/data) (gene locations derived from https://www.proteinatlas.org/)

Gene	Chromosome	Location	Class
MC1R	1	89,912,119	Melanin synthesis
SLC45A2/MATP	5	33,944,616	Melanosome biogenesis and trafficking
IRF4	6	391,739	Melanin synthesis
SNX13	7	17,790,761	Melanosome biogenesis and trafficking
SMARCA2	9	1,980,290	Melanocyte biogenesis and survival
VLDLR	9	2,621,834	Melanocyte biogenesis and survival
TYRP1	9	12,685,439	Melanin synthesis
TMEM38B	9	105,694,544	Melanosome biogenesis and trafficking
DDB1	11	61,299,451	Melanocyte biogenesis and survival
TYR	11	89,177,452	Melanin synthesis
KITLG	12	88,492,793	Melanocyte biogenesis and survival
OCA2	15	27,754,875	Melanosome biogenesis and trafficking
HERC2	15	28,111,040	Melanocyte biogenesis and survival
SLC24A5	15	48,120,972	Melanosome biogenesis and trafficking
MFSD12	19	3,538,261	Melanosome biogenesis and trafficking
TMEM38A	19	16,661,127	Melanosome biogenesis and trafficking
ASIP	20	34,194,569	Melanin synthesis

(d) Gender: The male population is more susceptible to MM than females in most of the world. Life risk for men is 1.5 times higher than that of women.

(e) Immunosuppression: This is a risk factor for MM that also reduces patient survival.

(f) Formerly removed MM: In patients with previous case history of MM, the risk for relapse of MM is 3–7%.

(g) Family history: 5–10% of MM appears in the 'high-risk' families. Familial form of MM is connected to multiple genes with both low and high penetrance. MC1R is the most commonly known low penetrance genes. Thus far, the high penetrance genes known are CDK4, CDKN2A, POT1, TERT, and BAP1. The most common mutation connected to the disease is the CDKN2A mutation, discovered in 2% of the MM patients.

UV radiations comprise of three set of wavelengths—ultraviolet C (UVC; 200–290 nm), ultraviolet B (UVB; 290–320 nm), and ultraviolet A (UVA; 320–400 nm), all of which have variable penetration and therefore have different effects on the skin. UVB plays a central role in the development of skin cancer since it causes sunburn and damages the epidermis. On the other hand, although UVA penetrates the skin deeper than UVB or UVC, it does not damage the epidermis considerably. UVC, however, penetrates the deeper layers of the skin limitedly. The direct consequence of UV exposure is the generation of DNA photoproducts, mainly cyclobutane pyrimidine dimers (CPD) and pyrimidine 6–4-pyrimidone

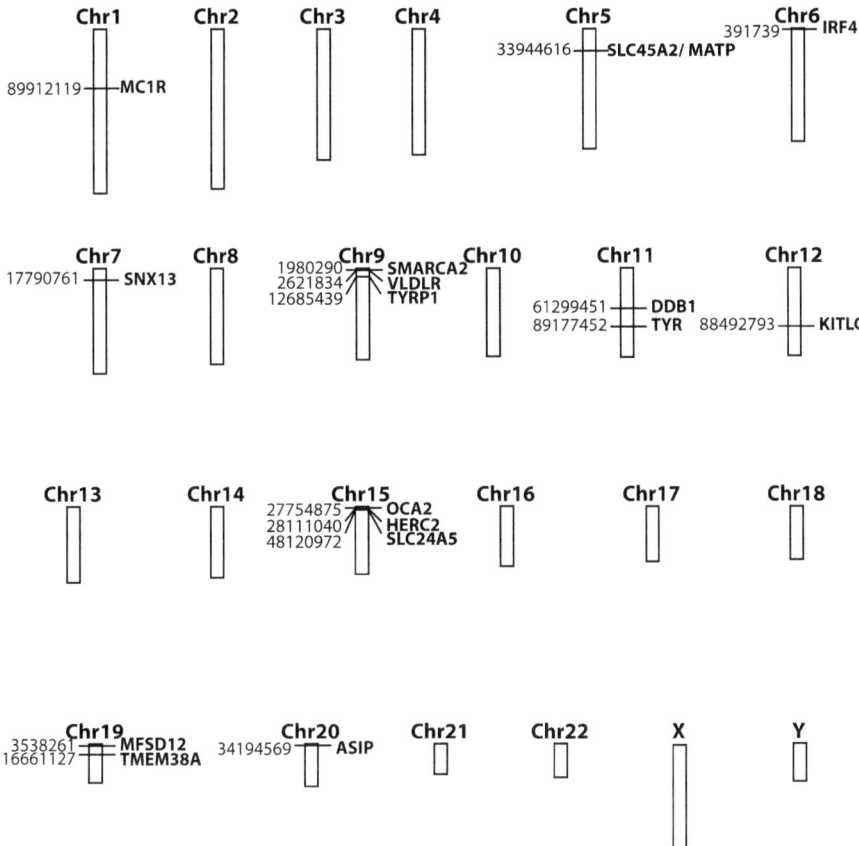

Fig. 3.10 Chromosome map of melanogenic genes susceptible to mutations (based on data from Table 3.3)

photoproducts (6-4PP). Additionally, UV-induced ROS indirectly cause oxidative DNA damage. UV-induced damage to cells and tissues thus includes DNA mutations and altered DNA integrity, changed transcription profile, and protein modification, which result in the dysregulation of the expression of multiple oncogenes and tumour suppressor genes. There are also frequent alterations in MAPK and PI3K/PTEN/AKT signaling pathways, thus leading to uncontrolled proliferations. The UV-induced DNA damage response pathway is modulated by the tumour suppressor p53, which functions in inducing cell cycle arrest, DNA repair, and apoptosis. p53 deletion drives UV-mediated mutagenesis in melanoma. Moreover, in response to UV, p53 also stimulates the proopiomelanocortin (POMC) promoter and induces the generation of melanocortin peptides including α-MSH. This is turn activates MC1R signaling. The MC1R–PTEN axis serves as a central regulator in response to UVB exposure in melanocytes. MC1R variants therefore are defective in association with PTEN following UV exposure, consequently failing to

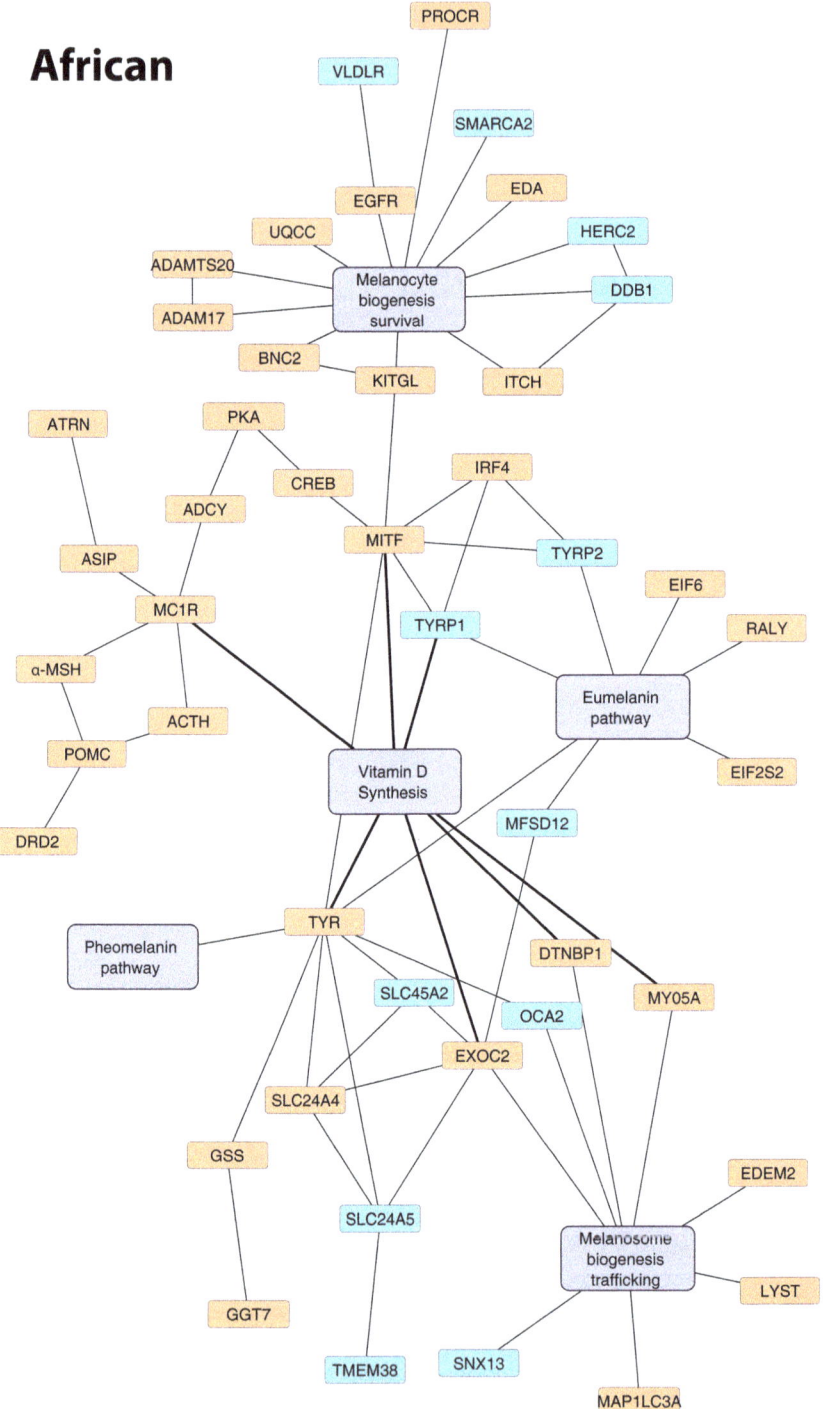

Fig. 3.11 Interaction networks of major melanogenic genes and gene polymorphism or changed gene expression that affect pigmentation in four ethnic skin types (Adapted from [21]). Affected genes are shown in blue

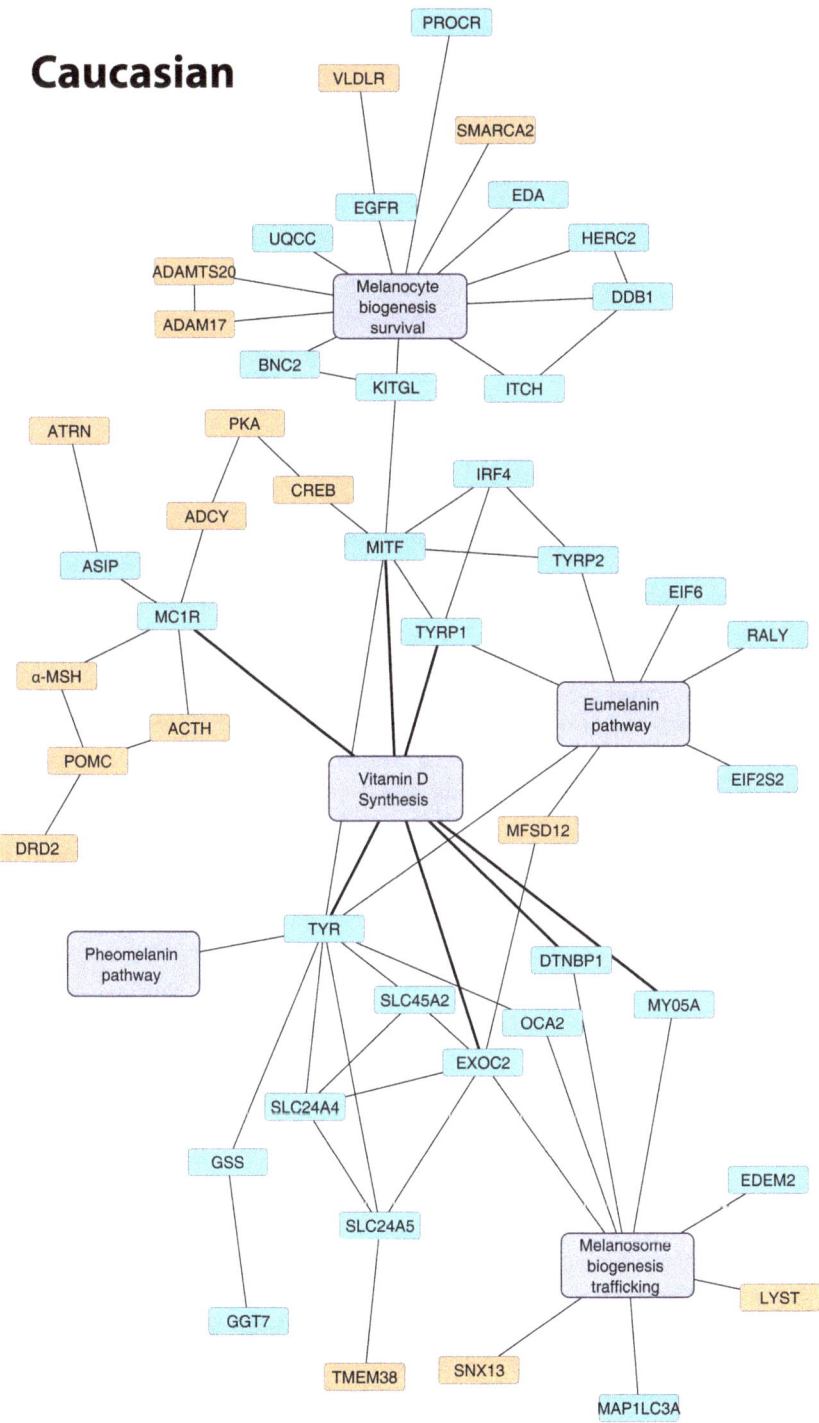

Fig. 3.11 (continued)

Fig. 3.12 Classification of skin cancer

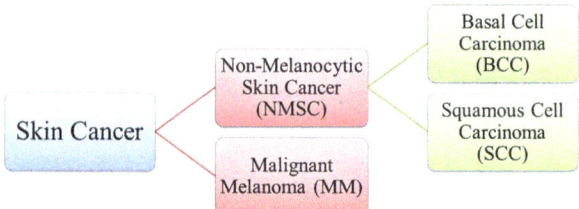

suppress the PI3K/AKT signaling pathway. This MC1R deficiency-induced elevation in PI3K/AKT signaling drives oncogenic transformation in melanoma [24]. The cross-talk between these pathways is represented in Fig. 3.13.

3.9 Photoprotective Role of Melanin

Epidemiological data strongly suggests an inverse correlation between skin pigmentation and incidence of UV-induced skin cancer which points towards a protective role of melanin. Out of the two types of melanin, eumelanin is generally accepted to be photoprotective. It acts as a physical barrier that scatters incident UV rays, as an absorbent filter that reduces the penetration of UV through the epidermis by 50–75% and also as a scavenger of ROS resulting from UV-induced cellular damage [6, 25]. Individuals with fair skin colour are at 70 times higher risk of developing skin cancer than individuals with dark skin colour because, dark skin having higher concentration of eumelanin than the fair skin, is better protected against UV-induced DNA and protein damage [6, 26]. What is striking is that melanin in dark skin is almost twice as effective as that found in fair skin in blocking UVB penetration. Furthermore, melanosomes once formed in the dark skin are resistant to (the type of UV that makes skin more prone to sunburn) degradation by lysosomal enzymes [27]. They remain intact throughout the epidermal layer and form a supranuclear shield or cap protecting the nucleus from UV-induced DNA damage [28]. On the contrary, melanosomes in fair skin get degraded easily and remain as melanin dust in the suprabasal layers, thus failing to protect the nucleus.

3.10 Deleterious Effects of Melanin

The protective role of melanin is discussed widely in the context of research that is related to pigmentation and skin cancer. However, melanin also has certain toxic effects especially after being exposed to UV radiation. In contrast to eumelanin, pheomelanin is weakly photoprotective against UV. It is also photolabile, undergoing extensive photodegradation by UVA and producing ROS like hydrogen peroxide and superoxide anions that react deleteriously with the DNA leading to mutations in the melanocytes (Fig. 3.14) [29, 30].

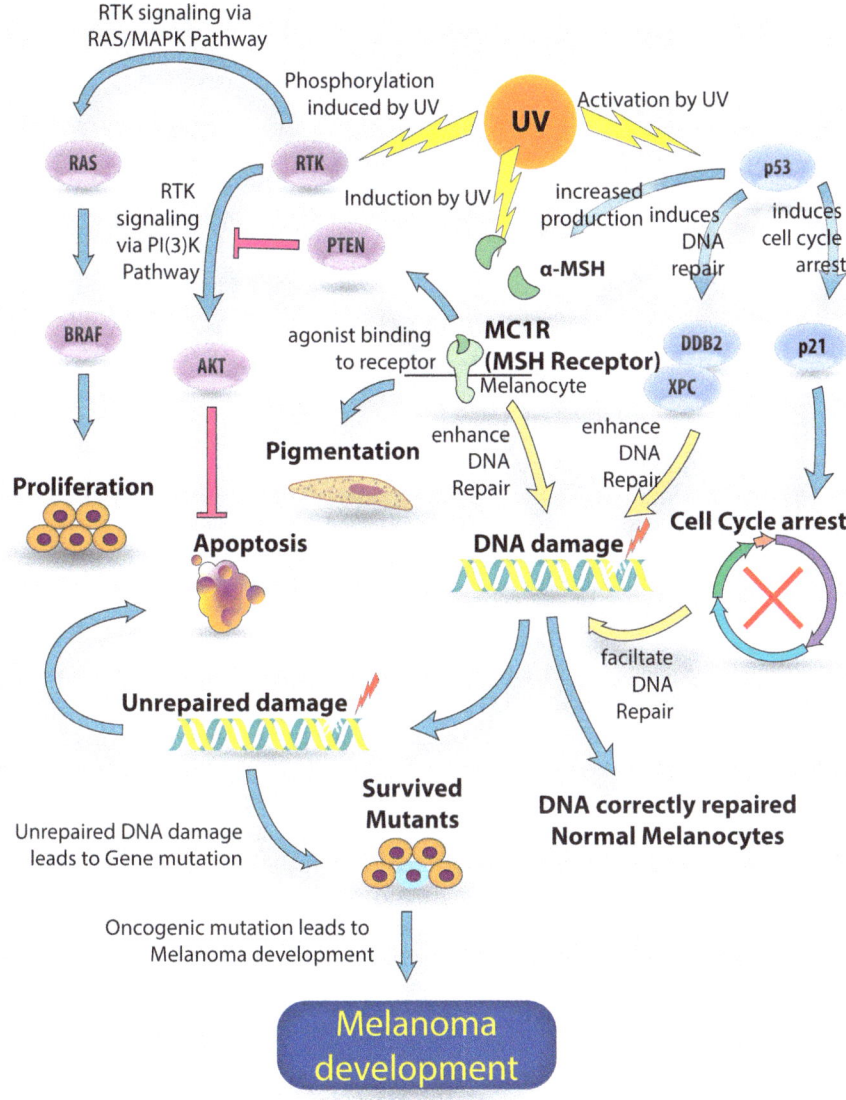

Fig. 3.13 Molecular mechanisms underlying the progression of UV-induced melanoma

UVA photoexcitation of benzothiazine chromophores within pheomelanin results in ROS generation from oxygen and modification of the pigment structural units with subsequent decrease in the photoprotective action as explained in the schematic above. Excited-state pheomelanin (singlet pheomelanin, [1]Pheomelanin) exhibiting an absorption maximum in the low energy red range of visible light decays to ground

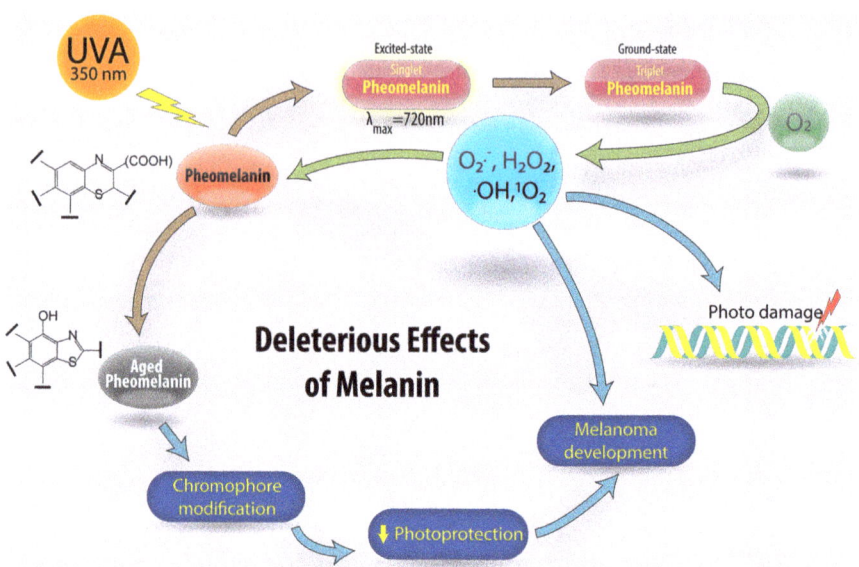

Fig. 3.14 Deleterious effect of pheomelanin

state (triplet pheomelanin, ^{3}Pheomelanin), a species capable of reducing molecular oxygen with production of ROS [31].

Pheomelanin synthesis and UV-mediated photo-oxidation also excessively depletes antioxidant reserves inside the cell adding to one of the other reasons that make its activity toxic to the cell (Fig. 3.15). Thus, increased pheomelanin, as in the fair skin individuals, photosensitizes DNA damage in lightly pigmented cells [25, 29, 31]. Additionally, pheomelanin increases the release of histamine, which contributes to the sun-induced erythema and oedema in fair skinned individuals [6]. Apart from these mechanisms, in vivo studies in mice have revealed that UV-irradiated melanin, particularly pheomelanin, photosensitizes adjacent epidermal cells to caspase-3 independent apoptosis and this occurs at a frequency greater than the normal apoptosis induced by direct UV absorption by DNA [32].

3.11   Conclusion

From the ongoing and available studies, we now understand that there exists a very narrow protective window of quality and quantity of melanin produced in an individual that confers resistance against developing skin cancers. Very low concentration of melanin does not prove beneficial as is exemplified by the high risk of skin cancer in albinos. On the other hand, excessive melanin, particularly pheomelanin, may become deleterious by photosensitizing the skin and thereby increasing the risk of skin cancer. This property, however, is highly contextual based on the ethnic group under consideration. This knowledge needs to be kept as a base for developing

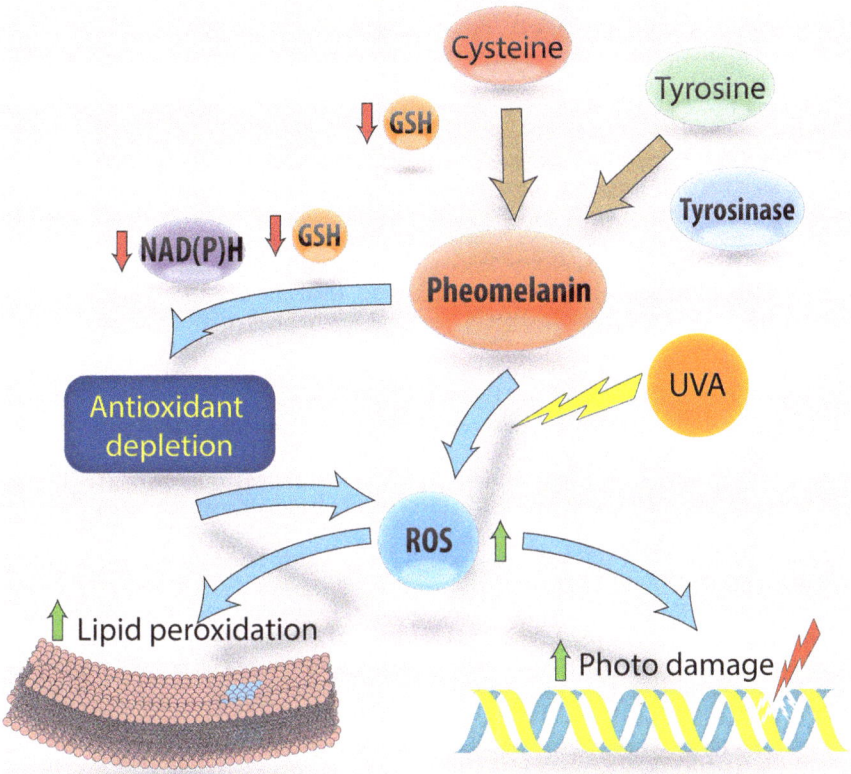

Fig. 3.15 Summary schematic of the role of pheomelanin in triggering oxidative stress under light exposure or dark conditions

various skin care cosmetics and treatments to skin cancer. Lately, the prominent shift in research interests observed in this regard is the use of natural plant extracts to safely increase pigmentation, independent of sun exposure for cosmetic reasons as well as to prevent skin cancer.

References

1. Arda O, Goksugur N et al (2014) Basic histological structure and functions of facial skin. Clin Dermatol 32(1):3–13
2. Moellmann G, McGuire J et al (1973) Ultrastructure and cell biology of pigment cells. Intracellular dynamics and the fine structure of melanocytes with special reference to the effects of MSH and cyclic AMP on microtubules and 10-nm filaments. J Biol Med 46(5):337–360
3. Tarnowski WM (1970) Ultrastructure of the epidermal melanocyte dense plate. J Invest Dermatol 55(4):265–268
4. Solano F (2014) Melanins: skin pigments and much more—types, structural models, biological functions, and formation routes. New J Sci 2014:498276

5. Breathnach AS, Nazzaro-Porro M et al (1991) Ultrastructure of melanocytes in chronically sun-exposed skin of elderly subjects. Pigment Cell Res 4(2):71–79
6. Brenner M, Hearing VJ (2008) The protective role of melanin against UV damage in human skin. Photochem Photobiol 84(3):539–549
7. Gilchrest BA, Park HY et al (1996) Mechanisms of ultraviolet light-induced pigmentation. Photochem Photobiol 63(1):1–10
8. Ali YH (2019) Proposed genetic classification for the skin types: Helmy's skin types classification. Plast Reconstr Surg Glob Open 7(4):e2130
9. Del Bino S, Duval C et al (2018) Clinical and biological characterization of skin pigmentation diversity and its consequences on UV impact. Int J Mol Sci 19(9):2668
10. McEvoy B, Beleza S et al (2006) The genetic architecture of normal variation in human pigmentation: an evolutionary perspective and model. Hum Mol Genet 15:176–181
11. Sturm RA (2009) Molecular genetics of human pigmentation diversity. Hum Mol Genet 18 (R1):9–17
12. Sulem P, Gudbjartsson DF et al (2007) Genetic determinants of hair, eye and skin pigmentation in Europeans. Nat Genet 39(12):1443–1452
13. Han J, Kraft P et al (2008) A genome-wide association study identifies novel alleles associated with hair color and skin pigmentation. PLoS Genet 4(5):e1000074
14. Bonilla C, Boxill LA et al (2005) The 8818G allele of the agouti signaling protein (ASIP) gene is ancestral and is associated with darker skin color in African Americans. Hum Genet 116 (5):402–406
15. Martin AR, Lin M et al (2017) An unexpectedly complex architecture for skin pigmentation in Africans. Cell 171(6):1340–1353
16. Crawford NG, Kelly DE et al (2017) Loci associated with skin pigmentation identified in African populations. Science 358(6365):8433
17. Norton HL, Kittles RA et al (2007) Genetic evidence for the convergent evolution of light skin in Europeans and East Asians. Mol Biol Evol 24(3):710–722
18. Basu Mallick C, Iliescu FM et al (2013) The light skin allele of SLC24A5 in South Asians and Europeans shares identity by descent. PLoS Genet 9(11):e1003912
19. Edwards M, Bigham A et al (2010) Association of the OCA2 polymorphism His615Arg with melanin content in east Asian populations: further evidence of convergent evolution of skin pigmentation. PLoS Genet 6(3):e1000867
20. Yang Z, Zhong H et al (2016) A genetic mechanism for convergent skin lightening during recent human evolution. Mol Biol Evol 33(5):1177–1187
21. Markiewicz E, Idowu OC (2020) Melanogenic difference consideration in ethnic skin type: a balance approach between skin brightening applications and beneficial Sun exposure. Clin Cosmet Investig Dermatol 13:215–232
22. Orthaber K, Pristovnik M et al (2017) Skin cancer and its treatment: novel treatment approaches with emphasis on nanotechnology. J Nanomater 2017:2606271
23. Domingues B, Lopes JM et al (2018) Melanoma treatment in review. Immunotargets Ther 7:35–49
24. Sun X, Zhang N et al (2020) Ultraviolet radiation and melanomagenesis: from mechanism to immunotherapy. Front Oncol 10:951
25. Kadekaro AL, Kavanagh RJ et al (2003) Cutaneous photobiology. The melanocyte vs. the sun: who will win the final round? Pigment Cell Res 16(5):434–447
26. Halder RM, Bang KM (1988) Skin cancer in blacks in the United States. Dermatol Clin 6 (3):397–405
27. Szabo G, Gerald AB et al (1969) Racial differences in the fate of melanosomes in human epidermis. Nature 222(5198):1081–1082
28. Kobayashi N, Nakagawa A et al (1998) Supranuclear melanin caps reduce ultraviolet induced DNA photoproducts in human epidermis. J Invest Dermatol 110(5):806–810

29. Hill HZ, Hill GJ (2000) UVA, pheomelanin and the carcinogenesis of melanoma. Pigment Cell Res 13(Suppl 8):140–144
30. Hill HZ, Li W et al (1997) Melanin: a two edged sword? Pigment Cell Res 10(3):158–161
31. Napolitano A, Panzella L et al (2014) Pheomelanin-induced oxidative stress: bright and dark chemistry bridging red hair phenotype and melanoma. Pigment Cell Melanoma Res 27 (5):721–733
32. Takeuchi S, Zhang W et al (2004) Melanin acts as a potent UVB photosensitizer to cause an atypical mode of cell death in murine skin. Proc Natl Acad Sci US A101(42):15076–15081

The Epidemiology of Skin Cancer Worldwide

4

Gurmanpreet Kaur and Nabiha Yusuf

Abstract

Skin cancer is rising at an alarming rate worldwide. The most common types of skin cancers, melanoma and non-melanoma are often seen in white population in the world. The geographical distribution for these cancers can be seen mainly in countries with this population. Among the non-melanoma skin cancers, basal cell carcinomas (BCC) have the highest incidence followed by squamous cell carcinomas (SCC). The incidence of melanoma is much lower than non-melanoma skin cancers but the mortality is high. Skin cancers cause a huge economic burden on the healthcare system so several countries employ public health measures for their prevention. In this chapter, we have discussed the global impact of melanoma and non-melanoma cancers along with other skin cancers. We have also discussed their etiology and strategies for prevention and treatment.

Keywords

Skin cancer · Epidemiology · Prevention

G. Kaur
Department of Epidemiology, School of Public Health, University of Alabama at Birmingham, Birmingham, AL, USA

N. Yusuf (✉)
Department of Epidemiology, School of Public Health, University of Alabama at Birmingham, Birmingham, AL, USA

Department of Dermatology, School of Medicine, University of Alabama at Birmingham, Birmingham, AL, USA
e-mail: nabihayusuf@uabmc.edu

© The Author(s), under exclusive license to Springer Nature Singapore Pte Ltd. 2021
A. Dwivedi et al. (eds.), *Skin Cancer: Pathogenesis and Diagnosis*,
https://doi.org/10.1007/978-981-16-0364-8_4

4.1 Introduction

Skin cancer is an abnormal growth of skin cells, which occurs as a result of mutation of DNA on exposure to ultraviolet (UV) and ionizing radiation, immunosuppression, viral infections, or elderly patients. There are different types of skin cancer depending on type of skin cell involved. Skin cancers can be classified into melanoma and non-melanoma skin cancers. Non-melanoma cancers can be further classified into basal cell carcinoma (BCC) and squamous cell carcinoma (SCC). Other types of skin cancers include cutaneous T-cell lymphoma, Merkel cell carcinoma, and Kaposi carcinoma [1]. According to the statistics from Skin Cancer Foundation, every third cancer is skin cancer. The depletion of ozone layer in the atmosphere has caused solar UV radiation to penetrate the earth's surface resulting in an increase in skin cancers all over the world. Skin pigmentation has a major role to play in the development of skin cancer and individuals with the Fitzpatrick skin type I–III are more prone to develop this cancer [2]. The incidence of skin cancer is very high in this population so it is important to study the epidemiological trends for effective control and management of this disease.

4.2 Melanoma

Melanoma arises due to uncontrolled proliferation of melanin producing cells [3–6]. It is mostly cutaneous in origin and can also arise from mucosal surfaces, uveal tract, and leptomeninges. It is the most lethal type of skin cancer as it accounts for majority of skin cancer deaths even though its incidence is lower than other skin cancers [7–9]. Melanoma is mostly reported in Caucasian populations as they have less protection from photodamage due to decreased melanin in their skin [8–10]. It costs enormous burden not only to the public health systems but also to the management of disease. Melanoma incidence is high in older adults but is also commonly seen in adolescents and young adults [8, 11]. Melanoma is ranked nineteenth for the most commonly occurring type of skin cancer. In 2018, around 300,000 cases of melanoma were reported and the top 20 countries that have the highest rates of melanoma are Australia, New Zealand, Norway, Denmark, Netherland, Sweden, Germany, Switzerland, Belgium, Slovenia, Luxembourg, Ireland, Finland, UK, Austria, France, the USA, Czech Republic, Canada, and Italy. The age-standardized rates per 100,000 of melanoma are higher among males in countries like Australia and New Zealand. Australia has the highest age-standardized rate of melanoma (33.6 per 100,000). It also has the highest age-standardized rate of melanoma in men (40.4 per 100,000). Denmark has the highest age-standardized rate of melanoma in women (33.1 per 100,000). Epidemiological approaches have helped to identify populations at risk and to provide them timely prevention, treatment, and management strategies [12].

4.3   Non-Melanoma Skin Cancer

Non-melanoma skin cancers comprise BCCs and SCCs. They are not lethal but their surgical excision can cause disfigurement. They are commonly seen on sun-exposed parts of the body. There seems to be clear relationship between the levels of UV radiation and incidence of skin cancers [2]. Non-melanoma skin cancer is the fifth most commonly occurring cancer in the world. In the year 2018, more than one million non-melanoma cases were reported. Globally, there is an underestimation of the incidence of non-melanoma skin cancer as some countries do not have cancer registries and some have incomplete registration or no records of cancer [13].

4.3.1   Basal Cell Carcinoma

Basal cell carcinoma (BCC) is the most common type of non-melanoma skin cancer, which occurs due to the uncontrolled growth of a basal cell. It destructs local skin cells but there is a lower rate of metastasis to skeletal and pulmonary sites. The lesions of BCC occur in an area that is more exposed to the sun like head or neck. The risk factors for BCCs are UV rays, age more than 50, chronic infection, light skin, and previous history. The lesions of BCCs look like elevated scars, red or pink patches, central indentations, ulcers which can be itchy, ooze out, or bleed. BCC is curable if diagnosed on time. BCC lesion can be dangerous or spread deep into skin, tissues, or bones if left untreated. The diagnosis and treatment of BCCs and SCCs have increased by 77% between 1994 and 2014. In Caucasians, there is a 30% higher lifetime risk of developing BCCs [14].

   The treatment of BCCs can be done with topical or oral medications, electrosurgery, radiation therapy, cryosurgery, laser surgery, Mohs surgery, or photodynamic therapy. The prognosis for BCCs is excellent but it can reoccur [15]. The primary tumor's nodular growth pattern without any free margins on subcutaneous fat, eyelid, or lip is treated with curettage. For low-risk lesions, curettage and electrodesiccation are effective. In well-defined BCCs with no infiltrations and sclerosis, cryotherapy with liquid nitrogen is performed, whereas it is contraindicated below the knee areas due to prolonged healing process. For face and scalp areas, the clearance rates are >98% if standardized cryotherapy and curettage are performed. To treat superficial BCCs photodynamic therapy (PDT) is an alternative approach but during the illumination phase pain is experienced and after PDT for 2–6 weeks, there is formation of crust and erosion. A clinical study done on 29 patients with topical application of 5-fluorouracil (5 FU) which is DNA-inhibitor twice a day for 12 weeks confirmed BCCs were treated. It has been reported in a retrospective study patients with BCCs were treated with 0.05% ingenol mebutate (derived from plant *Euphorbia peplus*) for 2–7 days. The BCCs that are not accessible with standard treatment are treated with radiotherapy, and the success rate is the same as we get by performing surgery. The studies have shown imiquimod, which is an immunomodulator when applied one time for 5 days has treated BCCs [16].

Annually, over four million cases of BCCs have been diagnosed in the USA. The incidence of BCC is 100 times more in older adults compared to younger ones [16]. An increase in trend of BCCs has been observed in countries like Canada, Finland, Australia, and the USA [17]. Geographical location has a big role to play in the incidence of BCCs, as places close to the equator have a higher incidence of BCCs [18, 19].

4.3.2 Squamous Cell Carcinoma

SCC is the most common type of skin cancer, which occurs as a result of the uncontrolled growth of a squamous cell. It can lead to 20% of skin malignancies and there are 14% chances that it can metastasize. In the USA, more than one million cases of SCCs are reported annually, and from the last three decades, its incidence has been increased by 200%. The studies have shown that every year there is a significant increase in new cases of SCCs in China. In Central Europe, every year incidence rate of SCCs increases by 5% [20]. Recent data suggests that there has been a plateau or decline in the incidence of SCCs, it has been stable in the USA and has increased in Germany from 2007 to 2015. The incident rates had a strong correlation with age. Germany had the highest mortality due to SCC, it was stable in Australia, and the data for mortality in the USA was not available [21]. The risk factors include exposure to UV rays, immunosuppression, chronic skin infections, previous history of skin cancer, xeroderma pigmentosa, HPV infection, and light skin complexion. The lesions look like ulcers, wart-like, red patches, and rolled up with central concavity. SCCs can occur in the area exposed to sun (head, neck) and genitals.

The treatment of SCCs can be done with topical medications, electrosurgery, radiation therapy, cryosurgery, laser surgery, Mohs surgery, or PDT. Around 95% of cases of SCCs can be detected at early stages but the remaining 5% cases are at an advanced stage which can be treated with immunotherapy. The drug nicotinamide decreases the risk of SCCs in people who are at high risk of getting it. The target drugs cetuximab and erlotinib attack the epidermal growth factor receptor (EGFR) protein produced by SCCs cells and relieve cancer. The other drugs that decrease the spread of SCC are cisplatin and 5-fluorouracil (FU). The programmed death (PD)-1inhibitors such as cemiplimab and pembrolizumab are effective in advanced SCCs. Radiation therapy is performed in the case of small SCCs in low-risk areas. The survival rates for SCCs are high [22].

4.3.3 Actinic Keratosis

Actinic keratosis (AK) is a scaly or crusty growth on the sun-damaged skin. AKs may progress to non-melanoma skin cancer (both BCCs and SCCs) so they are considered as an early warning sign for these cancers [23–26]. These lesions are an important target for the prevention of skin cancer using conventional treatment or alternate approaches [27]. Most of the data on AKs is from Australia and the USA. There is very limited data from Asia and Europe [22–27]. Patients with solid organ transplants are at increased risk of epithelial cancers, mainly squamous cell carcinomas, and their precursor lesions, which include actinic keratosis, warts, and parakeratosis. As patients with AKs have a high propensity to develop non-melanoma skin cancers, it is very important to identify and treat these patients so their AKs do not get converted into malignant lesions. Topical and systemic use of retinoids has been reported to treat these lesions [28]. PDT is widely used for the treatment of solid tumors including skin tumors. Emulsion from birch bark tree, an agent from North American traditional medicine, has been used for the treatment of actinic keratosis lesions [29]. In Australia, the topical application of latex from a flowering plant, *Euphorbia peplus L.* is used as a home-based remedy for actinic keratosis and skin cancer [30].

4.4 Merkel Cell Carcinoma

Merkel cell carcinoma (MCC) is a rare but aggressive type of skin cancer, which has high chances of reoccurrence and metastasis. Men have a high incidence of MCC compared to women (0.4–2.5 and 0.18–0.9 per 100,000). The age-adjusted rate of MCC is eight times more in white compared to black population (0.36–0.045 per 100,000). The factors that are responsible for increased risk of MCC are exposure to UV rays, immunosuppression, and a fair complexion. MCC tumor development is linked to the presence of clonally integrated Merkel cell polyomavirus (MCPyV) and/or mutations arising from exposure to UV radiation [31]. It can spread rapidly so it is very important to pay attention to the warning signs, which includes tender and asymptomatic lesions (not painful), lesion expands rapidly, immunosuppressed patient, age more than 50 years, and exposure to sunlight. The diagnosis and treatment of MCC are challenging as it can be misdiagnosed by the physician with cyst or hair follicle infection, appearance of it as painless lesion at mucosal sites such as mouth, nasal cavity, or throat, and 14% of MCC is undetectable as they appear on lymph nodes without any tumor. To know how much disease has spread (staging), sentinel lymph node biopsy is done. Depending on the stage of MCC, treatment is prescribed. The system that is used for MCC staging is TNM where T stands for original tumor size and its growth rate, N stands for to what extent cancer has spread to local lymph nodes, and N stands for its extent to other organs and distant lymph nodes. There is a 50% survival rate for MCC [32]. It has been observed in a study that more than half of cases in which a combination of etoposide and carboplatin was given have treated the tumor and distant metastatic disease [33]. A clinical trial done on a patient with a primary tumor of size >1 cm with carboplatin and etoposide has shown significant results. Another study done in Australia for local, advanced, and high-risk MCC with carboplatin at the same time with radiotherapy followed by three cycles of carboplatin and etoposide combination showed us a better regimen [34]. Recent advances in immunotherapy have provided valuable therapeutic options for patients with advanced or recurrent MCC.

4.5   Kaposi Sarcoma

Kaposi sarcoma (KS) is a rare type of cancer that occurs in cells lining blood vessels or lymph nodes. The lesions on the skin can appear as red or purple blotches. The lesions can also appear on the face, legs, groin area, lungs, liver, or digestive tract. It can cause difficulty in breathing (if developed in the lungs) or bleeding (if developed in the digestive tract). KS herpesvirus (KSHV, also known as HHV-8) is the causative agent for KS. After infection, the virus hijacks the cell machinery to evade the immune system and proliferate in the host cells. There are four different kinds of KS which are epidemic (AIDS-associated) KS (occurs in HIV-infected patient); classic Mediterranean KS (occurs in older population in the Middle East); endemic (African) KS (occurs in equatorial Africa and associated with herpesvirus); and iatrogenic KS (occurs in people with organ transplantation due to immunosuppression). Age standardized incidence rates of KS are much higher in sub-Saharan and Southern Africa (4.0 > 22.0 per 100,000) compared to North and South America, Europe (0.3–0.9 per 100,000), and rest of the world (<0.3 per 100,000). The seroprevalence rate of KSHV is <10% in Europe, Asia, and the USA compared to >40% in Sub-Saharan Africa [35].

The treatment of KS is by controlling underlying infections and immunodeficiency, radiation therapy, and chemotherapy [36]. DaunoXome, a daunorubicin citrate liposomal product is used for the treatment of AIDS-related KS (AIDS-KS). Combination antiretroviral therapy (cART) has been effective in 50% of cases of AIDS-KS. During this therapy immune system is reconstituted and HIV replication gets suppressed. Nelfinavir, an HIV protease inhibitor shows anti-KS activity. In transplant-related KS, immune reconstitution helps in the regression of KS as drugs as rapamycin/everolimus lead to a decrease in KS lesions. In addition, cytotoxic chemotherapy is considered as a standard treatment for KS. The VEGF-receptor inhibitors like bevacizumab and imatinib are effective in some of the patients, but not in all KS patients, which can be due to insufficient delivery of drugs to the lesion areas [37].

4.6   Cutaneous Lymphoma

Lymphoma is the cancer of white blood cells (lymphocytes) which are part of our immune system. Cutaneous lymphoma begins somewhere else in the body and then metastasize to the skin. There are two subtypes of cutaneous lymphoma: cutaneous T-cell lymphomas (CTCLs) and cutaneous B-cell lymphomas (CBCLs). CTCL is caused by expansion of malignant T-cells in the skin. CTCLs can spread to other body parts. The lesions are eczema-like dry, red, and itchy. They commonly occur on the armpits, neck, groin area, or face. CBCLs cause outgrowths in the skin and one or two other parts of the body. These nodules appear on the head, neck, legs, or back. Men are at more risk of developing skin lymphomas than women. The skin lymphomas can be diagnosed by performing a skin biopsy. The treatment includes topical medications, systematic medications, immunotherapy, chemotherapy, or stem cell transplant [38].

High incidence of age-standardized incidence of CTCL was reported higher in the USA compared to Europe and Asia. Among the subtypes of CTCL, mycosis fungoides (MF) was found to be the most common subtype (45%), followed by peripheral T-cell lymphoma (25%) and Sezary syndrome (SS) (1.3%), a particularly aggressive subtype of CTCL. The mean age at the time of diagnosis of CTCL is in the mid- to late-1950s. CTCL was reported to occur at a significantly higher rate in African-Americans compared to Caucasians. In a study from the USA, the age-adjusted incidence rates of CTCL were the highest among African-Americans (10.0/100,000 person-years) compared to non-Hispanic whites (8.1/100,000 person-years), Hispanic whites (5.1/100,000 person-years), and Asian/Pacific Islander (5.1/ 100,000 person-years) (10). The prognosis of CTCL was also reported to be worse in African-Americans [39].

4.7   Conclusions

The occurrence of skin cancer is highly associated with the skin color, exposure to sun, and geographical zone. In the USA, Australia, and European countries, there is a stabilization of mortality rates occurring due to melanoma but there is an increase in the incidence of skin cancer, possibly due to the depletion of ozone layer in the atmosphere and certain risky behaviors that involve exposure to UV and use of tanning beds. The prevention campaigns regarding early diagnosis and reducing the incidence have helped a lot in decreasing the trends of skin cancer. The increase in global trends of skin cancer shows that there is still an unmet need to control the incidence of skin cancer.

References

1. Types of skin cancer (2020) https://www.aad.org/public/diseases/skin-cancer/types/common/. Accessed 7 Nov 2020
2. Radiation: ultraviolet (UV) radiation and skin cancer (2020) https://www.who.int/news-room/q-a-detail/ultraviolet-(uv)-radiation-and-skin-cancer Accessed 7 Nov 2020
3. Lerner AB, McGuire JS (1964) Melanocyte-stimulating hormone and adrenocorticotrophic hormone. N Engl J Med 270(11):539–546
4. Abdel-Malek Z, Suzuki I, Tada A, Im S, Akcali C (2006) The melanocortin-1 receptor and human pigmentation. Ann N Y Acad Sci 885(1):117–133
5. Abdel-Malek Z, Swope V, Suzuki I, Akcali C, Harriger M, Boyce S et al (1995) Mitogenic and melanogenic stimulation of normal human melanocytes by melanotropic peptides. Proc Natl Acad Sci 92(5):1789–1793
6. Tsatmali M , Ancans J, Thody AJ (2002) Melanocyte function and its control by melanocortin peptides. https://journals.sagepub.com/doi/full/10.1177/002215540205000201. Accessed 7 Nov 2020
7. Linos E, Swetter S, Cockburn M, Colditz G, Clarke C (2009) Increasing burden of melanoma in the United States. J Investig Dermatol 129(7):1666–1674

8. Surveillance, Epidemiology, and End Results (SEER). Program cancer statistics review, 1975–2013, National Cancer Institute [Internet] Nov, 2015. [cited posted to the SEER web site, 2016 Apr]. SEER data submission. http://seer.cancer.gov/csr/1975_2013/. Accessed 7 Nov 2020

9. GLOBOCAN (2012) v1.0, Cancer Incidence and Mortality Worldwide: IARC Cancer Base No. 11 [Internet] 2013. [cited 2017 Apr 6]. http://globocan.iarc.fr. Accessed 7 Nov 2020

10. Brenner M, Hearing V (2007) The protective role of melanin against UV damage in human skin. Photochem Photobiol 84(3):539–549

11. Ballantine K, Watson H, Macfarlane S, Winstanley M, Corbett R, Spearing R et al (2017) Small numbers, big challenges: adolescent and young adult cancer incidence and survival in New Zealand. J Adolesc Young Adult Oncol 6(2):277–285

12. Matthews NH, Li WQ, Qureshi AA et al (2017) Epidemiology of melanoma. In: Ward WH, Farma JM (eds) Cutaneous melanoma: etiology and therapy. Codon Publications, Brisbane

13. Bray F, Ferlay J, Soerjomataram I, Siegel R, Torre L, Jemal A (2018) Global cancer statistics 2018: GLOBOCAN estimates of incidence and mortality worldwide for 36 cancers in 185 countries. CA Cancer J Clin 68(6):394–424

14. Samarasinghe V, Madan V, Lear J (2011) Focus on basal cell carcinoma. J Skin Cancer 2011:1–5

15. Basal Cell Carcinoma—The Skin Cancer Foundation (2020) https://www.skincancer.org/skin-cancer-information/basal-cell-carcinoma/. Accessed 7 Nov 2020

16. Scotto J, Fears TR, Fraumeni JF Jr, et al. (1983) Incidence of nonmelanoma skin cancer in the United States in collaboration with Fred Hutchinson Cancer Research Center. NIH publication No. 83–2433, U.S. Dept. of Health and Human Services, Public Health Service, National Institutes of Health, National Cancer Institute, Bethesda, MD, p 113

17. Wrone D, Swetter S, Egbert B, Smoller B, Khavari P (1996) Increased proportion of aggressive-growth basal cell carcinoma in the veterans affairs population of Palo Alto, California. J Am Acad Dermatol 35(6):907–910

18. Chuang T, Popescu A, Su W, Chute C (2020) Basal cell carcinoma. A population-based incidence study in Rochester, Minnesota. https://www.sciencedirect.com/science/article/abs/pii/019096229070056N. Accessed 7 Nov 2020

19. Reizner G, Chuang T, Elpern D, Stone J, Farmer E (2020) Basal cell carcinoma and keratoacanthoma in Hawaiians: an incidence report. https://pubmed.ncbi.nlm.nih.gov/8335736/. Accessed 7 Nov 2020

20. Voiculescu V, Calenic B, Ghita M, Lupu M, Caruntu A, Moraru L, Voiculescu S, Ion A, Greabu M, Ishkitiev N, Caruntu C (2020) From normal skin to squamous cell carcinoma: a quest for novel biomarkers. https://pubmed.ncbi.nlm.nih.gov/27642215/. Accessed 7 Nov 2020

21. Stang A, Khil L, Kajüter H, Pandeya N, Schmults C, Ruiz E, Karia P, Green A (2019) Incidence and mortality for cutaneous squamous cell carcinoma: comparison across three continents. J Eur Acad Dermatol Venereol 33(S8):6–10

22. Cancer.org (2020) Basal & squamous cell skin cancer chemo | non-melanoma chemo. https://www.cancer.org/cancer/basal-and-squamous-cell-skin-cancer/treating/systemic-chemotherapy.html. Accessed 7 Nov 2020

23. Sacar H, Sacar T (2009) Actinic keratosis. Anatol J Clin Investig 3:198–202

24. Strickland P, Vitasa B, West S, Rosenthal F, Emmett E, Taylor H (1989) Quantitative carcinogenesis in man: solar ultraviolet B dose dependence of skin cancer in Maryland watermen. JNCI J Natl Cancer Inst 81(24):1910–1913

25. Dziunycz P, Schuller E, Hofbauer G (2018) Prevalence of actinic keratosis in patients attending general practitioners in Switzerland. Dermatology 234(5–6):214–219

26. Frost G, Williams (1998) The prevalence and determinants of solar keratoses at a subtropical latitude (Queensland, Australia). Br J Dermatol 139(6):1033–1039

27. Trakatelli M, Barkitzi K, Apap C, Majewski S, De Vries E (2016) Skin cancer risk in outdoor workers: a European multicenter case-control study. J Eur Acad Dermatol Venereol 30:5–11

28. Ianhez M, Fleury Junior L, Miot H, Bagatin E (2013) Retinoids for prevention and treatment of actinic keratosis. An Bras Dermatol 88(4):585–593

29. Huyke C, Laszczyk M, Scheffler A, Ernst R, Schempp C (2006) Treatment of actinic keratoses with birch bark extract: a pilot study. JDDG 4(2):132–136

30. Ramsay J, Suhrbier A, Aylward J, Ogbourne S, Cozzi S, Poulsen M, Baumann K, Welburn P, Redlich G, Parsons P (2011) The sap from Euphorbia peplus is effective against human nonmelanoma skin cancers. Br J Dermatol 164(3):633–636

31. Schadendorf D, Lebbé C, zur Hausen A, Avril M, Hariharan S, Bharmal M, Becker J (2017) Merkel cell carcinoma: epidemiology, prognosis, therapy and unmet medical needs. Eur J Cancer 71:53–69

32. Harms KL, Healy MA, Nghiem P, Sober AJ, Johnson TM, Bichakjian CK et al (2016) Analysis of prognostic factors from 9387 Merkel cell carcinoma cases forms the basis for the new 8th edition AJCC staging system. Ann Surg Oncol 23(11):3564–3571

33. Iyer J, Blom A, Doumani R, Lewis C, Anderson A, Ma C et al (2014) Response rate and durability of chemotherapy for metastatic Merkel cell carcinoma among 62 patients. J Clin Oncol 32(15_suppl):9091–9091

34. Rabinowitz G (2017) Is this the end of cytotoxic chemotherapy in Merkel cell carcinoma? Onco Targets Ther 10:4803–4807

35. Cesarman E, Damania B, Krown SE, Martin J, Bower M, Whitby D (2019) Kaposi sarcoma. Nat Rev Dis Primers 5(1):9

36. Cancer.org (2020) Kaposi sarcoma stages. https://www.cancer.org/cancer/kaposi-sarcoma/detection-diagnosis-staging/staging.html. Accessed 7 Nov 2020

37. Schneider J, Dittmer D (2017) Diagnosis and treatment of Kaposi sarcoma. Am J Clin Dermatol 18(4):529–539

38. Sokołowska-Wojdyło M, Olek-Hrab K, Ruckemann-Dziurdzińska K (2015) Primary cutaneous lymphomas: diagnosis and treatment. Adv Dermatol Allergol 5:368–383

39. Ghazawi F, Alghazawi N, Le M, Netchiporouk E, Glassman S, Sasseville D, Litvinov I (2019) Environmental and other extrinsic risk factors contributing to the pathogenesis of cutaneous T cell lymphoma (CTCL). Front Oncol 9:300

UVR Induced Vitamin D Synthesis and Skin Cancer

5

Harshit Kumar Soni

Abstract

Ultraviolet radiation (UVR) is the major etiological agent for the development of skin cancers. UVR causes DNA damage and genetic mutations, which subsequently lead to skin cancer. On the other hand, exposure to UVR is required for the synthesis of vitamin D by skin. As per current data more than 50% of world's population is at risk of vitamin D deficiency. Vitamin D deficiency has been associated with increased risk of various cancers, autoimmune and infectious diseases. It has been reported that daily requirement of vitamin D cannot be fulfilled with the diet and sunlight is essential for maintaining the healthy levels of vitamin D in body. However, due to the risk of skin cancer and UVR exposure, a fine balance is needed for skin exposure as to fulfill the production of sufficient amount of vitamin D as well as prevent the skin malignancies. This book chapter reviews these aspects of role of UVR in skin cancer and vitamin D metabolism.

Keywords

Skin cancer · Melanoma · Non-melanoma · Ultraviolet radiation · Vitamin D · 25-hydroxyvitamin D3 · 7-dehydrocholesterol · Vitamin D metabolism

5.1 Introduction

Ultraviolet B (UVB) (280–315 nm) irradiation is a well-known cause for skin cancer. Upon exposure with UVB, DNA photoproduct—cyclobutane pyrimidine dimers (CPDs) are formed [1, 2]. They could lead to skin cancer causing mutation, if

H. K. Soni (✉)
Department of Zoology, Government Science College, Pandhurna, Madhya Pradesh, India

A. Dwivedi et al. (eds.), *Skin Cancer: Pathogenesis and Diagnosis*,
https://doi.org/10.1007/978-981-16-0364-8_5

not repaired [2]. In case of irreparable DNA damage, cells may go for apoptosis [3]. Furthermore, chronic UVR exposure might lead to the suppression of cell mediated immunity which could result into skin cancer outgrowth [4].

On the other hand, UVR from sunlight is also the major source for vitamin D [5]. Most land animals, including humans, use UVR for synthesis of previtamin D from its precursor 7-dehydrocholesterol (7-DHC) in skin cells.

Since UV exposure is important for the vitamin D synthesis, there is possibility of the link between melanoma and vitamin D. Seasonal melanoma fatality patterns showed that fatality rates are higher in winter than in summer [6]. Also, people with higher sun exposure history showed lower mortality from melanoma compared to the people with history of lower sun exposure [7]. Effect of sun exposure on vitamin D has also been shown to be very critical in providing protection against number of non-cutaneous cancers, including breast cancer, colon cancer, prostate cancer, and non-Hodgkin lymphoma [6, 8–11].

5.2   Vitamin D Synthesis and Metabolism

In course of evolution, aquatic animals took advantage of their calcium rich environment and used it to develop mineralized endoskeleton. However, when animals started living on land, they faced calcium deficient environment. Thus, their ability to photosynthesize vitamin D3 in their skin cells became extremely essential to optimal calcium absorption and maintain calcium homeostasis.

UVB radiation (wavelength range 290–315 nm) is able to penetrate the ozone layer. When skin is exposed to sunlight, this UVB radiation is absorbed by 7-dehydrocholesterol (7-DHC) in the skin cells [12–14]. This absorption excites the double bond and opens the B ring which results into conversion of a rigid steroid structure into a flexible molecule previtamin D3. Previtamin D3 found in two optical conformations: cis and trans. The cis conformation is thermodynamically less favorable and hence converted into vitamin D3. Once vitamin D is made, it must be converted into biologically inactive 25-hydroxyvitamin D3 (25(OH)D). It is major circulating form of the vitamin D, which is used to determine the vitamin D level in any person. This 25(OH)D is converted to biologically active form 1,25-dihydroxyvitamin D3 ($1,25(OH)_2$ D) in kidney via hydroxylation by hydroxyvitamin D-1α-hydroxylase (CYP27B1; 1-OHase) [15, 16]. $1,25(OH)_2$ D behaves like steroid hormone and interacts with vitamin D receptor (VDR) in nucleus of targeted tissues such as osteoblast cells of bone, renal tubular cells in kidney, and small intestine and thereby enhance the calcium absorption and reabsorption in intestine, bone, and kidney. $1,25(OH)_2$ D is an auto-regulated molecule. To control its own function, it activates the expression of 25 hydroxyvitamin D-24-hydroxylase (CYP24) [15–17]. CYP24 converts $1,25(OH)_2$ D into inactive, water soluble calcitroic acid, which then excreted in bile. There are evidences available that $1,25(OH)_2$ D exhibits photoprotective, anti-proliferative properties in keratinocytes, thus UVR has dual role [18]. On the one side, vitamin D synthesis is important to maintain the body health and onco-prevention, while on the other hand, it initiates mutation which could lead to the development of skin cancer. Hence, considering that photoproduction of vitamin D accounts for 90% of body's vitamin D requirements, a fine balance between sun exposure needed so that sufficient amount of vitamin D is produced while avoiding risk of skin cancer development.

5.3 UVR and Skin Cancer

Solar ultraviolet is composed of three parts—ultraviolet A (UVA; 315–400 nm), ultraviolet B (UVB; 280–315 nm), and ultraviolet C (UVC; less than 280 nm). UVC and most of the part of the UVB, up to 310 nm are blocked by ozone layer, while UVA reaches to earth. Remaining UVB is completely absorbed by epidermis and 50% of UVA reaches to the dermis [19]. The effect of UVA on human body includes skin aging, oxidative damage, and solar elastosis [19]. DNA present in epidermis showed decreasing absorption from UVB to UVA with the peak absorption showed at 260 nm [1, 20, 21]. Major damage to DNA due to UVB exposure is cycloaddition of the C5-C6 double bond of nearby pyrimidines, which results into the formation of the cyclobutane pyrimidine dimers (CPD), such as thymine dimers (TD). These dimers either repaired or if could not repaired, cells may undergo apoptosis [3] resulting in sun burn. If these dimers are not repaired, then they might lead to the initiating mutation for cutaneous cancer [2]. If this DNA damage avoids DNA repair or DNA damage occurs in the gene involved in DNA repair, proliferation, apoptosis, cell cycle control, or tumor inhibitory system, it may lead to the development of tumor growth [19]. As seen in the case of basal cell carcinoma (BCC) and squamous cell carcinoma (SCC), p53 a tumor suppressor gene and important transcriptional factor which regulates cell cycle and apoptosis exhibits a UVB induced point mutation. UVB induced mutation bears a signature trait of C to T or CC to TT transition associated with dipyrimidine site [22]. Furthermore, chromic UVR exposure to skin cells may lead to the suppression of cell-mediate immunity [4] which results into immune tolerance for immunogenic skin tumors. It has been found that excessive sun light exposure increases the risk of non-melanoma skin cancer, whereas occupational sun exposure decreases the risk of melanomas [23, 24]. This is achieved by the skin pigmentation. Skin pigmentation genes have evolved in such a way that they could minimize the damaging effect of sunlight exposure, while permit sufficient UVB penetration to skin in order to produce sufficient amount of vitamin D. It has been widely accepted that the risk of melanoma is calculated by the interplay between genetic factor of a person and its exposure to the sun light.

Majority of the reports, epidemiological and others, conclude that the sun exposure is responsible for the three most common types of skin cancer: BCC, SCC, and melanoma [25, 26]. However, multiple questions related to the UV exposure and skin cancer are still unanswered. The relationship between the cancer generation and wavelength of UV exposure (action spectrum) is not very well understood. Epidemiological data does not include the action of particular wavelength and corresponding malignancies. However, the well-established animal models do provide some insight for action spectrum. On the basis of animal model, it has been reported that the UVB region showed the maximum carcinogenicity [27, 28]. Nevertheless, the translation of these results from animal model to human has to be worked upon.

Another contesting issue is the local and systemic effect of sun exposure. BCC and SCC are most commonly occurred on the chronic sun exposed skin, but case control studies with melanoma failed to demonstrate any relationship between location of sun exposure and location of melanoma [29–31]. Also there have been active debate regarding the role of sun exposure in non-cutaneous malignancies. There have been a number of cancer sites that showed the latitude gradient, for which no possible explanation could be offered for.

5.4   Vitamin D and Skin Cancer

Keratinocytes are the only cells which exhibit and support complete vitamin D metabolism from 7-DHC to $1,25(OH)_2D$ [32, 33]. Furthermore, it has been observed that expression and level of vitamin D receptor (VDR) & $1,25(OH)_2D$ change with the differentiation status [34]. $1,25(OH)_2D$ induced keratinocytes differentiation suggests that $1,25(OH)_2D$ behaves as autocrine/ paracrine factor for keratinocytes differentiation [35]. $1,25(OH)_2D$ also induces calcium receptor (CaR) [36] and PLCγ [37] during differentiation process. Hence, $1,25(OH)_2D$ and calcium both act in a synergistic way to promote prodifferentiation effect. Therefore, any disturbance to the $1,25(OH)_2D$ mediated gene expression for differentiation may lead to the skin cancer.

Vitamin D receptor interacting protein (DRIP) and steroid receptor co-activators (SRC) are two major co-activation complexes which interact with VDR to induce the transcription of the differentiation markers in keratinocytes [38]. During early differentiation stage, it was DRIP, which majorly bind to VDR, while SRC complex majorly binds during late differentiation stage [39]. It was also found that Ras oncogene interacts with $1,25(OH)_2D$ and could contribute to the development of SCC and BCC [40–42].

UV radiation like other cellular stresses activates c-Jun NH2-terminal kinase (JNK) [43] and upregulates stress activated protein kinases (SAPKs) [44, 45]. This activation and upregulation promote apoptosis. It has been found that pre-treatment of keratinocytes 24 hrs. Prior to UVB radiation with pharmacological dosages of $1,25(OH)_2D$ (1 mM) reduces the rate of apoptosis [46]. Additionally, 30% reduction in the UVB stimulated JNK activation along with 90% inhibition in the mitochondrial cytochrome c release, have been reported. These findings showed that vitamin D protects UVB irradiated cells from apoptosis. However, this will lead to the concern that $1,25(OH)_2D$ might allow cells with DNA damage to survive, hence increases the risk of cancer [47]. This concern was tested by Gupta et al. [47]. They have reported that treatment of cells with physiological dose $(10^{-9}$ M) of 1,25 $(OH)_2D$, 24 hrs. Prior to irradiation showed dose-dependent increase of cell survival as well as dose-dependent decrease in the TD. It has also been observed that these effects can be reproduced by $1,25(OH)_2D$ treatment immediately post-UVB irradiation. Another important observation was corresponding increase in p53 with decreasing TD. It has been known that UV irradiation could increase the production of nitric oxide (NO) products [48]. These products could further increase the DNA damage by UVR [49] and inhibit CPD repair [50]. In cells treated with 1,25(OH)$_2$D, significant decrease in the levels of nitrites was also observed [47]. Hence it has been concluded from these experiments that treatment of 1,25(OH)$_2$D in cells could induce the expression of p53 and decrease the production of nitric oxide products, which ultimately results in the reduction of TD or DNA damage and improved DNA repair. Taken all these together, it can be inferred that 1,25(OH)$_2$D showed its photoprotective effect by reducing the cell apoptosis and improving the cell survival by enhancing the DNA damage repair. The series of other studies have been able to reproduce the photoprotective effect of 1,25(OH)$_2$D [51–54].

Apart from maintaining the mineral homeostasis, 1,25(OH)$_2$D also plays some non-canonical roles in external renal tissues. First evidence of synthesis of 1,25 (OH)$_2$D came from the experiment where vitamin D was administered to anephric patients. This led to significant increase of 1,25(OH)D serum level than those in the control group. This increase showed significant correlation with the precursor 25OHD levels [55]. This was further confirmed by a separate study where 25OHD was orally administered to uremic mongrel dogs and anephric patients. Here also, a significant correlation between serum level of 25OHD and 1,25(OH)$_2$D was observed [56]. The enzyme present in the extra renal tissue behaves in autocrine/paracrine way and acts locally. This complements the 1,25(OH)$_2$D produced by kidney [57]. This increase in the level of 1,25(OH)$_2$D in tissues can affect the gene expression that could suppress proliferation while promoting differentiation. These impacts on the gene expression are seen in various tissues such as prostate, breast, colon, bone, skin, and cells of immune system [58–61]. These findings of tissue specific regulations of proliferation and differentiation in extra renal tissues by 1,25 (OH)$_2$D directly linked the action of 1,25(OH)$_2$D in various cancers.

5.5   Conclusion

Considering the role of UVR in skin cancer, prevention programs and campaigns recommend protection and avoidance of sunlight [62]. In these campaigns, the beneficial effects of the sun lights have been completely overlooked. Experts agree that the daily requirement of vitamin cannot be obtained from the dietary sources to avoid all sun exposure. Hence, scientists are struggling on the recommendation of the amount of UVR which could facilitate the production of sufficient amount of vitamin D while preventing the skin malignancies higher exposure of the UVR.

References

1. Cadet J, Voituriez L, Grand A, Hruska FE, Vigny P, Kan LS (1985) Recent aspects of the photochemistry of nucleic acids and related model compounds. Biochimie 67(3–4):277–292. https://doi.org/10.1016/s0300-9084(85)80070-5
2. Setlow RB (1966) Cyclobutane-type pyrimidine dimers in polynucleotides. Science 153 (3734):379–386. https://doi.org/10.1126/science.153.3734.379
3. Smith ML, Chen IT, Zhan Q, O'Connor PM, Fornace AJ Jr (1995) Involvement of the p53 tumor suppressor in repair of u.v.-type DNA damage. Oncogene 10(6):1053–1059
4. Elsner P, Holzle E, Diepgen T, Grether-Beck S, Honigsmann H, Krutmann J et al (2007) Recommendation: daily sun protection in the prevention of chronic UV-induced skin damage. J German Soc Dermatol 5(2):166–173. https://doi.org/10.1111/j.1610-0387.2007.06099.x
5. Holick MF (2003) Evolution and function of vitamin D. Recent Results Cancer Res 164:3–28. https://doi.org/10.1007/978-3-642-55580-0_1
6. Boniol M, Armstrong BK, Dore JF (2006) Variation in incidence and fatality of melanoma by season of diagnosis in new South Wales, Australia. Cancer Epidemiol Biomarkers Prev 15 (3):524–526. https://doi.org/10.1158/1055-9965.EPI-05-0684
7. Berwick M, Armstrong BK, Ben-Porat L, Fine J, Kricker A, Eberle C et al (2005) Sun exposure and mortality from melanoma. J Natl Cancer Inst 97(3):195–199. https://doi.org/10.1093/jnci/dji019
8. Garland CF, Garland FC (1980) Do sunlight and vitamin D reduce the likelihood of colon cancer? Int J Epidemiol 9(3):227–231. https://doi.org/10.1093/ije/9.3.227
9. Garland FC, Garland CF, Gorham ED, Young JF (1990) Geographic variation in breast cancer mortality in the United States: a hypothesis involving exposure to solar radiation. Prev Med 19 (6):614–622. https://doi.org/10.1016/0091-7435(90)90058-r
10. Kricker A, Armstrong BK, Hughes AM, Goumas C, Smedby KE, Zheng T et al (2008) Personal sun exposure and risk of non-Hodgkin lymphoma: a pooled analysis from the Interlymph Consortium. Int J Cancer 122(1):144–154. https://doi.org/10.1002/ijc.23003
11. Luscombe CJ, French ME, Liu S, Saxby MF, Jones PW, Fryer AA et al (2001) Outcome in prostate cancer associations with skin type and polymorphism in pigmentation-related genes. Carcinogenesis 22(9):1343–1347. https://doi.org/10.1093/carcin/22.9.1343
12. Holick MF (2003) Vitamin D: a millenium perspective. J Cell Biochem 88(2):296–307. https://doi.org/10.1002/jcb.10338
13. Holick MF, MacLaughlin JA, Clark MB, Holick SA, Potts JT Jr, Anderson RR et al (1980) Photosynthesis of previtamin D3 in human skin and the physiologic consequences. Science 210 (4466):203–205. https://doi.org/10.1126/science.6251551
14. Holick MF, Tian XQ, Allen M (1995) Evolutionary importance for the membrane enhancement of the production of vitamin D3 in the skin of poikilothermic animals. Proc Natl Acad Sci U S A 92(8):3124–3126. https://doi.org/10.1073/pnas.92.8.3124
15. LJ DG (2001) Vitamin D: from photosynthesis, metabolism, and action to clinical applications. In: Endocrinology adult and pediatric: the parathyroid gland and bone metabolism, 6th edn. Elsevier, Amsterdam, pp 1009–1028
16. DeLuca HF (2004) Overview of general physiologic features and functions of vitamin D. Am J Clin Nutr 80(6 Suppl):1689S–1696S. https://doi.org/10.1093/ajcn/80.6.1689S
17. Holick MF (2007) Vitamin D deficiency. N Engl J Med 357(3):266–281. https://doi.org/10.1056/NEJMra070553
18. Sebag M, Henderson J, Rhim J, Kremer R (1992) Relative resistance to 1,25-dihydroxyvitamin D3 in a keratinocyte model of tumor progression. J Biol Chem 267(17):12162–12167
19. Rass K, Reichrath J (2008) UV damage and DNA repair in malignant melanoma and nonmelanoma skin cancer. Adv Exp Med Biol 624:162–178. https://doi.org/10.1007/978-0-387-77574-6_13

20. Ravanat JL, Douki T, Cadet J (2001) Direct and indirect effects of UV radiation on DNA and its components. J Photochem Photobiol B 63(1–3):88–102. https://doi.org/10.1016/s1011-1344(01)00206-8
21. de Gruijl FR, van Kranen HJ, Mullenders LH (2001) UV-induced DNA damage, repair, mutations and oncogenic pathways in skin cancer. J Photochem Photobiol B 63(1–3):19–27. https://doi.org/10.1016/s1011-1344(01)00199-3
22. Brash DE, Rudolph JA, Simon JA, Lin A, McKenna GJ, Baden HP et al (1991) A role for sunlight in skin cancer: UV-induced p53 mutations in squamous cell carcinoma. Proc Natl Acad Sci U S A 88(22):10124–10128. https://doi.org/10.1073/pnas.88.22.10124
23. Garland FC, White MR, Garland CF, Shaw E, Gorham ED (1990) Occupational sunlight exposure and melanoma in the U.S. navy. Arch Environ Health 45(5):261–267. https://doi.org/10.1080/00039896.1990.10118743
24. Kennedy C, Bajdik CD, Willemze R, De Gruijl FR, Bouwes Bavinck JN (2003) The influence of painful sunburns and lifetime sun exposure on the risk of actinic keratoses, seborrheic warts, melanocytic nevi, atypical nevi, and skin cancer. J Invest Dermatol 120(6):1087–1093. https://doi.org/10.1046/j.1523-1747.2003.12246.x
25. Elwood JM (1992) Melanoma and sun exposure: contrasts between intermittent and chronic exposure. World J Surg 16(2):157–165. https://doi.org/10.1007/BF02071515
26. Green A, MacLennan R, Youl P, Martin N (1993) Site distribution of cutaneous melanoma in Queensland. Int J Cancer 53(2):232–236. https://doi.org/10.1002/ijc.2910530210
27. Cole CA, Forbes PD, Davies RE (1986) An action spectrum for UV photocarcinogenesis. Photochem Photobiol 43(3):275–284. https://doi.org/10.1111/j.1751-1097.1986.tb05605.x
28. de Gruijl FR, Sterenborg HJ, Forbes PD, Davies RE, Cole C, Kelfkens G et al (1993) Wavelength dependence of skin cancer induction by ultraviolet irradiation of albino hairless mice. Cancer Res 53(1):53–60
29. Green A, Bain C, McLennan R, Siskind V (1986) Risk factors for cutaneous melanoma in Queensland. Recent Results Cancer Res 102:76–97. https://doi.org/10.1007/978-3-642-82641-2_6
30. Lee JA, Merrill JM (1970) Sunlight and the aetiology of malignant melanoma: a synthesis. Med J Aust 2(18):846–851
31. Weinstock MA, Colditz GA, Willett WC, Stampfer MJ, Bronstein BR, Mihm MC Jr et al (1991) Melanoma and the sun: the effect of swimsuits and a "healthy" tan on the risk of nonfamilial malignant melanoma in women. Am J Epidemiol 134(5):462–470. https://doi.org/10.1093/oxfordjournals.aje.a116117
32. Lehmann B, Genehr T, Knuschke P, Pietzsch J, Meurer M (2001) UVB-induced conversion of 7-dehydrocholesterol to 1alpha,25-dihydroxyvitamin D3 in an in vitro human skin equivalent model. J Invest Dermatol 117(5):1179–1185. https://doi.org/10.1046/j.0022-202x.2001.01538.x
33. Matsumoto K, Azuma Y, Kiyoki M, Okumura H, Hashimoto K, Yoshikawa K (1991) Involvement of endogenously produced 1,25-dihydroxyvitamin D-3 in the growth and differentiation of human keratinocytes. Biochim Biophys Acta 1092(3):311–318. https://doi.org/10.1016/s0167-4889(97)90006-9
34. Horiuchi N, Clemens TL, Schiller AL, Holick MF (1985) Detection and developmental changes of the 1,25-(OH)2-D3 receptor concentration in mouse skin and intestine. J Invest Dermatol 84(6):461–464. https://doi.org/10.1111/1523-1747.ep12272358
35. Hosomi J, Hosoi J, Abe E, Suda T, Kuroki T (1983) Regulation of terminal differentiation of cultured mouse epidermal cells by 1 alpha,25-dihydroxyvitamin D3. Endocrinology 113(6):1950–1957. https://doi.org/10.1210/endo-113-6-1950
36. Ratnam AV, Bikle DD, Cho JK (1999) 1,25 dihydroxyvitamin D3 enhances the calcium response of keratinocytes. J Cell Physiol 178(2):188–196. https://doi.org/10.1002/(SICI)1097-4652(199902)178:2<188::AID-JCP8>3.0.CO;2-4

37. Xie Z, Bikle DD (1997) Cloning of the human phospholipase C-gamma1 promoter and identification of a DR6-type vitamin D-responsive element. J Biol Chem 272(10):6573–6577. https://doi.org/10.1074/jbc.272.10.6573

38. Eelen G, Verlinden L, De Clercq P, Vandewalle M, Bouillon R, Verstuyf A (2006) Vitamin D analogs and coactivators. Anticancer Res 26(4A):2717–2721

39. Oda Y, Sihlbom C, Chalkley RJ, Huang L, Rachez C, Chang CP et al (2003) Two distinct coactivators, DRIP/mediator and SRC/p160, are differentially involved in vitamin D receptor transactivation during keratinocyte differentiation. Mol Endocrinol 17(11):2329–2339. https://doi.org/10.1210/me.2003-0063

40. Dlugosz A, Merlino G, Yuspa SH (2002) Progress in cutaneous cancer research. J Investig Dermatol Symp Proc 7(1):17–26. https://doi.org/10.1046/j.1523-1747.2002.19631.x

41. Spencer JM, Kahn SM, Jiang W, DeLeo VA, Weinstein IB (1995) Activated ras genes occur in human actinic keratoses, premalignant precursors to squamous cell carcinomas. Arch Dermatol 131(7):796–800

42. van der Schroeff JG, Evers LM, Boot AJ, Bos JL (1990) Ras oncogene mutations in basal cell carcinomas and squamous cell carcinomas of human skin. J Invest Dermatol 94(4):423–425. https://doi.org/10.1111/1523-1747.ep12874504

43. Huang C, Ma W, Ding M, Bowden GT, Dong Z (1997) Direct evidence for an important role of sphingomyelinase in ultraviolet-induced activation of c-Jun N-terminal kinase. J Biol Chem 272 (44):27753–27757. https://doi.org/10.1074/jbc.272.44.27753

44. Verheij M, Bose R, Lin XH, Yao B, Jarvis WD, Grant S et al (1996) Requirement for ceramide-initiated SAPK/JNK signalling in stress-induced apoptosis. Nature 380(6569):75–79. https://doi.org/10.1038/380075a0

45. Xia Z, Dickens M, Raingeaud J, Davis RJ, Greenberg ME (1995) Opposing effects of ERK and JNK-p38 MAP kinases on apoptosis. Science 270(5240):1326–1331. https://doi.org/10.1126/science.270.5240.1326

46. De Haes P, Garmyn M, Degreef H, Vantieghem K, Bouillon R, Segaert S (2003) 1,25-Dihydroxyvitamin D3 inhibits ultraviolet B-induced apoptosis, Jun kinase activation, and interleukin-6 production in primary human keratinocytes. J Cell Biochem 89(4):663–673. https://doi.org/10.1002/jcb.10540

47. Gupta R, Dixon KM, Deo SS, Holliday CJ, Slater M, Halliday GM et al (2007) Photoprotection by 1,25 dihydroxyvitamin D3 is associated with an increase in p53 and a decrease in nitric oxide products. J Invest Dermatol 127(3):707–715. https://doi.org/10.1038/sj.jid.5700597

48. Bruch-Gerharz D, Ruzicka T, Kolb-Bachofen V (1998) Nitric oxide in human skin: current status and future prospects. J Invest Dermatol 110(1):1–7. https://doi.org/10.1046/j.1523-1747.1998.00084.x

49. Suzuki T, Inukai M (2006) Effects of nitrite and nitrate on DNA damage induced by ultraviolet light. Chem Res Toxicol 19(3):457–462. https://doi.org/10.1021/tx050347l

50. Bau DT, Gurr JR, Jan KY (2001) Nitric oxide is involved in arsenite inhibition of pyrimidine dimer excision. Carcinogenesis 22(5):709–716. https://doi.org/10.1093/carcin/22.5.709

51. De Haes P, Garmyn M, Verstuyf A, De Clercq P, Vandewalle M, Degreef H et al (2005) 1,25-Dihydroxyvitamin D3 and analogues protect primary human keratinocytes against UVB-induced DNA damage. J Photochem Photobiol B 78(2):141–148. https://doi.org/10.1016/j.jphotobiol.2004.09.010

52. Dixon KM, Deo SS, Norman AW, Bishop JE, Halliday GM, Reeve VE et al (2007) In vivo relevance for photoprotection by the vitamin D rapid response pathway. J Steroid Biochem Mol Biol 103(3–5):451–456. https://doi.org/10.1016/j.jsbmb.2006.11.016

53. Dixon KM, Deo SS, Wong G, Slater M, Norman AW, Bishop JE et al (2005) Skin cancer prevention: a possible role of 1,25dihydroxyvitamin D3 and its analogs. J Steroid Biochem Mol Biol 97(1–2):137–143. https://doi.org/10.1016/j.jsbmb.2005.06.006

54. Wong G, Gupta R, Dixon KM, Deo SS, Choong SM, Halliday GM et al (2004) 1,25-Dihydroxyvitamin D and three low-calcemic analogs decrease UV-induced DNA damage via

the rapid response pathway. J Steroid Biochem Mol Biol 89(1–5):567–570. https://doi.org/10.1016/j.jsbmb.2004.03.072

55. Lambert PW, Stern PH, Avioli RC, Brackett NC, Turner RT, Greene A et al (1982) Evidence for extrarenal production of 1 alpha,25-dihydroxyvitamin D in man. J Clin Invest 69 (3):722–725. https://doi.org/10.1172/jci110501

56. Dusso A, Lopez-Hilker S, Rapp N, Slatopolsky E (1988) Extra-renal production of calcitriol in chronic renal failure. Kidney Int 34(3):368–375. https://doi.org/10.1038/ki.1988.190

57. Jones G (2007) Expanding role for vitamin D in chronic kidney disease: importance of blood 25-OH-D levels and extra-renal 1alpha-hydroxylase in the classical and nonclassical actions of 1alpha,25-dihydroxyvitamin D(3). Semin Dial 20(4):316–324. https://doi.org/10.1111/j.1525-139X.2007.00302.x

58. Fritsche J, Mondal K, Ehrnsperger A, Andreesen R, Kreutz M (2003) Regulation of 25-hydroxyvitamin D3-1 alpha-hydroxylase and production of 1 alpha,25-dihydroxyvitamin D3 by human dendritic cells. Blood 102(9):3314–3316. https://doi.org/10.1182/blood-2002-11-3521

59. Hewison M, Freeman L, Hughes SV, Evans KN, Bland R, Eliopoulos AG et al (2003) Differential regulation of vitamin D receptor and its ligand in human monocyte-derived dendritic cells. J Immunol 170(11):5382–5390. https://doi.org/10.4049/jimmunol.170.11.5382

60. Pillai S, Bikle DD, Elias PM (1988) 1,25-Dihydroxyvitamin D production and receptor binding in human keratinocytes varies with differentiation. J Biol Chem 263(11):5390–5395

61. Welsh J (2004) Vitamin D and breast cancer: insights from animal models. Am J Clin Nutr 80 (6 Suppl):1721S–1724S. https://doi.org/10.1093/ajcn/80.6.1721S

62. Reichrath J (2006) The challenge resulting from positive and negative effects of sunlight: how much solar UV exposure is appropriate to balance between risks of vitamin D deficiency and skin cancer? Prog Biophys Mol Biol 92(1):9–16. https://doi.org/10.1016/j.pbiomolbio.2006.02.010

The Role of Microbiome in the Induction, Diagnosis, and Therapy of Skin Cancer

6

Malini Kotak

Abstract

Tremendous advances have been made in understanding the structure of the human microbiome and its importance in health, homeostasis, and diseases. The human gut and skin microbiome have been implicated in conferring susceptibility and influencing response to therapy in several skin cancers. For certain cancers which have viral etiology, the oncogenic role of individual viruses is established and the detailed mechanism of tumorigenesis is elucidated. However, the role of bacteria in cutaneous cancers and the mechanism of carcinogenesis are not well understood. Potential associations between dysbiosis in skin microbial community composition, chronic inflammation, and skin malignancies are reported and implicated as drivers of carcinogenesis. Additionally, some studies also propose a beneficial role for skin microbiome in preventing tumor growth and providing immunity against some cancers. In spite of these recent advances there is a huge gap in our understanding of the relationship between microbiome and skin cancers, and attempts to bridge these gaps show great promise in advancing our knowledge of skin cancer and translation into therapies. Highlights of our current understanding regarding microbiome and its role in skin cancer initiation, diagnosis, and treatment will be discussed in this chapter.

Keywords

Microbiome · Cancer · Immune checkpoint blockade · Non-melanoma skin cancer · Melanoma · Kaposi sarcoma · Merkel cell carcinoma · Cutaneous squamous cell carcinoma

M. Kotak (✉)
ITC Life Sciences & Technology Center, ITC Ltd., Bangalore, India
e-mail: malini.kotak@itc.in

89

6.1   Skin Microbiome: Structure and Function

Microbiota is a sum total of all the diverse microorganisms that inhabit in and on the human body, while microbiome is the genetic material within these microbial communities [1]. The terminologies microbiome and microbiota are frequently used interchangeably. Approximately, a million microorganisms inhabit a square centimeter of human skin and these organisms vary across time, body site, and individuals [2]. In spite of these variabilities, the skin microbiome comprises of four dominant bacterial phyla the Actinobacteria, Proteobacteria, Firmicutes, and Bacteroidetes, which are relatively stable, while the other less abundant phyla account for the variability [3]. The skin is colonized by a wide range of commensal bacteria, viruses, and fungi, most of which are harmless and in certain instances perform important functions. Skin microbiome serve as a physical barrier and prevent the invasion of pathogenic microorganisms by competing for nutrients and space. Also, commensal bacteria of skin along with the skin itself produce antimicrobial peptides (AMPs), which directly kill the invading pathogens. Additionally, these microbes also play an important role in skin health by regulating cutaneous inflammatory and immune responses [4]. During neonatal life, the commensal skin microorganisms recruit regulatory T cells, which help the host in developing immune tolerance towards these commensal bacteria. They also promote interleukin 1 (IL-1) signaling and effector T cell functions, which suggests a role for these microbiota in driving or mediating inflammatory skin disorders. The skin microbiome plays an important role in training the innate and adaptive immune systems, while the immune system shapes and maintains the skin microbiome. The skin microbiome constantly interacts with the host immune system via secretion of metabolic by-products and this cross-talk is important for the maintenance of homeostasis, normal physiology, and disease processes. Any alteration or dysbiosis in the microbiome community composition leads to a shift in immune reaction and eventually results in the development of inflammation and cancer [5].

There are two main types of skin cancers: (1) Melanoma skin cancer and (2) Non-melanoma skin cancer (NMSC), out of which melanoma is a more serious type of skin cancer. NMSC can be further divided into Basal cell cancer (BCC) and Squamous cell cancer (SCC) depending upon the type of cells that undergo malignant transformation. In addition to these three skin cancers, which account for 99% of all skin cancer cases, there are other rare forms which will also be discussed.

6.2   Viral Oncogenesis and Skin Cancer

Globally, 10–15% of cancers are caused by oncovirus infections [6]. Several viruses are known to inhabit the healthy skin as resident commensals, but some of them are linked with malignancies including skin cancer [7, 8]. Oncoviruses cause tumorigenesis through both direct and indirect mechanisms. Viral-encoded proteins can directly act as oncogenes and drive cells to proliferate, leading to malignant transformation. Alternatively, cell transformation is mediated indirectly through insertional mutagenesis, inflammatory responses, evasion of apoptosis, and immune evasion [9–11]. Though human viruses are necessary causal agents for cancer, they are not sufficient and additional co-factors like immunosuppression and environmental mutagens are required for malignant transformation. Viral mediated skin cancers are induced by an interplay of three key factors: (1) oncoviruses, (2) ultraviolet radiation (UVR), and (3) immune suppression [12].

The oncoviruses Kaposi sarcoma herpesvirus/human herpesvirus 8 (KSHV/HHV8) and Merkel cell polyomavirus (MCPyV) are reported to have a causal association with NMSC Kaposi sarcoma (KS) and Merkel cell carcinoma (MCC), respectively [9, 13]. While an epidemiologic association between Human papillomavirus (HPV) and cutaneous Squamous Cell Carcinoma (cSCC) has been established so far [14]. Each of these three viruses and their role in the induction of carcinogenesis is discussed next.

6.2.1 Kaposi Sarcoma and Kaposi Sarcoma Herpesvirus/Human Herpesvirus 8

KS is a multifocal vascular proliferative disease of the skin, mucosa, and the viscera. KS is characterized by abnormal neoangiogenesis, inflammation, and proliferation of spindle shaped endothelial cells which are KS tumor cells. In 1994 Chang and Moore discovered KSHV in KS lesions from an AIDS patient, establishing it as causative agent for KS disease [15]. KSHV is double-stranded herpesvirus, member of the γ herpes virus subfamily and in normal population its infection is innocuous. However, in immunosuppressed patients, the virus is associated with several malignancies [16]. KSHV infects various cell types like endothelial cells, B cells, epithelial cells, dendritic cells, monocytes, and fibroblasts [17]. Epidemiologically KS can be classified in four clinical forms: classical KS, endemic (Africa) KS, immunosuppression (transplantation) iatrogenic KS, and epidemic (AIDS) KS. Prior infection with KSHV and co-factors like immunodeficiency, environmental, and genetic factors are required for the development of these four types of KS [18].

KSHV alternates between two distinct life cycles: latent and lytic. During latency the viral genome is maintained as an episome and passed on to the daughter cells promoting cell survival. The virus is activated in the lytic phase through the lytic switch gene, replication and transcription activator (RTA). During the lytic phase, the viral genome is replicated, and new virions are produced. KSHV undergoes lytic reactivation under certain environmental conditions like hypoxia, oxidative stress, presence of certain cytokines and co-infection with other viruses [19].

The mechanism by which KSHV infection leads to the development of KS is not yet understood. However, it is believed that KSHV encoded lytic and latent proteins, including 14 host homologues play a critical role in tumorigenesis [20, 21]. During latent infection, viral proteins like latency associated nuclear antigen (LANA), viral Cyclin (vCYC) and viral FLIP (vFLIP), kaposins, which are signaling proteins and several microRNAs (miRNAs) are expressed [22]. In addition, some transmembrane protein encoding genes like K1 and K15 and viral Interleukin 6 (vIL-6) are also expressed at low levels [22]. These proteins are expressed in most KSHV infected tumor cells and ensure viral maintenance by altering cell cycle regulation, promoting cell survival, proliferation, and inhibition of apoptosis. The modulation of cellular signaling pathways by these oncogenic proteins lead to cell transformation and immortalization and eventually, development of KS [23, 24].

The initial theory was that only the latent form of KSHV contributed to KS tumorigenesis as most KS lesions are latently infected [22]. However, it was later found that in most latently infected KS lesions, a small percentage of cells still undergo spontaneous lytic replication [20]. Also, KSHV lytic proteins like vIL-6 and viral Gprotein-coupled receptor (vGPCR) can induce expression of pro-inflammatory and angiogenic factors and contribute to tumorigenesis in a paracrine fashion [22]. Both lytic and latent proteins also inhibit host innate and adaptive immunity allowing the virus to survive for the entire life of an infected host. Thus, most likely, both the latent and lytic phases of the virus life cycle are involved in tumor initiation and progression, but unlike latent proteins that are expressed by all tumor cells lytic proteins are expressed by only a few tumor cells [22].

In addition, the KSHV encoded proteins like K15, K1, vGPCR, and vIL-6, modulate host cell signaling pathways like the phosphatidylinositol-3-kinase (PI3K)/AKT/mammalian target of rapamycin (PI3K/AKT/mTOR) pathway, the mitogen-activated protein kinase (MAPK) pathway, and the Nuclear factor -κB (NF-κB) pathway which allow cell survival, cell proliferation, and viral replication [22]. KSHV employs several immune evasion strategies to promote tumorigenesis. The virus encodes an arsenal of proteins which interfere with the complement system, downregulates cell surface MHC class I molecules, modulates Toll-like receptor pathways and viral chemokines (vCCL) to evade adaptive immunity [23].

Antibodies that recognize KSHV LANA are used in histopathology to confirm diagnosis of KS specifically those presenting with lesions that resemble other sarcomas. Although, LANA positivity confirms a KS diagnosis, negative stain may not rule out KS. Molecular diagnosis of KS by detecting KSHV DNA through PCR is highly sensitive but not widely used because of cost ineffectiveness [22]. Inhibitors of several KSHV proteins like vFLIP, vGPCR, and LANA can act as potential target for KS therapy, however, their testing is still in the experimental stage and will take several years before they become mainstream therapy [22].

While there is a large body of knowledge regarding the oncogenic properties of KSHV viral proteins, these are studied in cell culture models. Scientists are still struggling to confirm the oncogenic potential of these proteins in vivo using mouse models. The availability of good animal models can help in furthering our knowledge about the mechanisms of carcinogenesis and the development of therapy for KS.

6.2.2   Merkel Cell Carcinoma and Merkel Cell Polyomavirus

MCC is a rare and severe form of NMSC and generally arises in elderly and immunosuppressed populations who have diminished immune surveillance capacity. It is believed to originate from precursors of mechanoreceptor Merkel cells in the basal layer of the skin [25–27]. The majority of MCCs, approximately 80%, are caused by Merkel cell polyomavirus (MCPyV), while the remaining are associated with somatic mutations caused by UV-mediated DNA damage [28, 29]. Feng et al. established the causal association between MCPyV and MCC using digital transcriptome subtraction (DTS), which involves deep sequencing of tumor specimen and filtering out known human RNA sequences to identify potential viral transcripts. MCPyV-specific antibodies are found to be ubiquitously present in 60–80% human adults [30], suggesting that it may be part of the cutaneous microbiome [31]. Although the MCPyV infection is widespread, only a small population develops MCC.

Oncogenic transformation of MCPyV infection usually occurs as accident when the virus integrates into the host genome at a non-specific site and expresses two putative oncoproteins, the large T-antigen (LT) and small T-antigen (ST) [32]. In addition to integration of the viral genome into the host-genome, MCPyV-related oncogenesis requires truncation of LT to eliminate the virus' capability to replicate [28, 33]. These mutations eliminate the capacity of the viral DNA to replicate but it continues to express motifs that are capable of modulating the cell cycle and inducing uncontrolled proliferation. The probability of integration of viral genome in host genome and further acquiring a truncation mutation in LT is very low which might explain why MCC is rare.

Unlike virus-negative MCCs, virus-positive MCCs lack a UV mutational signature, have a low mutational burden and an absence of *TP53*, *RB1* mutations and loss of function mutations in genes involved in signaling pathways [32, 34]. Therefore, it is possible that in virus-positive MCCs, LT and ST heavily contribute to oncogenesis. In virus-positive MCC, binding of LT alters the RB1 protein, which is involved in tumor suppressive roles. As a result, RB1 is unable to repress E2F transcription factor, and cells are unable to arrest in the G1 [34]. The activity of p53 and several signaling pathways is reduced in virus-positive MCC but it is not clear whether LT, ST or insertion of MCPyV causes the reduction in this activity. ST has been reported to initiate MCC tumorigenesis through coexpression of the cell fate-determinant atonal bHLH transcription factor 1 (ATOH1) [35]. Lastly, MCC cells use immune escape strategies like inhibition of cellular immune responses via programmed cell death protein 1 (PD1) or defects in human leukocyte antigen (HLA) class I expression [34].

For diagnosis of MCC, positive staining for MCPyV LT probably strongly suggests a virus-positive MCC but negative staining does not necessarily rule it out. Studies to determine a prognostic impact of MCPyV in MCC pathogenesis have not reached a common conclusion but based on the largest epidemiologic study to date, the patients with virus-positive MCCs have a better prognosis [32]. Higher titers of antibodies to MCPyV capsid protein and the presence of anti-ST antibodies in the serum at diagnosis have been associated with favorable outcomes [32]. Recently, serology tests to measure T-antigen antibody levels are developed for disease monitoring in MCPyV-positive patients, however, they are not widely used.

The open questions in the field include questions regarding the biology of MCPyV infection, the precise mechanism of tumorigenesis, and immune escape mechanisms. Identification and a detailed understanding of tumor-promoting pathways will have direct implications on the development of therapy targeting virus-positive MCCs.

6.2.3 Cutaneous Squamous Cell Carcinoma and Human Papillomavirus

Papillomaviruses are small, double-stranded DNA viruses and till now more than 200 HPV types are known, the majority of which fall under the α, β,and γ genera [36]. HPVs are abundant in the general population as commensal residents, in fact more than 95% of all viral sequences detected in skin samples belong to the β and γ genera of papillomavirus family [37]. αHPV infect mucosal epithelium and are clearly associated with cervical, anal, and genital cancers and a subset of head and neck cancers [38]. β-HPV infect cutaneous epithelium and epidemiological and biological studies associate the combination of β-HPV and ultraviolet (UV) irradiation with development of cSCC, especially in immunosuppressed patients [39]. The first cutaneous β-HPVs were isolated from skin lesions of patients with a genetic disorder, epidermodysplasia verruciformis (EV). EV skin lesions evolve into SCC at UV-exposed body sites in approximately 30–60% of patients. Thus the evidence of association between β-HPV and cSSC was first established in EV patients. This association was further strengthened by the reports that the β-HPV was found in more than 80% of cSCCs in organ transplant patients with suppressed immune systems [40].

However, several studies have reported that not all cSCC skin lesions have β-HPV DNA, the viral load in cSCC is lower than that detected in the premalignant skin lesions actinic keratosis (AK), β-HPV genome does not integrate into DNA of host cancer cells and also it is transcriptionally inactive in cSCC lesions [40, 41]. Together these findings suggest a "hit-and-run" mode of carcinogenesis for β-HPVs in skin cancer. It is proposed that β-HPV facilitates the initiation of cSCC development but is not necessary for tumor maintenance [41]. In the absence of HPV infection, the UV-induced mutations are addressed by cell cycle arrest, DNA repair or apoptosis if there is irreparable damage. However, upon β-HPV infection, the expression of E6 and E7 oncoproteins deregulates the apoptosis and DNA repair machinery [41]. Additionally, β-HPV also target important cellular proteins, like pRb, p53, and Notch, resulting in unregulated cellular proliferation of mutated cells and accumulation of UV-induced mutations. Eventually, due to irreversible UV-induced DNA damage, the expression of viral genes becomes dispensable for cSCC maintenance. Therefore, Tommasino recently suggested UV as the driving force for cSCC and β-HPV as only a facilitator [41]. A recent provocative study by Strickley et al., however, proposes a beneficial role for commensal β-HPVs in SCC development. They show that β-HPV infection itself does not increase the risk of SCC but instead it is the loss of β-HPV-mediated T cell immunity that promotes cSCC in immunosuppressed patients [40].

Even though in vivo studies using experimental animals have provided strong evidence for the role of β-HPV in the development of cSCC and for a hit-and-run mechanism, the hypothesis needs to be validated in humans. Nevertheless, development of vaccines that target cutaneous HPVs are highly beneficial for immunosuppressed patients, which are at higher risk of NMSC development.

6.3 Bacterial Oncogenesis and Skin Cancer

Unlike viral oncogenesis where the role of individual viruses as causative agents is established and the detailed mechanism of tumorigenesis is elucidated, the potential contribution of bacteria in skin cancer is a topic of ongoing research. There is convincing evidence to suggest that dysbiosis in microbial skin communities promotes chronic inflammatory diseases which may eventually develop into cutaneous malignancies. Additionally, certain studies report the potential association of individual species of bacteria with certain skin cancers. However, the mechanistic insights into the role of skin microbiome in skin malignancies are still lacking and the ongoing studies to elucidate these roles are still in their infancy.

6.3.1 Skin Microbiome, Chronic Inflammatory Diseases, and Skin Cancer

Till date, there is no evidence of a causal association between a bacterial pathogen and the development of skin cancer. However, an indirect association can be made as the dysbiosis of skin microbiome is significantly associated with chronic inflammatory skin diseases like Atopic dermatitis (AD), Psoriasis, and Hidradenitis Suppurativa (HS) [42] and chronic inflammation is linked to the development and progression of several cancers including those of skin [43]. Dysbiosis and an abnormal colonization of skin by *Staphylococcus aureus* are hypothesized as key players in the development and increased severity of AD [42, 44]. An increased risk of developing cutaneous squamous cell carcinoma (cSCC) was observed in a retrospective case control study, for patients with AD [45]. Skin lesions in patients with psoriasis were reported to have an altered microbiome with reduced diversity and enrichment of *Firmicutes*-associated and *Actinobacteria*-associated microbiota, as compared to the healthy population [46]. An increased risk of melanoma and NMSC has been observed in patients with psoriasis [47]. An altered microbiome has been associated with HS, which is an inflammatory skin disease characterized by recurrent scarring, nodules, and tunnels in the intertriginous regions. The clinically non-affected axillary skin of HS patients had reduced microbiota resulting in less biofilm as compared to healthy controls [48]. HS has been reported to trigger the development of cSCC depending upon the duration of the inflammatory process [49, 50].

Although there is sufficient evidence to show that a dysbiosis of skin microbiome leads to or at least promotes inflammatory skin diseases, the underlying mechanism is still unclear. Dysbiosis between commensal and pathogenic microbiota results in compromised barrier function of the skin, leading to aberrant immune responses to commensal microbes and stabilization of a pro-inflammatory microbiota, which can eventually result into chronic inflammation [51]. The T cells that regulate chronic inflammation favor tumorigenesis by secreting pro-tumorigenic factors [IL-4, IL-6, IL-10, IL-13, and transforming growth factor (TGF)-β]. In NMSC, inflammation is a hallmark of tumorigenesis and several deregulated pathway together initiate malignant transformation [52].

6.3.2   Skin Microbiome and Skin Cancer

Because of an increased incidence of skin cancer among immunosuppressed patients, an infectious etiology has been postulated for a long time. The potential contribution of skin microbiome in skin cancer development is a topic of ongoing research as aforementioned. A strong relationship between melanoma development and changes in the diversity and composition of skin microbiome was recently reported by Mrazek et al. using a pig model [53]. A hospital based case control study comparing biopsies of NMSC, SCC, BCC, and Actinic keratosis (AK) with that from healthy skin of the same immunocompetent patients found a strong association between SCC and *S. aureus* [54]. A longitudinal study comparing the microbiome of SCC and AK lesions with that of photo damaged nonlesional control sites in patients with history of SCC showed significant association of *S. aureus* with lesional skin. *Propionibacterium* and *Malassezia* were found to be relatively more abundant in nonlesional photo damaged skin than in AK and SCC lesions. This finding strongly suggests the involvement of *S. aureus* in SCC etiology, and because SCC develops from AK, in AK to SCC progression [55]. These findings were further corroborated by a comparative study profiling the microbial community compositions of AK, SCC, and BCC from excised tumor specimens. They identified significantly different microbial community composition in skin tumors compared to normal skin and also between the different tumor entities, with prominent overabundance of *S. aureus* in SCCs [56].

The same study also reported a significant link between the overabundance of *S. aureus* and increased expression of *hBD-2* encoding AMP, human β-defensin-2 (hBD-2) in SCC tumors. They found that *S. aureus* induced *hBD-2* expression lead to increased tumor cell proliferation of cSCC tumor cells. Thus it can be inferred that adysbiosis in microbial community composition is associated with the development of SCC. In addition, the dysbiosis is characterized by an overabundance of *S. aureus* which promotes tumor growth through modulation of *hBD-2* expression [20]. AMPs like *hBD-2* are part of the innate immune system and are produced by epithelia and immune cells in response to specific microbes. AMPs are implicated in tumorigenesis as they affect tumor cell growth and migration which are both features of tumor progression [57, 58]. Bacteria can also contribute to carcinogenesis by modulating the tumor microenvironment through the immune system. In an animal model of keratinocyte skin cancer due to chronic inflammation, Hoste et al. showed that tumor formation can be driven by flagellin (the ligand for TLR-5) in wound-induced carcinogenesis [59].

In addition to producing tumor promoting metabolites, skin microbiome is also reported to produce metabolites that prevent tumor formation. Nakatsuji et al. reported that certain strains of *Staphylococcus epidermidis* produce a nucleobase analog called 6-N-hydroxyaminopurine (6-HAP) which has the capacity to inhibit DNA synthesis. Intravenous injections of 6-HAP slowed the growth of melanoma in the mice model. Additionally, the application of 6-HAP producing *S. epidermidis* to mouse skin reduced the incidence of tumors that are formed in response to ultraviolet radiation compared to the control strain that did not produce 6-HAP. This study proposes a beneficial role for skin microbiome in the host defense through suppression of tumor growth. It also suggests that the development of skin cancer due to dysbiosis is because of a loss of protective skin microbial communities rather than a gain of the detrimental communities [60].

The precise mechanisms elicited by the microbiome in the development of skin cancer remains to be revealed, although the future holds great promise for this fascinating field. The illumination of these mechanisms is bound to inspire further innovations in the therapy for skin cancer.

6.4   Gut Microbiome and Therapy for Melanoma

There is a large body of evidence that suggests that the gut microbiome may play a significant role in modulating the response to immune checkpoint blockade (ICB) therapy in melanoma patients. The initial association between the gut microbiome and response to ICB was first reported by two independent yet parallel studies by Vetizou et al. and Sivan et al. [61, 62]. Using murine models, they demonstrated that the gut microbiota composition affected the response to ICBs targeting the cytotoxic T lymphocyte antigen-4 (TLA-4) and programmed death receptor-1 (PD-1). Also, an alteration in the gut microbiome composition through either fecal microbiome transplant (FMT) or probiotic supplementation, to replicate the favorable gut microbiota, enhanced the response to ICB. These initial findings were further supplemented by several studies that substantiated the role for gut microbiota in shaping the patient response to ICB [63–67]. In order to understand the mechanism of this influence, two research groups focusing on patients with metastatic melanoma studied the gut microbiome composition of responders and non-responders to anti-PD-1 therapy [65, 66]. They identified a range of bacteria including Ruminococcus, Faecalibacteria, and Bifidobacteria as response-associated taxa. In light of these findings, there is an increasing interest in modulating the gut microbiome to improve the response to therapy. There are several approaches that can be implemented to alter the gut microbiome like FMT, prebiotics, probiotics, and targeted antibiotics [68].

References

1. Grice EA, Segre JA (2011) The skin microbiome. Nat Rev Microbiol 9:244–253
2. Grice EA, Kong HH, Renaud G et al (2008) A diversity profile of the human skin microbiota. Genome Res 18:1043–1050
3. Grice EA (2014) The skin microbiome: potential for novel diagnostic and therapeutic approaches to cutaneous disease. Semin Cutan Med Surg 33(2):98–103
4. Meisel JS, Sfyroera G, Bartow-McKenney C et al (2018) Commensal microbiota modulate gene expression in the skin. Microbiome 6(1):20
5. Balato A, Cacciapuoti S, Di Caprio R et al (2019) Human microbiome: composition and role in inflammatory skin diseases. Arch Immunol Ther Exp (Warsz) 67(1):1–18
6. Chen Y, Williams V, Filippova M, Filippov V, Duerksen-Hughes P (2014) Viral carcinogenesis: factors inducing DNA damage and virus integration. Cancer 6:2155–2186
7. Samimi M, Touzé A (2014) Viruses and skin cancers. Presse Med 43:e405–e411
8. Cyprian FS, Al-Farsi HF, Vranic S, Akhtar S, Al Moustafa AE (2018) Epstein–Barr virus and human papillomaviruses interactions and their roles in the initiation of epithelial-mesenchymal transition and cancer progression. Front Oncol 8(111):111
9. Kung HJ, Boerkoel C, Carter TH (1991) Retroviral mutagenesis of cellular oncogenes: a review with insights into the mechanisms of insertional activation. Curr Top Microbiol Immunol 171:1–25
10. Chatterjee M, Osborne J, Bestetti G et al (2002) Viral IL-6-induced cell proliferation and immune evasion of interferon activity. Science 298:1432–1435
11. Galluzzi L, Kepp O, Morselli E et al (2010) Viral strategies for the evasion of immunogenic cell death. J Intern Med 267:526–542
12. Arron ST, Jennings L, Nindl I et al (2011) Viral oncogenesis and its role in nonmelanoma skin cancer. Br J Dermatol 164(6):1201–1213
13. Minutilli E, Mulè A (2016) Merkel cell polyomavirus and cutaneous Merkel cell carcinoma. Future Sci OA 2(4):FSO155
14. Coggshall K, Brooks L, Nagarajan P, Arron ST (2019) The microbiome and its contribution to skin cancer. In: Robertson E (ed) Microbiome and cancer. Humana Press, Cham
15. Chang Y, Cesarman E, Pessin MS et al (1994) Identification of herpesvirus-like DNA sequences in AIDS-associated Kaposi's sarcoma. Science 266:1865–1869
16. Bouvard V, Baan R, Straif K et al (2009) A review of human carcinogens—part B: biological agents. Lancet Oncol 10(4):321–322
17. Bechtel JT, Liang Y, Hvidding J, Ganem D (2003) Host range of Kaposi's sarcoma- associated herpesvirus in cultured cells. J Virol 77:6474–6481
18. Douglas JL, Gustin JK, Moses AV, Dezube BJ, Pantanowitz L (2010) Kaposi sarcoma pathogenesis: a triad of viral infection, oncogenesis and chronic inflammation. Transl Biomed 1(2):172
19. Hu D, Wang V, Yang M et al (2015) Induction of Kaposi's sarcoma-associated Herpesvirus-encoded viral Interleukin-6 by X-Box binding protein 1. J Virol 90(1):368–378
20. Ganem D (2010) KSHV and the pathogenesis of Kaposi sarcoma: listening to human biology and medicine. J Clin Invest 120:939–949
21. Mesri EA, Feitelson MA, Munger K (2014) Human viral oncogenesis: a cancer hallmarks analysis. Cell Host Microbe 15:266–282
22. Cesarman E, Damania B, Krown SE et al (2019) Kaposi sarcoma. Nat Rev Dis Primers 5:9
23. Yan L, Majerciak V, Zheng ZM, Lan K (2019) Towards better understanding of KSHV life cycle: from transcription and posttranscriptional regulations to pathogenesis. Virol Sin 34 (2):135–161
24. Ariana G, Bravo C, Damania B (2019) In vivo models of Oncoproteins encoded by Kaposi's sarcoma-associated herpesvirus. J Virol 93(11):e01053–e01018
25. Becker JC, Stang A, Decaprio JA, Cerroni L, Lebbé C, Veness M, Nghiem P (2017) Merkel cell carcinoma. Nat Rev Dis Primers 3:17077

26. Drusio C, Becker JC, Schadendorf D, Ugurel S (2019) Merkel cell carcinoma. Hautarzt 70 (3):215–227
27. Jaeger T, Ring J, Andres C (2012) Histological, immunohistological, and clinicalfeatures of merkel cell carcinoma in correlation to Merkel cell polyomavirus status. J Skin Cancer 2012:983421
28. Feng H, Shuda M, Chang Y, Moore PS (2008) Clonal integration of a polyomavirus in human Merkel cell carcinoma. Science 319:1096–1100
29. Wong SQ, Waldeck K, Vergara IA, Schröder J, Madore J, Wilmott JS et al (2015) UV-associated mutations underlie the etiology of MCV-negative Merkel cell carcinomas. Cancer Res 75:5228–5234
30. Chang Y, Moore PS (2012) Merkel cell carcinoma: a virus-induced human cancer. Annu Rev Pathol 7:123–144
31. Foulongne V, Kluger N, Dereure O, Mercier G, Molès JP, Guillot B et al (2013) Merkel cell polyomavirus in cutaneous swabs. Emerg Infect Dis 16:685–687
32. Harms PW, Harms KL, Moore PS et al (2018) The biology and treatment of Merkel cell carcinoma: current understanding and research priorities. Nat Rev Clin Oncol 15(12):763–776
33. Shuda M, Feng H, Kwun HJ et al (2008) T antigen mutations are a human tumor-specific signature for Merkel cell polyomavirus. Proc Natl Acad Sci USA 105:16272–16277
34. Becker JC, Stang A, DeCaprio JA et al (2017) Merkel cell carcinoma. Nat Rev Dis Primers 3:17077
35. Verhaegen ME, Mangelberger D, Harms PW et al (2017) Merkel cell polyomavirus small T antigen initiates Merkel cell carcinoma-like tumor development in mice. Cancer Res 77 (12):3151–3157
36. Van Doorslaer K, Li Z, Xirasagar S et al (2017) The papillomavirus episteme: a major update to the papillomavirus sequence database. Nucleic Acids Res 45:D499–D506
37. Bzhalava D, Muhr LS, Lagheden C et al (2014) Deep sequencing extends the diversity of human papillomaviruses in human skin. Sci Rep 4:5807
38. Rollison D, Viarisio D, Amorrortu R, Gheit T, Tommasino M (2019) An emerging issue in oncogenic virology: the role of beta human papillomavirus types in the development of cutaneous squamous cell carcinoma. J Virol 93(7):e01003–e01018
39. Accardi R, Gheit T (2014) Cutaneous HPV and skin cancer. Presse Med 43:e435–e443
40. Strickley JD, Messerschmidt JL, Awad ME, Li T, Hasegawa T, Ha DT, Nabeta HW, Bevins PA, Ngo KH, Asgari MM et al (2019) Immunity to commensal papillomaviruses protects against skin cancer. Nature 575(7783):519–522
41. Tommasino M (2019) HPV and skin carcinogenesis. Papillomavirus Res 7:129–131
42. Nørreslet LB, Agner T, Clausen M (2020) The skin microbiome in inflammatory skin diseases. Curr Derm Rep 9:141–151
43. Tang L, Wang K (2016) Chronic inflammation in skin malignancies. J Mol Signal 11:2
44. Rodrigues HA (2017) The cutaneous ecosystem: the roles of the skin microbiome in health and its association with inflammatory skin conditions in humans and animals. Vet Dermatol 28 (1):60–e15
45. Cho JM, Davis DMR, Wetter DA, Bartley AC, Brewer JD (2018) Association between atopic dermatitis and squamous cell carcinoma: a case-control study. Int J Dermatol 57(3):313–316
46. Alekseyenko AV, Perez-Perez GI, De Souza A et al (2013) Community differentiation of the cutaneous microbiota in psoriasis. Microbiome 1(1):31
47. Egeberg A, Thyssen JP, Gislason GH, Skov L (2016) Skin cancer in patients with psoriasis. J Eur Acad Dermatol Venereol 30(8):1349–1353
48. Ring HC, Bay L, Kallenbach K et al (2017) Normal skin microbiota is altered in pre-clinical hidradenitis suppurativa. Acta Derm Venereol 97(2):208–213
49. Jourabchi N, Fischer AH, Cimino-Mathews A, Waters KM, Okoye GA (2017) Squamous cell carcinoma complicating a chronic lesion of hidradenitis suppurativa: a case report and review of the literature. Int Wound J 14(2):435–438

50. Samaras V, Rafailidis PI, Mourtzoukou EG, Peppas G, Falagas ME (2014) Chronic bacterial and parasitic infections and cancer: a review. J Infect Dev Ctries 4(5):267–281
51. Honda K, Littman DR (2016) The microbiota in adaptive immune homeostasis and disease. Nature 535:75–84
52. Neagu M, Constantin C, Caruntu C, Dumitru C, Surcel M, Zurac S (2019) Inflammation: a key process in skin tumorigenesis. Oncol Lett 17(5):4068–4084
53. Mrázek J, Mekadim C, Kučerová P et al (2019) Melanoma-related changes in skin microbiome. Folia Microbiol 64:435–442
54. Kullander J, Forslund O, Dillner J (2009) Staphylococcus aureus and squamous cell carcinoma of the skin. Cancer Epidemiol Biomark Prev 18(2):472–478
55. Wood DLA, Lachner N, Tan JM et al (2018) Natural history of actinic keratosis and cutaneous squamous cell carcinoma microbiomes. MBio 9(5):e01432–e01418
56. Madhusudhan N, Pausan MR, Halwachs B et al (2020) Molecular profiling of keratinocyte skin tumors links Staphylococcus aureus overabundance and increased human β-defensin-2 expression to growth promotion of squamous cell carcinoma. Cancers (Basel) 12(3):541
57. Niyonsaba F, Ushio H, Nakano N, Ng W, Sayama K, Hashimoto K, Nagaoka I, Okumura K, Ogawa H (2007) Antimicrobial peptides human beta-defensins stimulate epidermal keratinocyte migration, proliferation and production of proinflammatory cytokines and chemokines. J Investig Dermatol 127:94–604
58. Mburu YK, Abe K, Ferris LK, Sarkar SN, Ferris RL (2011) Human beta-defensin 3 promotes NF-kappaB-mediated CCR7 expression and anti-apoptotic signals in squamous cell carcinoma of the head and neck. Carcinogenesis 32:168–174
59. Hoste E, Arwert EN, Lal R et al (2015) Innate sensing of microbial products promotes wound-induced skin cancer. Nat Commun 6:5932
60. Nakatsuji T, Chen TH, Butcher AM et al (2018) A commensal strain of Staphylococcus epidermidis protects against skin neoplasia. Sci Adv 4(2):eaao4502
61. Sivan A, Corrales L, Hubert N et al (2015) Commensal bifidobacterium promotes antitumor immunity and facilitates anti-PD-L1 efficacy. Science 350(6264):1084–1089
62. Vetizou M, Pitt JM, Daillere R et al (2015) Anticancer immunotherapy by CTLA-4 blockade relies on the gut microbiota. Science 350(6264):1079–1084
63. Chaput N, Lepage P, Coutzac C et al (2017) Baseline gut microbiota predicts clinical response and colitis in metastatic melanoma patients treated with ipilimumab. Ann Oncol 28 (6):1368–1379
64. Frankel AE, Coughlin LA, Kim J et al (2017) Metagenomic shotgun sequencing and unbiased metabolomic profiling identify specific human gut microbiota and metabolites associated with immune checkpoint therapy efficacy in melanoma patients. Neoplasia 19(10):848–855
65. Gopalakrishnan V, Spencer C, Nezi L et al (2018) Gut microbiome modulates response to anti-PD-1 immunotherapy in melanoma patients. Science 359(6371):97–103
66. Matson V, Fessler J, Bao R et al (2018) The commensal microbiome is associated with anti-PD-1 efficacy in metastatic melanoma patients. Science 359(6371):104–108
67. Routy B, Le Chatelier E, Derosa L et al (2018) Gut microbiome influences efficacy of PD-1-based immunotherapy against epithelial tumors. Science 359(6371):91–97
68. Gopalakrishnan V, Helmink BA, Spencer CN, Reuben A, Wargo JA (2018) The influence of the gut microbiome on cancer, immunity, and cancer immunotherapy. Cancer Cell 33 (4):570–580

Skin Cancer: Molecular Biomarker for Diagnosis, Prognosis, Prevention, and Targeted Therapy

7

Sachchida Nand Pandey

Abstract

Skin malignancy is one of the most common cancer types in white population of world over. Occurrence of skin cancer, melanoma and non-melanoma skin cancers (NMSCs) are as yet rising. Early detection of melanoma and NMSCs are critical for clinical management and efficient therapy. However, conventional diagnostic biomarkers can frequently pretense a significant hurdle to early detection objective. Consequently, advance analytic tools and biomarkers are imperative to facilitating early recognition of skin cancer. Skin cancer initiated by consequence of genetic changes by UV exposure, which often call as a mutagenic risk factor. With increased sensitivity and specificity novel genetic testing techniques have improved recognition of molecular changes, which consequently uncovered its significance in diagnosis and prognosis of skin cancers. Early detection of genetic changes may be additive for selecting best treatment and further open avenues for discovering targeted therapies for skin malignancy. This book chapter on skin cancer consist the summary of possible molecular biomarkers uses in skin cancer advancement, metastasis, progression, prognosis and targeted therapy. In addition, it may be helpful to delineate the molecular alterations and its implications may posture for clinical management.

Keywords

Skin cancer · Biomarkers · Melanoma · Non-melanoma skin cancer · Prognosis · Diagnosis · Targeted therapy · UV exposure

S. N. Pandey (✉)
Department of Pathology, Muljibhai Patel Urological Hospital, Nadiad, Gujarat, India

© The Author(s), under exclusive license to Springer Nature Singapore Pte Ltd. 2021
A. Dwivedi et al. (eds.), *Skin Cancer: Pathogenesis and Diagnosis*,
https://doi.org/10.1007/978-981-16-0364-8_7

101

7.1   Introduction

Skin cancers comprise two groups; one melanoma and another are non-melanoma. In 2018, melanoma and non-melanoma accounted for 19th and fifth most commonly occurring skin cancer, respectively, worldwide [1]. White individuals relatively lack skin pigmentation might put them at higher risk for developing non-melanoma or melanoma skin cancers than individual with dark color. Skin cancer includes malignant melanoma (MM) and non-melanoma [basal cell carcinoma (BCC), squamous cell carcinoma (SCC), Merkel cell carcinoma (MCC), cutaneous lymphomas (CL), Kaposi sarcoma (KS)]. Skin cancers are huge health problem in many countries since its incidence is on rise [1]. The rise of skin cancer also increases the financial burden on the health. Skin cancers are highly preventable by avoiding the risk factor since ultraviolet (UV) radiation is well known risk factor. In addition, skin cancers are nearly curable if detected early. There is urgency to use appropriate skin cancer risk biomarkers to recognize persons in advance on possibility in emerging skin cancer. Skin type and number of nevi are known markers but focus is to enhance the sensitivity and specificity in early screening through the use of molecular biomarkers.

In addition to diagnosis and prevention, genetic alterations as biomarkers can be used in choosing appropriate treatment and developing targeted therapies for skin cancer. Better understanding of the molecular signatures essential in skin cancer pathogenesis has prompted the examination of skin cancer in better way with its prevention. In addition, new molecular signatures became the catalyst for discovery of targeted therapy. For example, the finding of ultraviolet radiation based biomarkers of skin cancer is now a fast growing and promising research field. Identified mechanism can also provide a novel target for therapy of skin cancer. Advances in genetic sequencing and high throughput molecular assay have provided the way to discover the novel biomarkers. These novel biomarkers may have the possibility in improving the skin cancer patient's clinical management.

Induction of suitable biomarkers panels in skin cancer's management will greatly assist the early diagnosis and personalized treatment for primary and relapsed tumors. Therefore, the aim of this chapter is not only to discuss the clinical uses of these biomarkers for skin cancer, but also provide information of novel biomarkers, which can provide a platform for advancement in skin cancer research. Here I also listed the molecular biomarkers still under research, which have potential to be added in skin cancer clinic in future to come.

7.2   Skin Phototype as Biomarkers in Skin Cancers

The incidences of BCC, SCC, and melanoma have been constantly increasing at a rate of 5–8% every year in whites [2–4]. However, incidence of skin cancer in black and brown remains constant [5]. Skin phototype is a hereditary susceptible biomarker which renders individuals with differential pigmentation has differential sensitivity to UV radiation. Solar sensitivity of human skin is depending on quality and quantity of melanin produced in epidermal melanocytes. Skin color sensitivity to UV radiation has been defined which ranges from type I, melano-compromised (no tanning), to type VI, melano-protected (black). A meta-analysis has shown two fold of relative risk of melanoma for skin type I in comparison to skin type IV [6]. The brown and black individuals (skin phototype V, VI) can tolerate sun exposure without greatly increasing risk of skin malignancy. Interestingly, people with skin phototype I and II (pale or freckled skin, blond or red hair, and blue eyes) have high risk for developing skin cancer, whereas people with phototype III and IV (dark hair and eyes) have medium risk of developing skin cancer [7].

Protective effect of melanin measured by minimal erythema dose (MED) determination between white and dark skin individuals indicated that dark skin was extremely protected from carcinogenesis [8–10]. Even less pigmented Asians have low rate of skin cancer [11]. Individuals with darker skin pigmentation protected from skin cancer risk may explain as skins with red pigments have higher risk of developing skin cancer. Individuals with MC1R mutations are prone to develop skin cancers which are independent of skin color including red hair phenotype [12, 13]. UV radiation induces the skin pigmentation through p53 protein expression, while absence of p53 inhibits the tanning response. The p53 protein expression induced through activation of proopiomelanocortin (POMC) gene [14]. POMC gene mutations are known to be involved in red color hair phenotype [15]. Ultraviolet A (UVA), wave length 320–400 nm, induces high single strand break in human melanocytes isolated from darker skin than white skin [16]. Following damage may occur through oxidative mechanisms and pronounced the role of UVA in melanoma causation [17].

7.3   Genetic Alterations as Biomarkers in Skin Cancers

Gold standard for diagnosis of skin cancer is examination of skin histology and architectural features. Histological examinations are always having issue with its subjectivity. Thickness and mitotic rate are usual characteristics of melanoma which may be inaccurate in diagnosis and prognosis. There is an urgent need of finding the novel detection method to know the diagnosis and prognosis. Detecting molecular biomarkers has emerged as an advanced form of diagnosis that guides therapeutic decisions and additive in diagnosis of histologically challenging cases. Recent decade, sequencing studies findings have strengthened the role of UV exposure in different mutations causes melanoma.

High throughput genome analysis has revealed a list of mutations, genes expression at single-base resolution across the genome causing the development of UV and non-UV associated melanomas [18–22]. In addition, comparative genomic hybridization (CGH) and fluorescence in situ hybridization (FISH) also have contributed in identifying the genetic alterations associated with skin cancer. Several diagnostic tests are under commercial use, designed with multiple genes pannel as DermTech, Inc. (Pigmented Lesion Assay), Castle Biosciences (DecisionDx-Melanoma), and Myriad Genetics (myPath Melanoma) [23, 24]. These biomarkers characterize the melanoma mutations, gene polymorphisms, signaling receptors, and melanin pigment.

7.4   Molecular Pathway Genes as Biomarkers

Melanoma generally initiated by mutations in signaling pathway genes important for cell survival. Particular signaling pathway gene, such as mitogen-activated protein kinase (MAPK), drives cell growth, apoptosis, differentiation, and proliferation [25, 26]. Mutations in genes of MAPK pathway initiates in augmentation of signaling which allows cells cycle malfunction results uninterepted cell growth. Growth factors bind to receptor tyrosine kinase (RTK) on cells surface to activate the MAPK pathway and ultimately stimulate the RAS's GTPase activity. The cascade of RAF, MEK, and ERK will be activated through defective MAPK pathway signals which allow them to enter into nucleus. This will activate the transcription factors promoting the cell cycle [27–29]. The PI3K/AKT pathway regulates cell growth and proliferation [30]. Direct stimulation of RAS or through binding of growth factors to RTK can activate PI3Ks signaling [31]. PI3K hence phosphorylates its substrate PIP2 on the cell surface into PIP3, and help to recruit and initiate AKT [32]. AKT promotes AKT related cell growth and survival through multiple effectors, such as mTOR, Bad, and Mdm2 [33]. Mutations in regulatory genes, oncogene and tumor suppressor gene PTEN, can be exclusive or it may found in addition to other mutations in melanoma cases [31]. On the contrary to cutaneous melanoma, uveal melanoma initiated from different sets of mutations beside the alteration in MAPK or PI3K/AKT pathways. Causative genes, GNAQ and GNA11, for uveal melanoma have most frequent mutations lead to alterations in the both pathways. The GNAQ and GNA11 genes encode the G-subunit of G proteins, keeping to a constitutively active GTP-bound state [34–36]. Presence of Hippo pathway may also increase the activity of GNAQ and GNA11 mutations activity. The Hippo pathway is known for its function in cell homeostasis and mammalian organ size. The Hippo pathway can regulate the size of heart, liver, and pancreas [37]. The expression level analysis of GNAQ or GNA11 may be a precious diagnostic tool in differentiating uveal melanoma from other types of melanoma and cancers [38]. Downstream activation of YAP/TAZ is driven by GNAQ and GNA11 mutations to initiate melanomagenesis [39]. Uveal melanomas are resultant of GNAQ/GNA11 mutations, followed by a secondary BSE event. The BSE even has been initiated by mutations in the genes BAP1, SF3B1, and EIF1AX [40, 41]. The list of molecular alterations and their implication is given in Table 7.1.

7.5   Molecular Biomarkers for Targeted Therapy

The most common BRAF mutation, V600E, directs the initiation of the MAPK pathway [42]. Load of BRAF and NRAS mutations in benign melanocytic nevi has been positively correlated with UV exposure [109]. There are several FDA-approv

Table 7.1 Summary of function, potential use as biomarkers, and known targeted therapies targeting melanoma mutations

Gene	Incidence and function	Potential as Biomarker	Targeted therapy	References
BRAF	40–60%, protein kinase along the MAPK pathway; most common mutation	Positive expression of V600E in the nucleus was correlated with worse tumor stage, lymph node metastasis, and depth of invasion in melanomas	Vemurafenib, dabrafenib, encorafenib	Davies et al. [42], Hauschild et al. [43], Pracht et al. [44], Melis et al. [45], Dummer et al. [46], Sarkisian and Davar [47], Abd Elmageed et al. [48]
NRAS	15–30%, GTPase with signal transduction along the MAPK and PI3K pathways	Mutation associated with shorter survival from metastatic melanomas	Phase II trials of FTIs, lonafarnib and tipifarnib (NCT00060125 and NCT00281957)	Smalley and Eisen [49], Lee et al. [50], Niessner et al. [51], Hodis et al. [52], Jakob et al. [53]
C-KIT	1–2%, growth factor-binding RTK; first signal along the MAPK and PI3K pathways	Mutations has been associated with worse survival of melanomas	Phase II trials of imatinib and nilotinib; phase II trial of regorafenib (NCT02501551)	Curtin et al. [54], Beadling et al. [55], Carvajal et al. [56], Pracht et al. [44], Carvajal et al. [57], Guo et al. [58], Ma et al. [59]
CDKN2A	25–40% (familial), encodes p16 and p14ARF to regulate cell cycle and apoptosis	Mutations are the most common alteration in hereditary melanoma	Phase II trial of CDK inhibitor, flavopiridol (NCT00005971)	Serrano et al. [60], Zhang et al. [61], Florell et al. [62], Burdette-Radoux et al. [63], Goldstein et al. [64], Aoude et al. [65], Soura et al. [66]
VDR	Active vitamin D birds to VDR and initiate downstream signal	Tumor propagation, mitotic rates, and survival time are inversely correlated with VDR protein expression	Vitamin D supplementation; phase II (ACTRN12609000351213) and phase III (NCT01748448) trials	Baker et al. [67], Demay et al. [68], Colnot et al. [69], Brozyna et al. [70], Brozyna et al. [71], Saw et al. [72], De Smedt et al. [73]
MC1R	Up to 60%, by interacting with ACTH and MSH it regulates melanogenesis	Mutations in CDKN2A gene increases its penetrance and melanoma risk	No	Fargnoli et al. [74], Tagliabue et al. [75], Raimondi et al. [76]
MITF 1	2% (familial), regulates involve in development and differentiation of melanocyte	Differentiating melanoma from histologically similar nonmelanocytic tumors	No	Price et al. [77], Bertolotto et al. [78], King et al. [79], Levy et al. [80], Yokoyama et al. [81], Naffouje et al. [82]

(continued)

Table 7.1 (continued)

Gene	Incidence and function	Potential as Biomarker	Targeted therapy	References
GNAQ/GNA11	80–90%, involved in the MAPK and PI3K pathways	Differentiating uveal melanoma from other types of melanoma and cancers	No	Landis et al. [34], Kalinec et al. [35], Van Raamsdonk et al. [83], Griewank et al. [38], Amaro et al. [36]
BAP1	8–50% (familial), Deubiquitinase involved in cell cycle progression	Differential in uveal and cutaneous melanoma cells	Phase II trial of PARP inhibitor, niraparib (NCT03207347)	Kalirai et al. [84], Pan et al. [85], Rai et al. [86], Garfield et al. [87], Vivet-Noguer et al. [88]
SF3B1	10–21%, splicing factor subunit	Good prognosis for uveal melanoma in younger patients	No	Dono et al. [89], Kumar et al. [90], Yavuzyigitoglu et al. [91], Alsafadi et al. [92], Robertson et al. [93], Smit et al. [94]
EIF1AX	13–21%, eukaryotic translation initiation factor that stabilizes ribosome	Associated with good prognosis	No	Chaudhuri et al. [95], Martin et al. [96], Dono et al. [89], Decatur et al. [97], Robertson et al. [93], Smit et al. [94]
CTLA4/PD-1/PD-L1	Downregulates the T cell immune response		Ipilimumab, pembrolizumab, and nivolumab	Fong and Small [98], Hodi et al. [99], Topalian et al. [100], Postow et al. [101]
Melanin	Pigment that scavenges free radicals	Differentiating melanoma from other tumors	No	Różanowska et al. [102], Slominski et al. [103], Slominski et al. [104]
TYR/TRP1/TRP2	Proteins associated with melanin synthesis	Low level of TRP1 protein is associated with high tumor stage and poor survival	No	Ito [105], Journe et al. [106], Slominski et al. [107]
HAPLN1	ECM component associated with age-related loss		No	Kaur et al. [108]

inhibitors of BRAF V600 mutations, are avilabe such as Dabrafenib, Vemurafenib and Encorafenib [43, 46, 47]. Although treating BRAF-mutant melanomas with BRAF inhibitors are efficacious, but through upregulation of RTKs or NRAS genes its develop resistance [110]. Therefore, long-term growth of melanoma can be suppressed by treating them by combined use of BRAF and MEK inhibitors (trametinib and cobimetinib). Furthermore, a combination therapy of encorafenib and binimetinib showed better efficacy in treating melanomas with BRAF mutation [46].

Mutation in NRAS gene reduces the GTPase activity, which activate the GTP-bound G protein for ultimate processing of the downstream signal. The association of NRAS with cumulative solar damage (CSD) of skin suggests that this mutagenesis is induced by UV irradiation [111]. NRAS expression level can be correlated with Infiltrating lymphocytes—lower grade tumor and a higher tumor stage [112]. Prognostic value of NRAS mutation is not clear enough but survival study of a large cohort shows shorter survival of melanoma with metastasis [53]. NRAS mutations are also reported in dysplastic nevi, melanocytic, and melanomas along BRAF mutations. This discrimination favour to NRAS as a diagnostic biomarker [109, 113]. Targeted therapy has shown limited effectiveness in melanomas with NRAS mutations. Direct targeting of NRAS mutations is difficult but it can be achieved by inhibiting the farnesylation and subsequent activation of NRAS [114, 115]. Drugs lonafarnib and Tipifarnib are farnesyltransferase inhibitors, which induce the apoptosis in melanoma cells [49, 51]. Recent research is targeting to treat the NRAS downstream signals. It has been shown that MEK inhibitors are potent in targeting NRAS mutants. Phase III trial of Binimetinib treatment in comparison to dacarbazine has shown improved survival and response in NRAS mutant melanomas [116]. Several clinical trials are ongoing phase to discover the feasibility of combination therapy of MEK inhibitors with PI3K, RAF along cell cycle inhibitors [115, 117–120].

A receptor tyrosine kinase, c-KIT binds to growth factors and trigger the MAP Kinase and PI3 Kinase pathways. c-KIT mutations are found in melanomas of different origins including mucosal, acral skin ones arising with CSD [54, 121].

c-KIT mutations have also been associated with worse survival [59]. Two C-KIT inhibitors, Imatinib and nilotinib, have been studied in melanoma. Imatinib has shown significant clinical response in tumors bearing c-KIT mutations and currently multiple phase -2 are ongoing [56, 122].

Immune checkpoint inhibitors have increasingly been used in melanoma therapy with significant number of immunotherapies approved for FDA for melanomas. Most of them work through the mechanism of augmenting host own anti-cancer immunity and thus clearing the cancer cells. Check point inhibitors, i.e. antibodies against T cell negative costimulatory molecules are major achievement in the area of melanoma in this decade. CTLA-4 antibodies (ipilimumab) and PD-1 antibodies (pembrolizumab, nivolumab) either alone or in combinations have shown effective against advanced stage melanoma ([99, 100, 123], and [101]). Treating with immunotherapy has shown significant potential. Tumor tissue specific expression of PD-L1 has been used as a predictive biomarker of treatment responsiveness against check point inhibitor of PD-1. Overexpression of PD-L1 has been reported in 45% of melanoma tumor samples and hence its expression is well associated with improved response rates to checkpoint therapy [124]. Therefore, identification of PD-L1 expression in tumors may serve as an effective first step in determining the best treatment option for the atient in personalized manner [125]. There is very limited amount of clinical data available regarding the expression of PD-1 and CTLA-4 on melanomas. As a conventional understanding, PD-1 expression has been studied well on immune cells, mainly on T cells to mount negative regulation or stopping T cell activation. PD-1 expression has been identified on melanoma cells. The PD-1 receptor has shown to promote growth of melanoma and also serve as biomarker for choice of therapy [126]. Parellel to PD-1 another negative costimulatory molecule known as CTLA-4 has also been found to be expressed on melanoma cells [127]. Again the expression of CTLA-4 serve as predictive biomarker for treatement in melanoma patients with check point inhibitor based therapies.

Nonmelanoma Skin Cancer (NMSC) type of cancers are of mild nature. Very limited data is available regarding their molecular mechanism. Molecular alterations are neither present nor uniform across all NMSCs. SCCs arise from a genetically predisposed clonal cell growth in contrast most of BCCs lack pre-existing genetic alterations. Genetic alterations accumulate and lead to pre-neoplastic lesions of Bowen disease (BD) or actinic keratosis (AK) and subsequently causes SCC [128]. These genetic alterations can cause multifocal development of SCCs too [129, 130]. Conventionally, several tumor suppressor genes and proto-oncogenes have been linked to BCC pathogenesis including the Sonic Hedgehog pathway (PTCH1 and SMO), the TP53 tumor suppressor gene, and RAS family members. Alterations associated with Sonic Hedgehog pathway have been shown to be associated with BCC carcinogenesis [131, 132]. SCCs carcinogenesis is also linked with several mutated genes [133]. Mutations of the tyrosine kinase receptors (epidermal growth factor receptor and fibroblast growth factor receptors) [134], cell cycle regulatory genes (TP53, CDKN2A/RB1, CCDN1, and MYC) [135, 136], RAS/MAPK and PI3K signaling pathways [134], genomic loci of squamous cell fate determination (TP63, SOX2, and NRF2) [137–139], and genes of squamous differentiation network (Notch and Fat1) [140, 141] have been implicated in SCC carcinogenesis. List of ongoing clinical trials are summarized in Table 7.2.

7.6   Epigenetic Biomarkers in Skin Cancers

Epigenetics also has significant contribution towards skin tumorigenesis and progression. Events such as alteration in promoter region methylation, histone related modification, and expression/alterations in various microRNAs are the major contributors towards tumerogenesis. Many of such epigenetic alterations have also served as biomarkers. Tumor biopsy as well as circulating DNA or circulating tumor cells can be used to explore such signatures and use them as biomarkers. Epigenetics based biomarkers have enormous potential to serve as biomarker in order to support

Table 7.2 List of molecular biomarkers based ongoing drug trials in skin cancers

Clinical trial	Trial phase	Biomarker	Therapies	Therapeutic context	Trail identifier
Open-label study, ASP-1929 with anti-PD1 in EGFR expressing solid tumors	1/2	EGFR expression positive	Cemiplimab, RM-1929	Advanced cutaneous squamous cell carcinoma	NCT04305795
SO-C101 and SO-with Pembro in adult patients in metastatic solid tumors	1	MSI-high/dMMR	Pembrolizumab, SO-C101	Solid tumor – metastatic	NCT04234113
MP0310 (AMG 506) in patients with advanced solid tumors	1	MSI-high/dMMR	MP0310	Solid tumor – metastatic	NCT04049903
LY3434172, a bispecific (PD-1 and PD-L1) antibody in advanced cancer	1	MSI-high/dMMR	LY3434172	Solid tumor – metastatic	NCT03936959
SL-279252 in advanced solid tumors or lymphomas	1	MSI-high/dMMR	SL-279252	Solid tumor - metastatic	NCT03894618
RP1 monotherapy and RP1 in combination with Nivolumab	1/2	MSI-high/dMMR	RP1, Nivolumab	Solid tumor - metastatic	NCT03767348
Combined therapy of Binimetinib and Encorafenib in adolescent melanoma patients (advanced tumors / or BRAF V600-mutant)	1	BRAF V600E BRAF V600K	Binimetinib, Encorafenib	Melanoma of unknown primary and squamous cell carcinoma	NCT03878719
Renal transplant patients with advance cancer treated with tacrolimus, Nivolumab, and Ipilimumab	1	MSI-high/dMMR	Prednisone, Ipilimumab, Nivolumab, tacrolimus	Metastatic solid tumor, basal cell carcinoma, melanoma, Merkel cell carcinoma, and squamous cell carcinoma	NCT03816332
CK-301 (Cosibelimab) as a single agent in advanced cancers	1	MSI-high/dMMR	Anti-PD-L1 monoclonal antibody CK-301	Hematological malignancies - relapse/ refractory therapy - non-cellular therapy, solid tumor -metastatic	NCT03212404
APL-501 in advanced, relapsed or recurrent solid tumors	1	MSI-high/dMMR and PD-L1 expression positive	Genolimzumab	Metastatic solid tumor	NCT03053466

overall patient management. Although several of them have been explored still, the clinical validation and their approval for clinical use is awaited.

Aberrant methylation in melanoma related gene can serve for early detection, progression, and as prognostic indicators in melanoma patients. A study has shown that RAS association domain family protein 1A (RASSF1A) inactivation is associated with melanoma [142]. RASSF1A impart pro-oncogenic properties such as migration, and metastasis [143]. Hypermethylation of RASSF1A has been shown to positively correlate with severity. Hence, RASSF1A may be a useful biomarker to track or predict melanoma progression [144]. Approximately 50% of Merkel cell carcinoma (MCC) cases were reported with promoter hypermethylation of RASSF1A gene [145].

In a detailed epistatic characterization study, methylation status of CpG islands in the promoter region of six tumor related genes involved in melanoma progression was studied along with a panel of methylated-in-tumor (MINT) non-coding genomic repeat sequences [144]. An increase in hypermethylation of tumor related genes was associated with increasing clinical tumor stage. Other studies specific to MINT loci have shown that there are hypermethylated CpG sites located in non-coding DNA regions exist in gastric system cancers [146, 147].

DNA hypomethylation lead to change in genetic make up through activation of endogenous retroviral elements, oncogene expression and overall chromosomal instability. An example for reactivation of genes is cancer testis genes, MAGE (melanoma antigen) family [148]. Aberrant expression of MAGE gene has been observed as secondary phenomenon to promoter hypomethylation [149]. Methylation of repetitive sequences and long interspersed nuclear element-1 (LINE-1) also represent the overall methylation status [150]. A study verified the LINE-1 methylation can be use as molecular marker of prognosis with stage IIIC melanoma patients showing LINE-1 hypomethylation with significant overall survival (OS) compared to those with hypermethylated LINE-1 [151].

DNMT3A and DNMT3B have been implicated in de novo methylation generation in previously unmethylated CpGs [151]. Unmethylation based alteration in expression has clinical significance. Expression level of these proteins significantly correlated stage of melanoma. Higher the expression of DNMT3B lower was the Over all survival specifically in advanced stage III melanoma patients suggesting that DNMT3 can be a potential biomarker for melanoma progression [152]. This data substantiates its use as drug target for therapy. DNMT inhibitors have been investigated in clinical trials, mainly small molecule based one with 5-aza-2′-deoxycytidine (decitabine) being one of them [143] with limited efficacy and high toxicity being reported at pre-clinical studies stage.

Further, the generalized demethylating agents are not the preferable treatment choices being able to cause global hypomethylation and activation of tumor proto-oncogenes [148]. Temozolomide (TMZ) which is a cancer chemodrug also downregulates the expression of DNA repair enzyme, known as methylguanine methyltransferase (MGMT). Its sensitivity has been correlated with methylation of the MGMT promoter [153]. In a clinical study chronic TMZ treatment in metastatic melanoma patients was assessed in conjunction with MGMT promoter methylation status. Extent of MGMT promoter methylation positively correlated with partial clinical response [153].

Clinical usage of various signature of histone modification such as methylation, acetylation, phosphorylation, sumoylation, uquitinylation as biomarkers are still ned to evolve till it reaches to clinics. Histone modifications based signatures may be potential genetics based biomarkers given that good clinical validation can be done for them [154–156]. Histone changes in malignant melanoma have been linked through the ability of cancer cells to escape the senescent phenotype. Uncontrolled cancer cell proliferation in melanoma has been shown to be correlated with level of expression of histone modifying enzymes [151, 157].

Enhancer of zeste homolog 2 (EZH2) is a histone-lysine N-methyltransferase enzyme, that participates in histone methylation and act as transcriptional repression. EZH2 expression level has been correlated with thicker primary melanomas occurrence. EZH2 have been associated with loss of p16 expression and high expression of Cyclin D1 [158]. In survival analysis, 5-year survival were observed in 48% of patients with high EZH2 expression where 71% among the patients with low EZH2 expression. EZH2 has been also implicated in downregulating the expression of tumor suppressor Rap1GAP [159] and p21 in melanoma [160].

Clinical usage of histone based biomarkers in melanoma is still not available. One of the major practical challenge towards it is lack of a cost effective and less turn around time based assays. Mass spectrometry have shown some ray of hope as compared to conventional genetics based techniques still being a multiste process and lab to lab variations makes it difficult to extrapolate to clinical applications. Research regarding epigenetic mechanism has attracted limited attention in past although, it is picking up with more technological advancements and availability of cost effective methodologies.

Epigenetic biomarkers in other skin cancers are limited. Summary of methylation studies in NMSCs are listed in Table 7.3. BCC and SCC represent the majority of skin cancer cases of NMSCs. Both of them are less aggressive than melanoma. NMSCs are well treated by surgical interventions and have good success rate. Limited epistatic signature based data sets are available for these skin cancer types.

Fragile histidine triad protein (FHIT) is an enzyme, encoded by the FHIT gene. FHIT promoter is methylation in BCC [174], Further, methylation of PTCH gene in BCC has shown to likely play a minor role in carcinogenesis [175]. Repression of BCL7a, PTPRG, TP73, and FAS through methylation has been observed in skin cancers with limited prevalence [149, 178, 179]. Less than half of the MCC patients has been observed with methylation in tumor suppressor gene p14 [180].

7.7   miRNAs as Biomarkers in Skin Cancer

MicroRNAs (miRNAs) are a noncoding RNA of small size involved in post-transcriptional regulation of gene expression through messenger RNA (mRNA) transcripts by base pairing with them and not allowing them to further translate in to proteins [181]. These miRNAs deregulations may trigger many disorders

Table 7.3 Methylation studies of NMSCs

Target Gene	Methylation status	Function alteration	References
SCC			
CDKN2A	Hypermethylated	Cell cycle deregulation	Brown et al. [161]
CDH1 and CDH13	Hypermethylated	Cellular environment deregulation	Takeuchi et al. [162], Chiles et al. [163], Murao et al. [164]
FOXE1, SFRPs and FRZB	Hypermethylated	Modulator of Wnt signaling	Liang et al. [165], Venza et al. [166], Darr et al. [167]
ASC, G0S2, miRNA-204 and DAPK1	Hypermethylated	Deregulation of apoptosis	Meier et al. [168], Li et al. [169], Toll et al. [170], Nobeyama et al. [171]
DSS1	Hypomethylation	Deregulated post translational protein modification	Venza et al. [172]
Global DNA	Hypomethylation	Restricted genomic silencing in benign SCC	Hervás-Marín et al. [173]
Global DNA	Hypermethylated	Extensive genomic silencing in aggressive SCC	Hervás-Marín et al. [173]
BCC			
FHIT promoter	Hypomethylation	DNA damage	Goldberg et al. [174]
PTCH promoter	Hypermethylated	Deactivation of tumor suppressor genes	Heitzer et al. [175]
MYCL2	Hypomethylated	Proto-oncogene activation	Darr et al. [167]
MCC			
p14-ARK, DUSP2, CDKN2A promoter	Hypermethylated	Tumor suppressor genes get deactivated	Greenberg et al. [176], Harms et al. [177]

[182, 183]. miRNAs can serve as potential therapeutic targets as well diagnostic and/or prognostic biomarkers [184, 185].

Alterations in the miRNA-processing enzyme DICER have been identified [186]. miRNAs interact with microphthalmia-associated transcription factor in melanocytes [187]. There are more than 800 miRNAs reported in cells and their expression has been shown to fluctuate during tumorigenesis stages. In melanoma, miR-21, miR-125b, miR-150, miR-155, miR-205, and miR-211 miRNAs were shown to have prognostic value. It led to exploration of targeted therapy [188]. miRNA capable of causing dysregulation in essential pathways involved in melanoma tumourogenesis such as RAS/MAPK pathway, the MITF pathway,

PI3K-AKT pathway. Such events may offer miRNA based diagnosis, prognosis, and molecular targeted therapy [189, 190].

7.8 miRNA in Tissues of Melanoma

Within the tumor mocroenvironment of melanomas, miR-221 and miR-222 were found to be abnormally expressed with capability of downregulating c-KIT receptor and p27Kip expression, respectively [191]. Further, miR-205 downregulation is correlated with lower survival in melanoma patients. Based on such effects, miR-205 is considered as "tumor suppressor miRNA" in melanoma [192]. A reduced expression of miR-29c was also correlated with metastatic melanoma. miR-29c expression level has shown to be strongly linked with the overall survival of melanoma patients [152]. miR-10b has been shown to increased in primary melanoma tissues, and metastatic sites as well. Coexpression of multiple miRNAs has also been explored as biomarker. miR-10b along with miR-200b has prognostic value for aggressive melanomas [193]. Another micro-RNA, miR-203 expression was found to be associated with tumor thickness, stage, and reduced overall survival [194].

It has been demonstrated that miR-155 induce tyrosinase-related protein 1 (TYRP1) mRNA degradation in metastatic tissues of melanoma, TYRP1 mRNA inversely correlated with miR-155 expression [195]. Another study has shown a new target, a protein kinase WEE1 against miRNA155 in link to metastasis [196].

Metatherian (MTDH) is a type-two transmembrane protein containing an extracellular lung homing domain. It is the direct target of miR-675, therefore, miR-675 can be further developed as a potential therapeutic target [197]. miR-135b with target gene, tumor suppressor kinase 2 (LATS2) has altered expression in melanoma cell lines. This molecular phenomenon involved in LATS2 mediated pro-oncogenic effects needs to be deciphered [198]. Panels of tissue miRNAs have also been used as strategy to define more sensitive biomarker. A set of four miRNAs including miR-125b, miR-182, miR-200c which were under expressed, and miR-205 with over expression, has been correlated with shorter survival. Such panel of defined miRNAs can be useful for identifying high-risk patients [199]. Another panel including miR-10b, miR-16, and miR-21 in melanoma was associated with poor prognosis. These studies are suggesting the need of detailed characterization of several miRNAs and establish their prognostic potential [200].

A microarray study of melanoma tissue and peritumoral region has revealed more than 140 differentially expressed miRNAs. Highest over expression was observed for hsa-miR-146a-5p. It can target almost 40 genes [201]. Upon cross validation of the array data, five miRNAs (miR-142-5p, miR-150-5p, miR-342-3p, miR-155-5p, and miR-146b-5p) showed reproducible results with clinical patient prognosis [202].

7.9   Circulating miRNAs in Melanoma

Taking tissue biopsy can enhance the morbidity risks in an invasive procedure [203], failure rate in small tumors [204]. This procedure may relatively expensive and limit the availability of accessible sample. miRNA circulating in peripheral blood can avoid the need of tissue biopsy. Circulating miRNA based assays hence have an advantage in the clinical setting. Moreover, circulating miRNA also shows better stability over tissue derived biomarkers [205, 206] so it provides advantages over tissue biopsy for monitoring the changes in miRNA expression throughout a patient's treatment. [207], demonstrated the potential as a non-invasive detection biomarker and its capability in differentiating between in situ and invasive melanoma using miR-221 expression in the serum from 90 melanoma patients along with eight postoperative recurrence sera. This miRNA identification in circulation has also confirmed the prior miR-221/222 identification in melanoma tissue [191]. A study screen out three circulating miRNA miR-199a-5p, miR-33a, and miR-424 of prognostic value in melanoma with ability to differentiate between the recurrence-risk levels among patients [208]. miR-16 circulating levels in melanoma patients correlated with tumor thickness, ulceration, stage, proliferation potential along with predicting patients' survival [209, 210]. Low level of miR-206 predicted melanoma metastasis and a significantly shorter overall survival [211].

Peripheral blood based markers including circulating tumor cells (CTCs), cell-free circulating tumor DNA (ctDNA), and circulating miRNAs (cmiRNA) in combination can provide a wide range of information about stages III and IV melanoma patients along with proposing individualized therapy. In this regard massive parallel sequencing (MPS) can be molecular assays to predict powerful biomarkers [212]. Aberrant activation of circulating miRNA, let-7a and b, miR-148, miR-155, miR-182, miR-200c, miR-211, miR-214, miR-221, and miR-222 were found to linked with melanoma associated molecular changes in genes NRAS, microphthalmia-associated transcription factor, receptor tyrosine kinase c-KIT, and AP-2 transcription factor. It can be aid of potential biomarkers and may provide potential target for targeted therapy [213].

Panel of several miRNA based biomarkers present in serum have shown better prognosis than other biochemichal markers such as lactate dehydrogenase (LDH) and S100B. These panels in combination can well predict progression, recurrence, and survival and early relapse [210]. Although more standardization and clinical validation is required to establish them in clinics [214].

7.10   miRNA Differentiating Melanoma from Non-Melanoma Skin Cancers

Discrimination between non-melanoma skin cancers and melanoma site serve as comparative controls in clinical settings. One such comparative study found upregulation of miR-21 and miR-155 which was found associated cell division and tissue thickness at tumor site [215]. In another study, miR-21 was found to increase from dysplastic nevi to melanomas. The expression levels were also found to correlate with Breslow index, clinical stage, and shorter overall survival [216]. miRNA miR-15b expressed differentiallyin malignant versus benign melanocytes [217]. Xu et al. [218] found an improved three miRNAs panels (miR-200c, miR-205, and miR-211) in differentiating between primary and metastatic melanomas. Further, miR-106b over expression was found to be correlated with Breslow index which is an index of that how much the melanoma has invaded the host [219].

7.11   miRNA Profile in Therapy Resistant Melanoma

Treatment resistance is a common phenomenon associated with almost all the therapies being offered to melanoma patients. Having biomarkers to predict evolution of treatment resistance, opting best therapeutic options, etc. is badly needed for clinical management of the patients. Comparing profiles of resistant vs responsive tumors can provide lead in this direction. Some such studies are available including miRNAs (miR-92a-1-5p, miR-708-5p) and genes (*DOK5* and *PCSK2*). Drug resistance in melanoma may involve a set of miRNAs that regulate particular genes and ultimately causes drug resistance [220]. BRAF/MEK inhibitors resistant melanoma cell lines expresses low miR-579-3p [221]. Involvement of miRNAs in the chemoresistance in melanoma cells is also reported. Low levels of miR-211 have been shown in chemoresistance cancer cells and found to be linked DNA hypermethylation in tumor tissues. Reversing the DNA hypermethylation increases miR-211 levels and makes cancer cells chemosensitive [222]. Resistance to MAK inhibitors has been linked with miR-214. The over expression of miR-214 has been related pro-tumorigenic characteristics including cancer cell division, migration and decreases sensitivity towards MAPK inhibitor therapies [223].

7.12   miRNAs as Predictor of Therapeutic Efficacy

If well validated biomarkers will be available forpredicting theraputic efficacy it will allow not only save the patients for side effects but will end up having appropriate cost effective therapy for them. Several miRNAs have been explored for this objective under various clinical studies. Panels of miRNAs have been related to MDSCs induction making the local tumor microenvironment highly immunosuppressive along with development of checkpoint inhibitor therapy resistance. These miRNAs were also found increased in blood CD14+ cells and in tumor tissues, and correlated with MDSC infiltrates. These finding established the rationale to test miRNAs in circulating MDSCs as a specific lineage for therapy efficacy [224]. miRNA profiling of melanoma patients at baseline and during resistant state under BRAF and MEK inhibitors therapies led to identification miR-126-3p expression [225]. Exploration and validation of such miRNAs either alone or in combination can provide help in patient stratification and other clinical benefits.

7.13   miRNAs Status in Non-Melanoma Skin Cancers

The miR-205 has been associated with desmoplasia, perineural invasion, and infiltrative pattern. The miR-203 shows tissue characteristics for favorable prognosis in SCC [226]. In CSCC samples miR-221 targeting *PTEN* gene. Anti-miR-221 based therapeutic approaches have been tested in SCC treatment [227]. A bunch of miRNAs with oncogenic functions and miRNAs as tumor suppressors are implicated in SCC. They regulate pro-oncogenic traits including cell cycle dysregulation/excessive cell division, epithelial–mesenchymal transition for metastasis, and stem cell formation [228]. Cutaneous T cell lymphoma (CTCL) progression has been characterized by aberrant miRNAs, therefore miRNA guided therapy would be an opportunity [229]. Mycosis fungoides (MF) is one of the most common type of CTCL with around 30% of patients with aggressive form of disease [230]. Reference [231] characterized in detail the miRNAs, DICER, and DROSHA, in such patients. Decrease in DROSHA expression turned out as independent predictor of advanced stages. Further, a panel of three-miRNA comprising miR-106b-5p, miR-148a-3p, and miR-338-3p, correlated with clinical progression. This panel could also discriminate between patients based on the risk levels [232]. Merkel cells that reside in the basal epithelial layer are subjected to malignant transformation, probably induced by Merkel cell polyomavirus infection.

Merkel cell polyomavirus infection in basal layer cells leads to malignant transformation and was found in 90% of MCC [233]. Early metastasis and recurrence are key characteristic of them. Atonal homolog 1 (*ATOH1*) expression, which is a tumor suppressor gene, has been implicated in disease pathogenesis hence, therapeutic strategy using antisense oligonucleotides or miRNAs are tested preclinically [234]. *ATOH1* null cell lines reduced miR-375 expression leading to the loss of metastatic potential. Such promising approach can be further developed as target therapy for MCC [235].

7.14   Biophysical Biomarkers in Skin Cancer

Raman spectroscopy (RS) can be a useful tool for clinical diagnosis of skin cancer by discovery of newer biomolecules which can serve as biomarker or drug targets. RS is highly sensitive method and it can well discriminate between malignant melanoma and benign pigmented lesion [236–238]. Malignant melanoma can be discriminated from pigmented lesions with 100% sensitivity and specificity [239, 240]. [241] demonstrated the ability of RS method towards analyzing the biochemical composition of skin cancers. These findings can be extrapolated to develop biomarkers. Major biomolecules identified in this exercise are collagen and triolein. RS method successfully detects and differentiates the various forms of skin cancers among themselves as well as from normal skin tissue [242]. RS has high molecular specificity without doing invasive process it can provide precise result with sample preparation requirement [243].

7.15   Conclusions

There is urgent need of early diagnosis, relevant biomarkers, targeted therapies, resistance, and responsiveness predictors for skin cancers being one of the aggressive forms of cancers. Molecular profiling for identification of novel biomarkers and their clinical validation is need of the time. The molecular events associated with complex processes of oncogenesis include genetic alterations, epigenetic changes; miRNAs are gaining increased importance recently. These molecular biomarkers could be important for diagnosis/prognosis, therapy monitoring, and targeted therapy. Overcoming to some issues regarding sensitivity and specificity of molecular biomarkers, for example, determining circulating miRNAs, we will be able to make it robust. In addition, emerging molecular assay to determine the biomarkers could overcome these bottlenecks. Overall research for hunting biomarkers has adopting approach with acceptable sensitivity and specific so that they can be translated in clinics with confidence.

References

1. Bray F, Ferlay J, Soerjomataram I, Siegel RL, Torre LA, Jemal A (2018) Global cancer statistics 2018: GLOBOCAN estimates of incidence and mortality worldwide for 36 cancers in 185 countries. CA Cancer J Clin 68(6):394–424
2. Armstrong BK, Kricker A (1995) Skin cancer. Dermatol Clin 13:583–594
3. Gloster HM Jr, Brodland DG (1996) The epidemiology of skin cancer. Dermatol Surg 22:217–226
4. Hall HI, Miller DR, Rogers JD, Bewerse B (1999) Update on the incidence and mortality from melanoma in the United States. J Am Acad Dermatol 40:35–42
5. Brenner M, Hearing VJ (2008) The protective role of melanin against UV damage in human skin. Photochem Photobiol 84(3):539–549
6. Gandini S, Sera F, Catarzzuzza MS, Pasquini P, Abeni D, Boyle P, Melchi CF (2005) Meta-analysis of risk factors for cutaneous melanoma: I.Common and atypical naevi. Eur J Cancer 41:28–44
7. Wheless L, Ruczinski I, Alani RM et al (2009) The association between skin characteristics and skin cancer prevention behaviors. Cancer Epidemiol Biomark Prev 18(10):2613–2619
8. Kollias N, Sayre RM, Zeise L, Chedekel MR (1991) Photoprotection by melanin. J Photochem Photobiol B 9:135–160
9. Halder RM, Bang KM (1988) Skin cancer in blacks in the United States. Dermatol Clin 6:397–405
10. Kaidbey KH, Agin PP, Sayre RM, Kligman AM (1979) Photoprotection by melanin--a comparison of black and Caucasian skin. J Am Acad Dermatol 1:249–260
11. Armstrong BK, Kricker A (2001) The epidemiology of UV induced skin cancer. J Photochem Photobiol B 63:8–18
12. Kennedy C, Jter H, Berkhout M, Gruis N, Bastiaens M, Bergman W, Willemze R, Bavinck JN (2001) Melanocortin 1 receptor (MC1R) gene variants are associated with an increased risk for cutaneous melanoma which is largely independent of skin type and hair color. J Invest Dermatol 117:294–300
13. Scott MC, Wakamatsu K, Ito S, Kadekaro AL, Kobayashi N, Groden J, Kavanagh R, Takakuwa T, Virador V, Hearing VJ, Abdel-Malek ZA (2002) Human melanocortin 1 receptor variants, receptor function and melanocyte response to UV radiation. J Cell Sci 115:2349–2355

14. Cui R, Widlund HR, Feige E, Lin JY, Wilensky DL, Igras VE, D'Orazio J, Fung CY, Schanbacher CF, Granter SR, Fisher DE (2007) Central role of p53 in the suntan response and pathologic hyperpigmentation. Cell 128:853–864

15. Krude H, Biebermann H, Luck W, Horn R, Brabant G, Gruters A (1998) Severe early-onset obesity, adrenal insufficiency and red hair pigmentation caused by POMC mutations in humans. Nat Genet 19:155–157

16. Wenczl E, Van der Schans GP, Roza L, Kolb RM, Timmerman AJ, Smit NP, Pavel S, Schothorst AA (1998) (Pheo)melanin photosensitizes UVA-induced DNA damage in cultured human melanocytes. J Invest Dermatol 111:678–682

17. Hill HZ, Hill GJ (2000) UVA, pheomelanin and the carcinogenesis of melanoma. Pigment Cell Res 13:140–144

18. Dawes JM, Antunes-Martins A, Perkins JR, Paterson KJ, Sisignano M, Schmid R, Rust W, Hildebrandt T, Geisslinger G, Orengo C, Bennett DL, McMahon SB (2014) Genome-wide transcriptional profiling of skin and dorsal root ganglia after ultraviolet-B-induced inflammation. PLoS One 9(4):e93338

19. Cassarino DS, Lewine N, Cole D, Wade B, Gustavsen G (2014) BudgetImpactAnalysisofaNovelGene expression assay for the diagnosis of malignant melanoma. J Med Econ 17:782–791

20. Berger AC, Davidson RS, Poitras JK, Chabra I, Hope R, Brackeen A, Johnson CE, Maetzold DJ, Middlebrook B, Oelschlager KM et al (2016) Clinical impact of a 31-gene expression profile test for cutaneous melanoma in 156 prospectively and consecutively tested patients. Curr Med Res Opin 32:1599–1604

21. Hayward NK, Wilmott JS, Waddell N, Johansson PA, Field MA, Nones K, Patch AM, Kakavand H, Alexandrov LB, Burke H et al (2017) Whole-genome landscapes of major melanoma subtypes. Nature 545:175–180

22. Premi S, Han L, Mehta S, Knight J, Zhao D, Palmatier MA, Kornacker K, Brash DE (2019) Genomic sites hypersensitive to ultraviolet radiation. Proc Natl Acad Sci U S A 116 (48):24196–24205

23. Ferris LK, Jansen B, Ho J, Busam KJ, Gross K, Hansen DD, Alsobrook JP 2nd, Yao Z, Peck GL, Gerami P (2017) Utility of a noninvasive 2-gene molecular assay for cutaneous melanoma and Effect on the decision to biopsy. JAMA Dermatol 153:675–680

24. Lee JJ, Lian CG (2019) Molecular testing for cutaneous melanoma: an update and review. Arch Pathol Lab Med 143:811–820

25. Blanchard DA, Mouhamad S, Auredou M-T, Pesty A, Bertoglio J, Leca G, Vazquez A (2000) Cdk2 associates with MAP kinase in vivo and its nuclear translocation is dependent on MAP kinase activation in Il-2-dependent kit 225 T lymphocytes. Oncogene 19:4184–4189

26. Raman M, Chen W, Cobb MH (2007) Differential regulation and properties of Mapks. Oncogene 26:3100–3112

27. Dent P, Haser W, Haystead TA, Vincent LA, Roberts TM, Sturgill TW (1992) Activation of mitogen-activated protein kinase by V-Raf in Nih 3t3 cells and in vitro. Science 257:1404–1407

28. Burotto M, Chiou VL, Lee J-M, Kohn EC (2014) The Mapk pathway across different malignancies: a new perspective. Cancer 120:3446–3456

29. Leonardi GC, Falzone L, Salemi R, Zanghì A, Spandidos DA, McCubrey JA, Candido S, Libra M (2018) Cutaneous melanoma: From pathogenesis to therapy (review). Int J Oncol 52:1071–1080

30. Yuan TL, Cantley LC (2008) PI3K pathway alterations in Cancer: variations on a theme. Oncogene 27:5497–5510

31. Rodriguez-Viciana P, Warne PH, Dhand R, Vanhaesebroeck B, Gout I, Fry MJ, Waterfield MD, Downward J (1994) Phosphatidylinositol-3-OH kinase as a direct target of Ras. Nature 370:527–532

32. De Luca A, Maiello MR, D'Alessio A, Pergameno M, Normanno N (2012) The RAS/RAF/ MEK/ERK and the PI3K/AKT signalling pathways: role in cancer pathogenesis and implications for therapeutic approaches. Expert Opin Ther Targets 16(Suppl 2):S17–S27

33. Mayo LD, Donner DB (2001) A phosphatidylinositol 3-kinase/AKT pathway promotes translocation of MDM2 from the cytoplasm to the nucleus. Proc Natl Acad Sci U S A 98:11598–11603

34. Landis CA, Masters SB, Spada A, Pace AM, Bourne HR, Vallar L (1989) GTPase inhibiting mutations activate the alpha chain of Gs and stimulate adenylyl cyclase in human pituitary Tumours. Nature 340:692–696

35. Kalinec G, Nazarali AJ, Hermouet S, Xu N, Gutkind JS (1992) Mutated alpha subunit of the Gq protein induces malignant transformation in NIH 3T3 cells. Mol Cell Biol 12:4687–4693

36. Amaro A, Gangemi R, Piaggio F, Angelini G, Barisione G, Ferrini S, Pfeffer U (2017) The biology of uveal melanoma. Cancer Metastasis Rev 36:109–140

37. George NM, Day CE, Boerner BP, Johnson RL, Sarvetnick NE (2012) Hippo signaling regulates pancreas development through inactivation of yap. Mol Cell Biol 32:5116–5128

38. Griewank KG, Schilling B, Scholz SL, Metz CH, Livingstone E, Sucker A, Moller I, Reis H, Franklin C, Cosgarea I et al (2016) Oncogene status as a diagnostic tool in ocular and cutaneous melanoma. Eur J Cancer 57:112–117

39. Yu FX, Luo J, Mo JS, Liu G, Kim YC, Meng Z, Zhao L, Peyman G, Ouyang H, Jiang W et al (2014) Mutant Gq/11 promote uveal melanoma tumorigenesis by activating YAP. Cancer Cell 25:822–830

40. Field MG, Durante MA, Anbunathan H, Cai LZ, Decatur CL, Bowcock AM, Kurtenbach S, Harbour JW (2018) Punctuated evolution of canonical genomic aberrations in uveal melanoma. Nat Commun 9:116

41. Jager MJ, Shields CL, Cebulla CM, Abdel-Rahman MH, Grossniklaus HE, Stern M-H, Carvajal RD, Belfort RN, Jia R, Shields JA et al (2020) Uveal melanoma. Nat Rev Dis Prim 6:24

42. Davies H, Bignell GR, Cox C, Stephens P, Edkins S, Clegg S, Teague J, Woendin H, Garnett MJ, Bottomley W et al (2002) Mutations of the Braf gene in human cancer. Nature 417:949–954

43. Hauschild A, Grob JJ, Demidov LV, Jouary T, Gutzmer R, Millward M, Rutkowski P, Blank CU, Miller WH Jr, Kaempgen E et al (2012) Dabrafenib in Braf-mutated metastatic melanoma: a multicentre, open-label, phase 3 randomised controlled trial. Lancet 380:358–365

44. Pracht M, Mogha A, Lespagnol A, Fautrel A, Mouchet N, Le Gall F, Paumier V, Lefeuvre-Plesse C, Rioux-Leclerc N, Mosser J et al (2015) Prognostic and predictive values of oncogenic BRAF, NRAS, C-KIT and MITF in cutaneous and mucous melanoma. J Eur Acad Dermatol Venereol 29:1530–1538

45. Melis C, Rogiers A, Bechter O, van den Oord JJ (2017) Molecular genetic and immunotherapeutic targets in metastatic melanoma. Virchows Arch 471:281–293

46. Dummer R, Ascierto PA, Gogas HJ, Arance A, Mandala M, Liszkay G, Garbe C, Schadendorf D, Krajsova I, Gutzmer R et al (2018) Encorafenib plus Binimetinib versus Vemurafenib or Encorafenib in patients with Braf-mutant melanoma (Columbus): a multicentre, open-label, randomised phase 3 trial. Lancet Oncol 19:603–615

47. Sarkisian S, Davar D (2018) Mek inhibitors for the treatment of NRAS mutant melanoma. Drug Des Dev Ther 12:2553–2565

48. Abd Elmageed ZY, Moore RF, Tsumagari K, Lee MM, Sholl AB, Friedlander P, Al-Qurayshi Z, Hassan M, Wang AR, Boulares HA et al (2018) Prognostic role of Braf (V600e) cellular localization in melanoma. J Am Coll Surg 226:526–537

49. Smalley KSM, Eisen TG (2003) Farnesyl transferase inhibitor Sch66336 is cytostatic, pro-apoptotic and enhances Chemosensitivity to cisplatin in melanoma cells. Int J Cancer 105:165–175

50. Lee JH, Choi JW, Kim YS (2011) Frequencies of BRAF and NRAS mutations are different in histological types and sites of origin of cutaneous melanoma: a meta-analysis. Br J Dermatol 164:776–784
51. Niessner H, Beck D, Sinnberg T, Lasithiotakis K, Maczey E, Gogel J, Venturelli S, Berger A, Mauthe M, Toulany M et al (2011) The farnesyl transferase inhibitor Lonafarnib inhibits MTOR signaling and enforces Sorafenib-induced apoptosis in melanoma cells. J Investig Dermatol 131:468–479
52. Hodis E, Watson IR, Kryukov GV, Arold ST, Imielinski M, Theurillat JP, Nickerson E, Auclair D, Li L, Place C et al (2012) A landscape of driver mutations in melanoma. Cell 150:251–263
53. Jakob JA, Bassett RL Jr, Ng CS, Curry JL, Joseph RW, Alvarado GC, Rohlfs ML, Richard J, Gershenwald JE, Kim KB et al (2012) NRAS mutation status is an independent prognostic factor in metastatic melanoma. Cancer 118:4014–4023
54. Curtin JA, Busam K, Pinkel D, Bastian BC (2006) Somatic activation of KIT in distinct subtypes of melanoma. J Clin Oncol 24:4340–4346
55. Beadling C, Jacobson-Dunlop E, Hodi FS, Le C, Warrick A, Patterson J, Town A, Harlow A, Cruz F 3rd, Azar S et al (2008) KIT gene mutations and copy number in melanoma subtypes. Clin Cancer Res 14:6821–6828
56. Carvajal RD, Antonescu CR, Wolchok JD, Chapman PB, Roman R-A, Teitcher J, Panageas KS, Busam KJ, Chmielowski B, Lutzky J et al (2011) KIT as a therapeutic target in metastatic melanoma. JAMA 305:2327–2334
57. Carvajal RD, Lawrence DP, Weber JS, Gajewski TF, Gonzalez R, Lutzky J, O'Day SJ, Hamid O, Wolchok JD, Chapman PB et al (2015) Phase II study of Nilotinib in melanoma harboring KIT alterations following progression to prior KIT inhibition. Clin Cancer Res 21:2289–2296
58. Guo J, Carvajal RD, Dummer R, Hauschild A, Daud A, Bastian BC, Markovic SN, Queirolo P, Arance A, Berking C et al (2017) Efficacy and safety of Nilotinib in patients with KIT-mutated metastatic or inoperable melanoma: final results from the global, single-arm Phase II TEAM. Trial Ann Oncol 28:1380–1387
59. Ma X, Wu Y, Zhang T, Song H, Jv H, Guo W, Ren G (2017) The clinical significance of C-KIT mutations in metastatic Oral mucosal melanoma in China. Oncotarget 8:82661–82673
60. Serrano M, Hannon GJ, Beach D (1993) A new regulatory motif in cell-cycle control causing specific inhibition of cyclin D/CDK4. Nature 366:704–707
61. Zhang Y, Xiong Y, Yarbrough WG (1998) ARF promotes MDM2 degradation and stabilizes P53: ARF-INK4A locus deletion impairs both the Rb and P53 tumor suppression pathways. Cell 92:725–734
62. Florell SR, Meyer LJ, Boucher KM, Porter-Gill PA, Hart M, Erickson J, Cannon-Albright LA, Pershing LK, Harris RM, Samlowski WE et al (2004) Longitudinal assessment of the nevus phenotype in a melanoma kindred. J Investig Dermatol 123:576–582
63. Burdette-Radoux S, Tozer RG, Lohmann RC, Quirt I, Ernst DS, Walsh W, Wainman N, Colevas AD, Eisenhauer EA (2004) Phase II trial of Flavopiridol, a cyclin dependent kinase inhibitor, in untreated metastatic malignant melanoma. Investig New Drugs 22:315–322
64. Goldstein AM, Chan M, Harland M, Hayward NK, Demenais F, Timothy Bishop D, Azizi E, Bergman W, Bianchi-Scarra G, Bruno W et al (2007) Features associated with germline CDKN2A mutations: a Genomel study of melanoma-prone families from three continents. J Med Genet 44:99–106
65. Aoude LG, Wadt KAW, Pritchard AL, Hayward NK (2015) Genetics of familial melanoma: 20 years after CDKN2A. Pigment Cell Melanoma Res 28:148–160
66. Soura E, Eliades PJ, Shannon K, Stratigos AJ, Tsao H (2016) Hereditary melanoma: update on syndromes and management: genetics of familial atypical multiple mole melanoma syndrome. J Am Acad Dermatol 74:395–410

67. Baker AR, McDonnell DP, Hughes M, Crisp TM, Mangelsdorf DJ, Haussler MR, Pike JW, Shine J, O'Malley BW (1988) Cloning and expression of full-length CDNA encoding human vitamin D receptor. Proc Natl Acad Sci U S A 85:3294–3298
68. Demay MB, Kiernan MS, DeLuca HF, Kronenberg HM (1992) Sequences in the human parathyroid hormone gene that bind the 1,25-Dihydroxyvitamin D3 receptor and mediate transcriptional repression in response to 1,25-Dihydroxyvitamin D3. Proc Natl Acad Sci U S A 89:8097–8101
69. Colnot S, Lambert M, Blin C, Thomasset M, Perret C (1995) Identification of DNA sequences that bind retinoid X Receptor-1,25(oh)2d3-receptor heterodimers with high affinity. Mol Cell Endocrinol 113:89–98
70. Brozyna AA, Jozwicki W, Janjetovic Z, Slominski AT (2011) Expression of vitamin D receptor decreases during progression of pigmented skin lesions. Hum Pathol 42:618–631
71. Brozyna AA, Józwicki W, Slominski AT (2014) Decreased VDR expression in cutaneous melanomas as marker of tumor progression: new data and analyses. Anticancer Res 34:2735–2743
72. Saw RPM, Armstrong BK, Mason RS, Morton RL, Shannon KF, Spillane AJ, Stretch JR, Thompson JF (2014) Adjuvant therapy with high dose vitamin d following primary treatment of melanoma at high risk of recurrence: a placebo controlled randomised phase II trial (Anzmtg 02.09 Mel-D). BMC Cancer 14:780
73. De Smedt J, Van Kelst S, Boecxstaens V, Stas M, Bogaerts K, Vanderschueren D, Aura C, Vandenberghe K, Lambrechts D, Wolter P et al (2017) Vitamin D supplementation in cutaneous malignant melanoma outcome (Vidme): a randomized controlled trial. BMC Cancer 17:562
74. Fargnoli MC, Gandini S, Peris K, Maisonneuve P, Raimondi S (2010) MC1R variants increase melanoma risk in families with CDKN2A mutations: a meta-analysis. Eur J Cancer 46:1413–1420
75. Tagliabue E, Gandini S, Bellocco R, Maisonneuve P, Newton-Bishop J, Polsky D, Lazovich D, Kanetsky PA, Ghiorzo P, Gruis NA et al (2018) Mc1r variants as melanoma risk factors independent of at-risk phenotypic characteristics: a pooled analysis from the M-skip project. Cancer Manag Res 10:1143–1154
76. Raimondi S, Sera F, Gandini S, Iodice S, Caini S, Maisonneuve P, Fargnoli MC (2008) MC1R variants, melanoma and red hair color phenotype: a meta-analysis. Int J Cancer 122:2753–2760
77. Price ER, Horstmann MA, Wells AG, Weilbaecher KN, Takemoto CM, Landis MW, Fisher DE (1998) Alpha-melanocyte-stimulating hormone signaling regulates expression of Microphthalmia, a gene deficient in Waardenburg syndrome. J Biol Chem 273:33042–33047
78. Bertolotto C, Abbe P, Hemesath TJ, Bille K, Fisher DE, Ortonne JP, Ballotti R (1998) Microphthalmia gene product as a signal transducer in camp-induced differentiation of melanocytes. J Cell Biol 142:827–835
79. King R, Googe PB, Weilbaecher KN, Mihm MC Jr, Fisher DE (2001) Microphthalmia transcription factor expression in cutaneous benign, malignant melanocytic, and nonmelanocytic tumors. Am J Surg Pathol 25:51–57
80. Levy C, Khaled M, Fisher DE (2006) MITF: master regulator of melanocyte development and melanoma oncogene. Trends Mol Med 12:406–414
81. Yokoyama S, Woods SL, Boyle GM, Aoude LG, MacGregor S, Zismann V, Gartside M, Cust AE, Haq R, Harland M et al (2011) A novel recurrent mutation in MITF predisposes to familial and sporadic melanoma. Nature 480:99–103
82. Naffouje S, Naffouje R, Bhagwandin S, Salti GI (2015) Microphthalmia transcription factor in malignant melanoma predicts occult sentinel lymph node metastases and survival. Melanoma Res 25:496–502
83. Van Raamsdonk CD, Griewank KG, Crosby MB, Garrido MC, Vemula S, Wiesner T, Obenauf AC, Wackernagel W, Green G, Bouvier N et al (2010) Mutations in GNA11 in uveal melanoma. N Engl J Med 363:2191–2199

84. Kalirai H, Dodson A, Faqir S, Damato BE, Coupland SE (2014) Lack of Bap1 protein expression in uveal melanoma is associated with increased metastatic risk and has utility in routine prognostic testing. Br J Cancer 111:1373–1380

85. Pan H, Jia R, Zhang L, Xu S, Wu Q, Song X, Zhang H, Ge S, Leon Xu X, Fan X (2015) BAP1 regulates cell cycle progression through E2F1 target genes and mediates transcriptional silencing via H2A Monoubiquitination in uveal melanoma cells. Int J Biochem Cell Biol 60:176–184

86. Rai K, Pilarski R, Boru G, Rehman M, Saqr AH, Massengill JB, Singh A, Marino MJ, Davidorf FH, Cebulla CM et al (2017) Germline BAP1 alterations in familial uveal melanoma. Genes Chromosom Cancer 56:168–174

87. Garfield EM, Walton KE, Quan VL, VandenBoom T, Zhang B, Kong BY, Isales MC, Panah E, Kim G, Gerami P (2018) Histomorphologic Spectrum of germline-related and sporadic Bap1-inactivated melanocytic tumors. J Am Acad Dermatol 79:525–534

88. Vivet-Noguer R, Tarin M, Roman-Roman S, Alsafadi S (2019) Emerging therapeutic opportunities based on current knowledge of uveal melanoma biology. Cancers 11:1019

89. Dono M, Angelini G, Cecconi M, Amaro A, Esposito AI, Mirisola V, Maric I, Lanza F, Nasciuti F, Viaggi S et al (2014) Mutation frequencies of GNAQ, GNA11, BAP1, SF3B1, EIF1AX and TERT in uveal melanoma: detection of an activating mutation in the TERT gene promoter in a single case of uveal melanoma. Br J Cancer 110:1058–1065

90. Kumar R, Taylor M, Miao B, Ji Z, Njauw JCN, Jönsson G, Frederick DT, Tsao H (2015) BAP1 has a survival role in cutaneous melanoma. J Investig Dermatol 135:1089–1097

91. Yavuzyigitoglu S, Koopmans AE, Verdijk RM, Vaarwater J, Eussen B, Van Bodegom A, Paridaens D, Kiliç E, de Klein A (2016) Rotterdam ocular melanoma study group. Uveal melanomas with SF3B1 mutations: a distinct subclass associated with late-onset metastases. Ophthalmology 123:1118–1128

92. Alsafadi S, Houy A, Battistella A, Popova T, Wassef M, Henry E, Tirode F, Constantinou A, Piperno-Neumann S, Roman-Roman S et al (2016) Cancer-associated Sf3b1 mutations affect alternative splicing by promoting alternative Branchpoint usage. Nat Commun 7:10615

93. Robertson AG, Shih J, Yau C, Gibb EA, Oba J, Mungall KL, Hess JM, Uzunangelov V, Walter V, Danilova L et al (2017) Integrative analysis identifies four molecular and clinical subsets in uveal melanoma. Cancer Cell 32:204–220

94. Smit KN, Jager MJ, de Klein A, Kiliⵏ E (2019) Uveal melanoma: towards a molecular understanding. Prog Retin Eye Res 75:100800

95. Chaudhuri J, Si K, Maitra U (1997) Function of eukaryotic translation initiation factor 1a (EIF1A) (formerly called EIF-4C) in initiation of protein synthesis. J Biol Chem 272:7883–7891

96. Martin M, Maßhöfer L, Temming P, Rahmann S, Metz C, Bornfeld N, van de Nes J, Klein-Hitpass L, Hinnebusch AG, Horsthemke B et al (2013) Exome sequencing identifies recurrent somatic mutations in EIF1AX and SF3B1 in uveal melanoma with Disomy 3. Nat Genet 45:933–936

97. Decatur CL, Ong E, Garg N, Anbunathan H, Bowcock AM, Field MG, Harbour JW (2016) Driver mutations in uveal melanoma: associations with gene expression profile and patient outcomes. JAMA Ophthalmol 134:728–733

98. Fong L, Small EJ (2008) Anti-cytotoxic T-lymphocyte Antigen-4 antibody: the first in an emerging class of immunomodulatory antibodies for Cancer treatment. J Clin Oncol 26:5275–5283

99. Hodi FS, O'Day SJ, McDermott DF, Weber RW, Sosman JA, Haanen JB, Gonzalez R, Robert C, Schadendorf D, Hassel JC et al (2010) Improved survival with Ipilimumab in patients with metastatic melanoma. N Engl J Med 363:711–723

100. Topalian SL, Sznol M, McDermott DF, Kluger HM, Carvajal RD, Sharfman WH, Brahmer JR, Lawrence DP, Atkins MB, Powderly JD et al (2014) Survival, durable tumor remission, and long-term safety in patients with advanced melanoma receiving Nivolumab. J Clin Oncol 32:1020–1030

101. Postow MA, Callahan MK, Wolchok JD (2015) Immune checkpoint blockade in Cancer therapy. J Clin Oncol 33:1974–1982
102. Rózanowska M, Sarna T, Land EJ, Truscott TG (1999) Free radical scavenging properties of melanin interaction of Eu- and Pheo-melanin models with reducing and Oxidising radicals. Free Radic Biol Med 26:518–525
103. Slominski A, Tobin DJ, Shibahara S, Wortsman J (2004) Melanin pigmentation in mammalian skin and its hormonal regulation. Physiol Rev 84:1155–1228
104. Slominski RM, Zmijewski MA, Slominski AT (2015) The role of melanin pigment in melanoma. Exp Dermatol 24:258–259
105. Ito S (2003) The IFPCS presidential lecture: a Chemist's view of Melanogenesis. Pigment Cell Res 16:230–236
106. Journe F, Id Boufker H, Van Kempen L, Galibert MD, Wiedig M, Salès F, Theunis A, Nonclercq D, Frau A, Laurent G et al (2011) TYRP1 Mrna expression in melanoma metastases correlates with clinical outcome. Br J Cancer 105:1726–1732
107. Slominski A, Zmijewski MA, Pawelek J (2012) L-tyrosine and L-Dihydroxyphenylalanine as hormone-like regulators of melanocyte functions. Pigment Cell Melanoma Res 25:14–27
108. Kaur A, Ecker BL, Douglass SM, Kugel CH, Webster MR, Almeida FV, Somasundaram R, Hayden J, Ban E, Ahmadzadeh H et al (2019) Remodeling of the collagen matrix in aging skin promotes melanoma metastasis and affects immune cell motility. Cancer Discov 9:64–81
109. Colebatch AJ, Ferguson P, Newell F, Kazako SH, Witkowski T, Dobrovic A, Johansson PA, Saw RPM, Stretch JR, McArthur GA et al (2019) Molecular genomic profiling of melanocytic nevi. J Investig Dermatol 139:1762–1768
110. Amann VC, Ramelyte E, Thurneysen S, Pitocco R, Bentele-Jaberg N, Goldinger SM, Dummer R, Mangana J (2017) Developments in targeted therapy in melanoma. Eur J Surg Oncol 43:581–593
111. Van't Veer LJ, Burgering BM, Versteeg R, Boot AJ, Ruiter DJ, Osanto S, Schrier PI, Bos JL (1989) N-Ras mutations in human cutaneous melanoma from sun-exposed body sites. Mol Cell Biol 9:3114–3116
112. Thomas NE, Edmiston SN, Alexander A, Groben PA, Parrish E, Kricker A, Armstrong BK, Anton-Culver H, Gruber SB, From L (2015) Et al. association between Nras and Braf mutational status and melanoma-specific survival among patients with higher-risk primary melanoma. JAMA Oncol 1:359–368
113. Melamed RD, Aydin IT, Rajan GS, Phelps R, Silvers DN, Emmett KJ, Brunner G, Rabadan R, Celebi JT (2017) Genomic characterization of dysplastic nevi unveils implications for diagnosis of melanoma. J Investig Dermatol 137:905–909
114. Hancock JF, Magee AI, Childs JE, Marshall CJ (1989) All Ras proteins are Polyisoprenylated but only some are Palmitoylated. Cell 57:1167–1177
115. Boespflug A, Caramel J, Dalle S, Thomas L (2017) Treatment of NRAS-mutated advanced or metastatic melanoma: rationale, current trials and evidence to date. Ther Adv Med Oncol 9:481–492
116. Dummer R, Schadendorf D, Ascierto PA, Arance A, Dutriaux C, Di Giacomo AM, Rutkowski P, Del Vecchio M, Gutzmer R, Mandala M et al (2017) Binimetinib versus Dacarbazine in patients with advanced Nras-mutant melanoma (nemo): a multicentre, open-label, randomised, phase 3 trial. Lancet Oncol 18:435–445
117. Posch C, Moslehi H, Feeney L, Green GA, Ebaee A, Feichtenschlager V, Chong K, Peng L, Dimon MT, Phillips T et al (2013) Combined targeting of MEK and PI3K/mTOR effector pathways is necessary to effectively inhibit NRAS mutant melanoma in vitro and in vivo. Proc Natl Acad Sci U S A 110:4015–4020
118. Weisberg E, Nonami A, Chen Z, Liu F, Zhang J, Sattler M, Nelson E, Cowens K, Christie AL, Mitsiades C et al (2015) Identification of WEE1 as a novel therapeutic target for mutant Ras-driven acute leukemia and other malignancies. Leukemia 29:27–37
119. Vu HL, Aplin AE (2016) Targeting mutant NRAS signaling pathways in melanoma. Pharmacol Res 107:111–116

120. Nakagawa N, Kikuchi K, Yagyu S, Miyachi M, Iehara T, Tajiri T, Sakai T, Hosoi H (2019) Mutations in the RAS pathway as potential precision medicine targets in treatment of rhabdo-myosarcoma. Biochem Biophys Res Commun 512:524–530
121. Slipicevic A, Herlyn M (2015) KIT in melanoma: many shades of gray. J Investig Dermatol 135:337–338
122. Guo J, Si L, Kong Y, Flaherty KT, Xu X, Zhu Y, Corless CL, Li L, Li H, Sheng X et al (2011) Phase II,open-label, single-arm trial of imatinib mesylate in patients with metastatic melanoma harboring C-kit mutation or amplification. J Clin Oncol 29:2904–2909
123. Wolchok JD, Kluger H, Callahan MK, Postow MA, Rizvi NA, Lesokhin AM, Segal NH, Ariyan CE, Gordon RA, Reed K et al (2013) Nivolumab Plus Ipilimumab in Advanced Melanoma. N Engl J Med 369:122–133
124. Postow MA, Cardona DM, Taube JM, Anders RA, Taylor CR, Wolchok JD, Callahan MK, Curran MA, Lesokhin AM, Grosso JF et al (2014) Peripheral and tumor immune correlates in patients with advanced melanoma treated with Nivolumab (anti-Pd-1, Bms-936558, Ono-4538) monotherapy or in combination with Ipilimumab. J Transl Med 12:O8
125. Topalian SL, Taube JM, Anders RA, Pardoll DM (2016) Mechanism-driven biomarkers to guide immune checkpoint blockade in Cancer therapy. Nat Rev Cancer 16:275–287
126. Kleffel S, Posch C, Barthel SR, Mueller H, Schlapbach C, Guenova E, Elco CP, Lee N, Juneja VR, Zhan Q et al (2015) Melanoma cell-intrinsic PD-1 receptor functions promote tumor growth. Cell 162:1242–1256
127. Zhang B, Dang J, Ba D, Wang C, Han J, Zheng F (2018) Potential function of CTLA-4 in the Tumourigenic capacity of melanoma stem cells. Oncol Lett 16:6163–6170
128. Samarasinghe V, Madan V (2012) Nonmelanoma skin cancer. J Cutan Aesthet Surg 5:3
129. McGillis ST, Fein H (2004) Topical treatment strategies for non-melanoma skin cancer and precursor lesions. Semin Cutan Med Surg 23:174–183
130. Christensen SR (2018) Recent advances in field cancerization and management of multiple cutaneous squamous cell carcinomas [version 1; referees: 2 approved]. F1000Research 7: F1000
131. Reifenberger J, Wolter M, Knobbe CB, Köhler B, Schönicke A, Scharwächter C, Kumar K, Blaschke B, Ruzicka T, Reifenberger G (2005) Somatic mutations in the PTCH, SMOH, SUFUH and TP53 genes in sporadic basal cell carcinomas. Br J Dermatol 152:43–51
132. Pellegrini C, Maturo MG, Di Nardo L, Ciciarelli V, Gutiérrez García-Rodrigo C, Fargnoli MC (2017) Understanding the molecular genetics of basal cell carcinoma. Int J Mol Sci 18:2485
133. Dotto GP, Rustgi AK (2016) Squamous cell cancers: a unified perspective on biology and genetics. Cancer Cell 29:622–637
134. Lawrence MS, Sougnez C, Lichtenstein L, Cibulskis K, Lander E, Gabriel SB, Getz G, Ally A, Balasundaram M, Birol I et al (2015) Comprehensive genomic characterization of head and neck squamous cell carcinomas. Nature 517:576–582
135. Freed-Pastor WA, Prives C (2012) Mutant p53: one name, many proteins. Genes Dev 26:1268–1286
136. Muller PAJ, Vousden KH (2014) Mutant p53 in cancer: new functions and therapeutic opportunities. Cancer Cell 25:304–317
137. Crum CP, McKeon FD (2010) p63 in epithelial survival, germ cell surveillance, and neoplasia. Annu Rev Pathol Mech Dis 5:349–371
138. Weina K, Utikal J (2014) SOX2 and cancer: current research and its implications in the clinic. Clin Transl Med 3:19
139. Schäfer M, Werner S (2015) Nrf2—a regulator of keratinocyte redox signaling. Free Radic Biol Med 88:243–252
140. Kopan R, Ilagan MXG (2009) The canonical notch signaling pathway: unfolding the activation mechanism. Cell 137:216–233
141. Sadeqzadeh E, De Bock CE, Thorne RF (2014) Sleeping giants: emerging roles for the fat Cadherins in health and disease. Med Res Rev 34:190–221

142. Hoon DS, Spugnardi M, Kuo C, Huang SK, Morton DL, Taback B (2004) Profiling epigenetic inactivation of tumor suppressor genes in tumors and plasma from cutaneous melanoma patients. Oncogene 23:4014–4022
143. Schinke C, Mo Y, Yu Y, Amiri K, Sosman J, Greally J et al (2010) Aberrant DNA methylation in malignant melanoma. Melanoma Res 20:253–265
144. Tanemura A, Terando AM, Sim MS, van Hoesel AQ, de Maat MF, Morton DL et al (2009) CpG island methylator phenotype predicts progression of malignant melanoma. Clin Cancer Res 15:1801–1807
145. Helmbold P, Lahtz C, Enk A, Herrmann-Trost P, Marsch W, Kutzner H et al (2009) Frequent occurrence of RASSF1A promoter hypermethylation and Merkel cell polyomavirus in Merkel cell carcinoma. Mol Carcinog 48:903–909
146. Kusano M, Toyota M, Suzuki H, Akino K, Aoki F, Fujita M et al (2006) Genetic, epigenetic, and clinicopathologic features of gastric carcinomas with the CpG island methylator phenotype and an association with Epstein-Barr virus. Cancer 106:1467–1479
147. Toyota M, Ahuja N, Ohe-Toyota M, Herman JG, Baylin SB, Issa JP (1999) CpG island methylator phenotype in colorectal cancer. Proc Natl Acad Sci U S A 96:8681–8686
148. Howell PM Jr, Liu S, Ren S, Behlen C, Fodstad O, Riker AI (2009) Epigenetics in human melanoma. Cancer Control 16:200–218
149. van Doorn R, Gruis NA, Willemze R, van der Velden PA, Tensen CP (2005) Aberrant DNA methylation in cutaneous malignancies. Semin Oncol 32:479–487
150. Fazzari MJ, Greally JM (2010) Introduction to epigenomics and epigenome-wide analysis. Methods Mol Biol 620:243–265
151. Sigalotti L, Fratta E, Bidoli E, Covre A, Parisi G, Colizzi F et al (2011) Methylation levels of the "long interspersed nucleotide element-1" repetitive sequences predict survival of melanoma patients. J Transl Med 9:78
152. Nguyen T, Kuo C, Nicholl MB, Sim MS, Turner RR, Morton DL et al (2011) Downregulation of microRNA-29c is associated with hypermethylation of tumor-related genes and disease outcome in cutaneous melanoma. Epigenetics 6:388–394
153. Rietschel P, Wolchok JD, Krown S, Gerst S, Jungbluth AA, Busam K et al (2008) Phase II study of extended-dose temozolomide in patients with melanoma. J Clin Oncol 26:2299–2304
154. Kondo Y (2009) Epigenetic cross-talk between DNA methylation and histone modifications in human cancers. Yonsei Med J 50:455–463
155. Ausio J, Abbott DW (2002) The many tales of a tail: carboxyl-terminal tail heterogeneity specializes histone H2A variants for defined chromatin function. Biochemistry 41:5945–5949
156. Bonenfant D, Coulot M, Towbin H, Schindler P, van Oostrum J (2006) Characterization of histone H2A and H2B variants and their post-translational modifications by mass spectrometry. Mol Cell Proteomics 5:541–552
157. Willis-Martinez D, Richards HW, Timchenko NA, Medrano EE (2010) Role of HDAC1 in senescence, aging, and cancer. Exp Gerontol 45:279–285
158. Bachmann IM, Halvorsen OJ, Collett K, Stefansson IM, Straume O, Haukaas SA et al (2006) EZH2 expression is associated with high proliferation rate and aggressive tumor subgroups in cutaneous melanoma and cancers of the endometrium, prostate, and breast. J Clin Oncol 24:268–273
159. Zheng H, Gao L, Feng Y, Yuan L, Zhao H, Cornelius LA (2009) Down-regulation of RAP1GAP via promoter hypermethylation promotes melanoma cell proliferation, survival, and migration. Cancer Res 69:449–457
160. Fan T, Jiang S, Chung N, Alikhan A, Ni C, Lee CC et al (2011) EZH2-dependent suppression of a cellular senescence phenotype in melanoma cells by inhibition of p21/CDKN1A expression. Mol Cancer Res 9:418–429
161. Brown VL, Harwood CA, Crook T, Cronin JG, Kelsell DR, Proby CM (2004) p16INK4a and p14ARF tumor suppressor genes are commonly inactivated in cutaneous squamous cell carcinoma. J Invest Dermatol 122:1284–1292

162. Takeuchi T, Liang SB, Matsuyoshi N, Zhou S, Miyachi Y, Sonobe H, Ohtsuki Y (2002) LossofT-cadherin (CDH13, H-cadherin) expression in cutaneous squamous cell carcinoma. Lab Investig 82:1023–1029

163. Chiles MC, Ai L, Zuo C, Fan CY, Smoller BRE (2003) Cadherin promoter Hypermethylation in Preneoplastic and neoplastic skin lesions. Mod Pathol 16:1014–1018

164. Murao K, Kubo Y, Ohtani N, Hara E, Arase S (2006) Epigeneticabnormalitiesincutaneoussquamouscell carcinomas: frequent inactivation of the RB1/p16 and p53 pathways. Br J Dermatol 155:999–1005

165. Liang J, Kang X, Halifu Y, Zeng X, Jin T, Zhang M, Luo D, Ding Y, Zhou Y, Yakeya B et al (2015) Secreted frizzled-related protein promotors are hypermethylated in cutaneous squamous carcinoma compared with normal epidermis. BMC Cancer 15:641

166. Venza I, Visalli M, Tripodo B, DeGrazia G, Loddo S, Teti D, Venza M (2010) FOXE1isatargetforaberrant methylation in cutaneous squamous cell carcinoma. Br J Dermatol 162:1093–1097

167. Darr OA, Colacino JA, Tang AL, McHugh JB, Bellile EL, Bradford CR, Prince MP, Chepeha DB, Rozek LS, Moyer JS (2015) Epigenetic alterations in metastatic cutaneous carcinoma. Head Neck 37:994–1001

168. Meier K, Drexler SK, Eberle FC, Lefort K, Yazdi AS (2016) SilencingofASCincutaneoussquamouscell carcinoma. PLoS One 11:e0164742

169. Li L, Jiang M, Feng Q, Kiviat NB, Stern JE, Hawes S, Cherne S, Lu H (2015) AberrantMethylationChanges detected in cutaneous squamous cell carcinoma of immunocompetent individuals. Cell Biochem Biophys 72:599–604

170. Toll A, Salgado R, Espinet B, Díaz-Lagares A, Hernández-Ruiz E, Andrades E, Sandoval J, Esteller M, Pujol RM, Hernández-Muñoz I (2016) MiR-204 silencing in intraepithelial to invasive cutaneous squamous cell carcinoma progression. Mol Cancer 15:1

171. Nobeyama Y, Watanabe Y, Nakagawa H (2017) SilencingofG0/G1switchgene2incutaneoussquamouscell carcinoma. PLoS One 12:e0187047

172. Venza M, Visalli M, Catalano T, Beninati C, Teti D, Venza I (2017) DSS1promoterhypomethylationand overexpression predict poor prognosis in melanoma and squamous cell carcinoma patients. Hum Pathol 60:137–146

173. Hervás-Marín D, Higgins F, Sanmartín O, López-Guerrero JA, Bañó MC, Igual JC, Quilis I, Sandoval J (2019) Genome wide DNA methylation profiling identifies specific epigenetic features in high-risk cutaneous squamous cell carcinoma. PLoS One 14:e0223341

174. Goldberg M, Rummelt C, Laerm A, Helmbold P, Holbach LM, Ballhausen WG (2006) Epigenetic silencing contributes to frequent loss of the fragile histidine triad tumour suppressor in basal cell carcinomas. Br J Dermatol 155:1154–1158

175. Heitzer E, Bambach I, Dandachi N, Horn M, Wolf P (2010) PTCH promoter methylation at low level in sporadic basal cell carcinoma analysed by three different approaches. Exp Dermatol 19:926–928

176. Greenberg ES, Chong KK, Huynh KT, Tanaka R, Hoon DSB (2014) Epigeneticbiomarkersinskincancer. Cancer Lett 342:170–177

177. Harms PW, Harms KL, Moore PS, DeCaprio JA, Nghiem P, Wong MKK, Brownell I (2018) Thebiology and treatment of Merkel cell carcinoma: current understanding and research priorities. Nat Rev Clin Oncol 15:763–776

178. Jones CL, Wain EM, Chu CC, Tosi I, Foster R, McKenzie RC et al (2010) Downregulation of Fas gene expression in Sezary syndrome is associated with promoter hypermethylation. J Invest Dermatol 130:1116–1125

179. Wu J, Wood GS (2010) Reduction of Fas/CD95 promoter methylation, upregulation of Fas protein, and enhancement of sensitivity to apoptosis in cutaneous T-cell lymphoma. Arch Dermatol 147:443–449

180. Lassacher A, Heitzer E, Kerl H, Wolf P (2008) p14ARF hypermethylation is common but INK4a-ARF locus or p53 mutations are rare in Merkel cell carcinoma. J Invest Dermatol 128:1788–1796

181. Caron MP, Bastet L, Lussier A, Simoneau-Roy M, Masse E, Lafontaine DA (2012) Dual-acting riboswitch control of translation initiation and mRNA decay. Proc Natl Acad Sci U S A 109:E3444–E3453
182. Cretoiu D, Xu J, Xiao J, Cretoiu SM (2016) Telocytes and their extracellular vesicles-evidence and hypotheses. Int J Mol Sci 17:1322
183. Cretoiu D, Xu J, Xiao J, Suciu N, Cretoiu SM (2016) Circulating MicroRNAs as potential molecular biomarkers in pathophysiological evolution of pregnancy. Dis Markers 2016:3851054
184. Horsham JL, Ganda C, Kalinowski FC, Brown RA, Epis MR, Leedman PJ (2015) MicroRNA-7: a miRNA with expanding roles in development and disease. Int J Biochem Cell Biol 69:215–224
185. Monroig-Bosque Pdel C, Rivera CA, Calin GA (2015) MicroRNAs in cancer therapeutics: "from the bench to the bedside". Expert Opin Biol Ther 15:1381–1385
186. de Unamuno B, Palanca S, Botella R (2015) Update on melanoma epigenetics. Curr Opin Oncol 27:420–426
187. Leibowitz-Amit R, Sidi Y, Avni D (2012) Aberrations in the micro-RNA biogenesis machin-ery and the emerging roles of micro-RNAs in the pathogenesis of cutaneous malignant melanoma. Pigment Cell Melanoma Res 25:740–757
188. Latchana N, Ganju A, Howard JH, Carson WE III (2016) MicroRNA dysregulation in melanoma. Surg Oncol 25:184–189
189. Segura MF, Greenwald HS, Hanniford D, Osman I, Hernando E (2012) MicroRNA and cutaneous melanoma: from discovery to prognosis and therapy. Carcinogenesis 33:1823–1832
190. Greenberg E, Nemlich Y, Markel G (2014) MicroRNAs in cancer: lessons from melanoma. Curr Pharm Des 20:5246–5259
191. Felicetti F, Errico MC, Bottero L, Segnalini P, Stoppacciaro A, Biffoni M et al (2008) The promyelocytic leukemia zinc finger-microRNA-221/−222 pathway controls melanoma pro-gression through multiple oncogenic mechanisms. Cancer Res 68:2745–2754
192. Hanna JA, Hahn L, Agarwal S, Rimm DL (2012) In situ measurement of miR-205 in malignant melanoma tissue supports its role as a tumor suppressor microRNA. Lab Investig 92:1390–1397
193. Saldanha G, Elshaw S, Sachs P, Alharbi H, Shah P, Jothi A et al (2016) microRNA-10b is a prognostic biomarker for melanoma. Mod Pathol 29:112–121
194. Wang K, Zhang ZW (2015) Expression of miR-203 is decreased and associated with the prognosis of melanoma patients. Int J Clin Exp Pathol 8:13249–13254
195. El Hajj P, Gilot D, Migault M, Theunis A, Van Kempen LC, Sales F et al (2015) SNPs at miR-155 binding sites of TYRP1 explain discrepancy between mRNA and protein and refine TYRP1 prognostic value in melanoma. Br J Cancer 113:91–98
196. DiSano JA, Huffnagle I, Gowda R, Spiegelman VS, Robertson GP, Pameijer CR (2019) Loss of miR-155 upregulates WEE1 in metastatic melanoma. Melanoma Res 29:216–219
197. Liu K, Jin J, Rong K, Zhuo L, Li P (2018) MicroRNA675 inhibits cell proliferation and invasion in melanoma by directly targeting metadherin. Mol Med Rep 17:3372–3379
198. Hu Y, Wang Q, Zhu XH (2019) MiR-135b is a novel oncogenic factor in cutaneous melanoma by targeting LATS2. Melanoma Res 29:119–125
199. Sanchez-Sendra B, Martinez-Ciarpaglini C, Gonzalez-Munoz JF, Murgui A, Terradez L, Monteagudo C (2018) Downregulation of intratumoral expression of miR-205, miR-200c and miR-125b in primary human cutaneous melanomas predicts shorter survival. Sci Rep 8:17076
200. Sabarimurugan S, Madurantakam Royam M, Das A, Das S, K M, G., and Jayaraj, R. (2018) Systematic review and meta-analysis of the prognostic significance of miRNAs in melanoma patients. Mol Diagn Ther 22:653–669
201. Aksenenko M, Palkina N, Komina A, Tashireva L, Ruksha T (2019) Differences in microRNA expression between melanoma and healthy adjacent skin. BMC Dermatol 19:1

202. Jayawardana K, Schramm SJ, Tembe V, Mueller S, Thompson JF, Scolyer RA et al (2016) Identification, review, and systematic crossvalidation of microRNA prognostic signatures in metastatic melanoma. J Invest Dermatol 136:245–254

203. Young AL, Malik HZ, Abu-Hilal M, Guthrie JA, Wyatt J, Prasad KR et al (2007) Large hepatocellular carcinoma: time to stop preoperative biopsy. J Am Coll Surg 205:453–462

204. Corcoran NM, Hovens CM, Hong MK, Pedersen J, Casey RG, Connolly S et al (2011) Underestimation of Gleason score at prostate biopsy reflects sampling error in lower volume tumours. BJU Int 109(5):660–664

205. Ho AS, Huang X, Cao H, Christman-Skieller C, Bennewith K, Le QT et al (2010) Circulating miR-210 as a novel hypoxia marker in pancreatic Cancer. Transl Oncol 3:109–113

206. Mitchell PS, Parkin RK, Kroh EM, Fritz BR, Wyman SK, Pogosova-Agadjanyan EL et al (2008) Circulating microRNAs as stable blood-based markers for cancer detection. Proc Natl Acad Sci U S A 105:10513–10518

207. Kanemaru H, Fukushima S, Yamashita J, Honda N, Oyama R, Kakimoto A et al (2011) The circulating microRNA-221 level in patients with malignant melanoma as a new tumor marker. J Dermatol Sci 61:187–193

208. Friedman EB, Shang S, De Miera EV, Fog JU, Teilum MW, Ma MW et al (2012) Serum microRNAs as biomarkers for recurrence in melanoma. J Transl Med 10:155. https://doi.org/10.1186/1479-5876-10-155

209. Guo S, Guo W, Li S, Dai W, Zhang N, Zhao T et al (2016) Serum miR-16: a potential biomarker for predicting melanoma prognosis. J Invest Dermatol 136:985–993

210. Stark MS, Klein K, Weide B, Haydu LE, Pflugfelder A, Tang YH et al (2015) The prognostic and predictive value of melanoma-related microRNAs using tissue and serum: a microRNA expression analysis. EBioMedicine 2:671–680

211. Tian R, Liu T, Qiao L, Gao M, Li J (2015) Decreased serum microRNA-206 level predicts unfavorable prognosis in patients with melanoma. Int J Clin Exp Pathol 8:3097–3103

212. Huang SK, Hoon DS (2016) Liquid biopsy utility for the surveillance of cutaneous malignant melanoma patients. Mol Oncol 10:450–463

213. Mirzaei H, Gholamin S, Shahidsales S, Sahebkar A, Jaafari MR, Mirzaei HR et al (2016) MicroRNAs as potential diagnostic and prognostic biomarkers in melanoma. Eur J Cancer 53:25–32

214. Polini B, Carpi S, Romanini A, Breschi MC, Nieri P, Podesta A (2019) Circulating cell-free microRNAs in cutaneous melanoma staging and recurrence or survival prognosis. Pigment Cell Melanoma Res 32:486–499

215. Grignol V, Fairchild ET, Zimmerer JM, Lesinski GB, Walker MJ, Magro CM, Kacher JE, Karpa VI, Clark J, Nuovo G, Lehman A, Volinia S, Agnese DM, Croce CM, Carson WE 3rd. (2011) miR-21 and miR-155 are associated with mitotic activity and lesion depth of borderline melanocytic lesions. Br J Cancer 105(7):1023–1029

216. Jiang L, Lv X, Li J, Li J, Li X, Li W, Li Y (2012) The status of microRNA-21 expression and its clinical significance in human cutaneous malignant melanoma. Acta Histochem 114 (6):582–588

217. Satzger I, Mattern A, Kuettler U, Weinspach D, Voelker B, Kapp A, Gutzmer R (2010) MicroRNA-15b represents an independent prognostic parameter and is correlated with tumor cell proliferation and apoptosis in malignant melanoma. Int J Cancer 126(11):2553–2562

218. Xu Y, Brenn T, Brown ER, Doherty V, Melton DW (2012) Differential expression of microRNAs during melanoma progression: miR-200c, miR-205 and miR-211 are downregulated in melanoma and act as tumour suppressors. Br J Cancer 106(3):553–561

219. Lin N, Zhou Y, Lian X, Tu Y (2015) Expression of microRNA-106b and its clinical significance in cutaneous melanoma. Genet Mol Res 14(4):16379–16385

220. Kozar I, Cesi G, Margue C, Philippidou D, Kreis S (2017) Impact of BRAF kinase inhibitors on the miRNomes and transcriptomes of melanoma cells. Biochim Biophys Acta Gen Subj 1861(11 Pt B):2980–2992

221. Fattore L, Mancini R, Acunzo M, Romano G, Laganà A, Pisanu ME, Malpicci D, Madonna G, Mallardo D, Capone M, Fulciniti F, Mazzucchelli L, Botti G, Croce CM, Ascierto PA, Ciliberto G (2016) miR-579-3p controls melanoma progression and resistance to target therapy. Proc Natl Acad Sci U S A 113(34):E5005–E5013
222. Li N, Liu Y, Pang H, Lee D, Zhou Y, Xiao Z (2019) Methylation-mediated silencing of MicroRNA-211 decreases the sensitivity of melanoma cells to cisplatin. Med Sci Monit 25:1590–1599
223. Prabhakar K, Rodríguez CI, Jayanthy AS, Mikheil DM, Bhasker AI, Perera RJ, Setaluri V (2019) Role of miR-214 in regulation of β-catenin and the malignant phenotype of melanoma. Mol Carcinog 58(11):1974–1984
224. Huber V, Vallacchi V, Fleming V, Hu X, Cova A, Dugo M, Shahaj E, Sulsenti R, Vergani E, Filipazzi P, De Laurentiis A, Lalli L, Di Guardo L, Patuzzo R, Vergani B, Casiraghi E, Cossa M, Gualeni A, Bollati V, Arienti F, De Braud F, Mariani L, Villa A, Altevogt P, Umansky V, Rodolfo M, Rivoltini L (2018) Tumor-derived microRNAs induce myeloid suppressor cells and predict immunotherapy resistance in melanoma. J Clin Invest 128 (12):5505–5516
225. Caporali S, Amaro A, Levati L, Alvino E, Lacal PM, Mastroeni S, Ruffini F, Bonmassar L, Antonini Cappellini GC, Felli N, Carè A, Pfeffer U, D'Atri S (2019) miR-126-3p down-regulation contributes to dabrafenib acquired resistance in melanoma by up-regulating ADAM9 and VEGF-A. J Exp Clin Cancer Res 38(1):272
226. Cañueto J, Cardeñoso-Álvarez E, García-Hernández JL, Galindo-Villardón P, Vicente-Galindo P, Vicente-Villardón JL, Alonso-López D, De Las RJ, Valero J, Moyano-Sanz E, Fernández-López E, Mao JH, Castellanos-Martín A, Román-Curto C, Pérez-Losada J (2017) MicroRNA (miR)-203 and miR-205 expression patterns identify subgroups of prognosis in cutaneous squamous cell carcinoma. Br J Dermatol 177(1):168–178
227. Gong ZH, Zhou F, Shi C, Xiang T, Zhou CK, Wang QQ, Jiang YS, Gao SF (2019) miRNA-221 promotes cutaneous squamous cell carcinoma progression by targeting PTEN. Cell Mol Biol Lett 24:9
228. García-Sancha N, Corchado-Cobos R, Pérez-Losada J, Cañueto J (2019) MicroRNA dysregulation in cutaneous squamous cell carcinoma. Int J Mol Sci 20(9):2181. https://doi.org/10.3390/ijms20092181
229. Kohnken R, Mishra A (2019) MicroRNAs in cutaneous T-cell lymphoma: the future of therapy. J Invest Dermatol 139(3):528–534
230. Willemze R, Jaffe ES, Burg G, Cerroni L, Berti E, Swerdlow SH, Ralfkiaer E, Chimenti S, Diaz-Perez JL, Duncan LM, Grange F, Harris NL, Kempf W, Kerl H, Kurrer M, Knobler R, Pimpinelli N, Sander C, Santucci M, Sterry W, Vermeer MH, Wechsler J, Whittaker S, Meijer CJ (2005) WHO-EORTC classification for cutaneous lymphomas. Blood 105(10):3768–3785
231. Gambichler T, Salveridou K, Schmitz L, Käfferlein HU, Brüning T, Stockfleth E, Sand M, Lang K (2019) Low Drosha protein expression in cutaneous T-cell lymphoma is associated with worse disease outcome. J Eur Acad Dermatol Venereol 33(9):1695–1699
232. Lindahl LM, Besenbacher S, Rittig AH, Celis P, Willerslev-Olsen A, Gjerdrum LMR, Krejsgaard T, Johansen C, Litman T, Woetmann A, Odum N, Iversen L (2018) Prognostic miRNA classifier in early-stage mycosis fungoides: development and validation in a Danish nationwide study. Blood 131(7):759–770
233. Feng H, Shuda M, Chang Y, Moore PS (2008) Clonal integration of a polyomavirus in human Merkel cell carcinoma. Science 319(5866):1096–1100
234. Krejcí K, Zadrazil J, Tichý T, Horák P, Ciferská H, Hodulová M, Zezulová M, Zlevorová M (2010) Kozní karcinom z Merkelových bunek [Merkel cell skin carcinoma]. Klin Onkol 23 (4):210–217
235. Fan K, Gravemeyer J, Ritter C, Rasheed K, Gambichler T, Moens U, Shuda M, Schrama D, Becker JC (2020) MCPyV large T antigen-induced atonal homolog 1 Is a lineage-dependency oncogene in merkel cell carcinoma. J Invest Dermatol 140(1):56–65

236. Gniadecka M, Philipsen PA, Sigurdsson S, Wessel S, Nielsen OF, Christensen DH, Hercogova J, Rossen K, Thomsen HK, Gniadecki R, Hansen LK, Wulf HC (2004) Melanoma diagnosis by Raman spectroscopy and neural networks: structure alterations in proteins and lipids in intact cancer tissue. J Invest Dermatol 122(2):443–449

237. Lui H, Zhao J, McLean D, Zeng H (2012) Real-time Raman spectroscopy for in vivo skin cancer diagnosis. Cancer Res 72(10):2491–2500

238. Lim L, Nichols B, Migden MR, Rajaram N, Reichenberg JS, Markey MK, Ross MI, Tunnell JW (2014) Clinical study of noninvasive in vivo melanoma and nonmelanoma skin cancers using multimodal spectral diagnosis. J Biomed Opt 19(11):117003

239. Sharma M, Marple E, Reichenberg J, Tunnell JW (2014) Design and characterization of a novel multimodal fiber-optic probe and spectroscopy system for skin cancer applications. Rev Sci Instrum 85(8):083101

240. Zhao J, Lui H, Kalia S, Zeng H (2015) Real-time Raman spectroscopy for automatic in vivo skin cancer detection: an independent validation. Anal Bioanal Chem 407(27):8373–8379

241. Feng X, Moy AJ, Nguyen HTM, Zhang Y, Zhang J, Fox MC, Sebastian KR, Reichenberg JS, Markey MK, Tunnell JW (2018) Raman biophysical markers in skin cancer diagnosis. J Biomed Opt 23(5):1–10

242. Lieber CA, Majumder SK, Ellis DL, Billheimer DD, Mahadevan-Jansen A (2008) In vivo nonmelanoma skin cancer diagnosis using Raman microspectroscopy. Lasers Surg Med 40 (7):461–467

243. Pence I, Mahadevan-Jansen A (2016) Clinical instrumentation and applications of Raman spectroscopy. Chem Soc Rev 45(7):1958–1979

Therapeutics Intervention of Skin Cancer in the OMICS Era

Deepti Chopra, Shruti Goyal, Saroj Amar, Ankit Verma, Saumya Shukla, Sunil Kumar Patel, Sarika Yadav, Ajeet K. Srivastav, Jyoti Singh, and Divya Dubey

---

D. Chopra (✉) · S. Goyal · S. Shukla · J. Singh · D. Dubey
Systems Toxicology and Health Risk Assessment Group, CSIR-Indian Institute of Toxicology Research (CSIR-IITR), Vishvigyan Bhawan, Lucknow, Uttar Pradesh, India

S. Amar
Oak Ridge Institute for Science and Education, Oak Ridge, TN, USA

School of Bioengineering and Biosciences, Lovely Professional University, Phagwara, Punjab, India

A. Verma
Department of Life Sciences and the National Institute for Biotechnology in the Negev, Ben Gurion University of Negev, Beer Sheva, Israel

S. K. Patel
Systems Toxicology and Health Risk Assessment Group, CSIR-Indian Institute of Toxicology Research (CSIR-IITR), Vishvigyan Bhawan, Lucknow, Uttar Pradesh, India

Academy of Scientific and Innovative Research, AcSIR Headquarters, CSIR-HRDC Campus, Sector 19, Ghaziabad, Uttar Pradesh, India

S. Yadav
Food, Drugs and Chemical Toxicology Group, CSIR-Indian Institute of Toxicology Research (CSIR-IITR), Vishvigyan Bhawan, Lucknow, Uttar Pradesh, India

Academy of Scientific and Innovative Research, AcSIR Headquarters, CSIR-HRDC Campus, Sector 19, Ghaziabad, Uttar Pradesh, India

A. K. Srivastav
Systems Toxicology and Health Risk Assessment Group, CSIR-Indian Institute of Toxicology Research (CSIR-IITR), Vishvigyan Bhawan, Lucknow, Uttar Pradesh, India

PEE SAFE™, AVP-R&D-Compliances, Redcliffe Hygiene Pvt. Ltd., 456-457, Ground Floor, Udyog Vihar, Phase-III, Gurugram, Haryana, India

Abstract

In the past, many attempts were made to solve the molecular mechanisms of cancer biology using a single OMICS approach through transcriptomics or proteomics for screening gene-level cancer-specific mutations, changed epigenetic profile, or varied mRNA and protein expressions. Apart from the contribution of these approaches in the identification of cancer-related mutations, alterations, these have lacked in establishing a direct link between molecular signatures and phenotypic examination of cancer hallmarks. Nevertheless, multi-OMICS approaches will reveal the underlying complex molecular mechanism of cancer hallmark stages like metastasis and angiogenesis. These approaches can very well be used to analyze cellular response to various cancer treatment therapies as well as find out molecular candidates having the potential to diagnose or cure. This chapter deals with applications of diverse OMICS approaches in the varied and dynamic field of cancer biology and also confers how these multi-OMICS approaches can be decisive in the personalized medicine field. The unified experimental data along with computational or mathematical data models have been accumulated in the Cancer Genome Atlas (TCGA) consortium, which further with the multi-OMICS approach will provide an opportunity to deal with the cancer cells complexity. This chapter will encourage the readers to integrate these OMICS approaches together to analyze the oncogenesis at different cellular, molecular, and system basis.

Keywords

Genomics · Proteomics · Transcriptomics · OMICS · Radiomics · Microbiomics

8.1   Introduction to OMICS

The term OMIC has now become the focus for all the fields involving biomolecular studies of RNA, DNA, protein, lipids, and their metabolites. The need of the hour in healthcare is the "omics revolution" which assures an enriched knowledge to alter cure through integrating the information with the personalized matching of patient's molecular data. The finding of cancer features requires molecular modification at multiple molecular levels like genomic, epigenomic, transcriptomic, proteomic, and metabolomic. Multi-OMICS-based approaches involve high-throughput interfaces that assist the analysis of genome, transcriptome, proteome, epigenome, and metabolome in a global-unbiased manner. OMICS-based approaches are now being exploited to understand the complex biological systems and find out the molecular markers fundamental to intricate cellular phenotypes [1, 2].

The known biomolecular studies information of different multifactorial diseases along with OMICS have raised hopes that in the coming decade there will be a better therapeutic prediction for likely molecular targets of cancer and their related cure. These varied molecular classes and their broad-spectrum data will provide the

Table 8.1 Examples of molecular species testing important to clinical practice or oncology research [6]

Molecular species	Alteration of interest	Abnormality in cancer	Example
RNA	Change in gene expression	Induction	*PI3K, AKT*
		Repression	*CDKN1A*
	Gene expression profiling	Distinct co-expression patterns	Luminal A versus triple-negative breast cancer
	Gene mutation	Missense	*TP53. KRAS*
		Nonsense	BRCA2
DNA	Gene copy number variation	Amplification	*HER2, MYC*
		Loss of heterozygosity	*APC, PTEN*
Karyotype	Chromosomal translocation	9:22	Chronic myeloid leukemia
	Chromosomal deletion	3p21	Small cell lung cancer
Protein	Change in protein expression	Upregulation	*ERK*
		Downregulation	*pRb*
Lipid	Change in (extra)cellular lipids	Increase	Phosphatidylcholine
		Reduction	Phosphatidylethanolamine

requisite disease-related information that will be helpful in the prediction of probable molecular targets of anticancer therapies [3, 4]. The already known biomarkers will help in achieving these goals [5]. Few examples of molecular species important to recent oncology-related research or clinical practices are given in Table 8.1.

Varied OMICS approaches developed will help to unravel the complex biological systems at a different gene, RNA, and protein biomolecular levels. The current advancement in multi-OMICS techniques is a choice medium to study the peculiar and complex cellular functions that are placed in the core of complex diseases such as cancer [1]. Each OMICS techniques are vital to interpreting the intricate phenotypes. The future advancement of the multi-OMICS approach would involve the decrease in sample processing or measurement period and increase in reproducibility of results to decisively ascertain these approaches in medical settings for conclusive findings and prediction of cancer.

8.2 Application of OMICS in Skin Cancer Therapy

8.2.1 Genomics Approach in Skin Cancer Therapy

Cancer cells secrete the biomarker material via different mechanisms for their detection. These biomarkers may be identified in the blood or tissues. It shows that unique disease in the body secretes specific types of informative markers.

Single-nucleotide polymorphisms (SNPs) are significantly used for genomics approaches for cancer therapy. The presence of SNPs as markers in disease conditions may assist the identification of abnormal genes at increased risk for cancers. Besides, SNP genetic results may explore specific genetic profiles that play a key role in drug efficacy and toxicity. DNA and tissue microarray techniques have the power to change the future concern of cancer therapy. Next-generation sequencing (NGS) is another technique for genomics that provides the correct understanding of the structure of the cancer genome and identifies differentially expressed genes that will be useful for target cancer therapy.

Many studies have been done to understand cancer biology and its related therapy that are originated from the accumulation of genomic alterations, including base substitutions, small insertions, and deletions, and chromosomal rearrangements [7]. For example, the Philadelphia chromosome was studied in chronic myelogenous leukemia (CML) cells which shows the translocation of chromosome between 9 and 22 [8] Genome sequencing study reported the presence of 360 exonic mutations, 165 genomic rearrangements, and 323 segments of changes in copy number per tumor, and loss-of-function mutations in lung squamous cell carcinoma (LSCC) that may be targeted for therapy [9].

The application of NGS technologies is to develop the full story of mutated cancer genes. It accelerates the research of new targeted drugs and has a positive impact on understanding cancer biology and increases the new input of PPPM in cancer. For example, in the tumorigenesis process, gene fusions play an important role that was developed from chromosome translocation. Kinase and transcription factors act as a common fusion gene and play the main role in tumorigenesis and metastasis. So it is a new insight to focus the study of the development of PPM in cancer [10].

From the NGS study, it is clear that kinase inhibitors may provide a meaningful impact on cancer cells. In the study, it is published that a pan-NTRK as well as ALK and ROS1 tyrosine kinase inhibitor, entrectinib, has been found successful therapy for a single patient with SC, which highlighted the potential role of kinase inhibitor in treating of ETV6-NTRK3 fusion gene-associated cancers.

In 2005 in the USA, the National Cancer Institute developed The Cancer Genome Atlas (TCGA) project, which plays a major role in sequencing all cancer genomes and their aberrations. This genome sequencing data are now easily accessible for the research of human tumors.

Both SNP and NGS genomics technologies in combination could be a key element to rapidly develop approaches to test individual cancer patients for specific therapeutic targets.

8.2.2 Proteomics Approach in Skin Cancer Therapy

Proteomics is a rapidly growing field in molecular biology that is helpful for systemic high-throughput approach for protein expression analysis and function under given conditions. So it would be helpful to explain the metastatic cancer mechanisms. As a result, it provides a therapeutic approach and clinical analysis of cancer. Protein changes mainly include gain- or loss-of-function mechanisms via, for example, protein–protein interaction or post-translational modification may contribute to the specific drug target of cancer.

It is known that glycosylated proteins play a major role in the cancer diagnostic approach. MS-based proteomics can separate and identify large numbers of glycosylated proteins qualitatively and quantitatively, which shows a great hallmark for the development of novel cancer biomarkers. In recent time, the glycoproteomics technique has been highlighted and frequently used in cancer research. For example, it is reported that in each subtype of lung cancer there is an increase in the level of the fucosylated haptoglobin (HP) with the addition of three α-2, 6-linked sialic acids that were measured by MS-based glycoproteomics [11]. This specific study can be used as a potential glycobiomarker for lung cancer diagnosis and therapy.

In addition to glycosylation of proteins, other post-translational modifications (PTMs) such as phosphorylation also play an active role as biomarkers in skin cancer diagnosis and therapy. The study on phosphoprotein secretomes showed a set of novel breast cancer subtype-specific phosphopeptides for the therapeutics approach.

Nitration of protein tyrosine is another important PTM mechanism, which alters the chemical properties of tyrosine amino acid and ultimately protein functions [12] that also act as a target for therapy. It is well reported that in human astrocytomas, nitration of 18 proteins and 20 tyrosine was discovered via 2DGE-based nitroproteomics, which are linked to a series of biological processes such as drug therapy and signal transduction. This research is helpful for the discovery of new biomarkers for its early detection and effective therapeutic targets [13].

Auto-antibodies are another useful biomarker of some diseases, in specific cancer. Le Naour et al. reported in their study that there is a presence of auto-antibodies in hepatocellular carcinoma which is detected by 2DGE of cultured cells and tumor tissues, followed by immunoblotting. That finding may be helpful in diagnosis for high-risk subjects [14].

Overall MS-based proteomics and pathway analysis tools have become an essential approach in cancer therapy.

8.2.3 Transcriptomics Approach in Skin Cancer Therapy

Since cancers arise from the collection of genomic mutations and epigenetic alterations that alter gene function and expression thus transcriptomics approach can play important role in the early prediction of malignancy. There is convincing scientific evidence that skin carcinoma is caused mainly by the interplay between genetic factors and environmental UV radiation [15–17]. An efficient approach is required to illustrate the spectrum of skin cancer-associated mRNA alterations through the integration of transcriptomic and bioinformatics via genomic data science.

The major risk factor associated with melanoma and non-melanoma skin cancers is UV radiation. UV radiation is not only responsible for UV signature mutation but also induces substantial transcriptional instability in the case of skin cancer [18]. A study showed that the major etiological factor in photo-induced skin cancer is transcriptional instability of skin cancer genes as well as UV induced permanent alteration of mRNA sequence of human skin squamous cell carcinomas [18]. RNA-Seq studies by Shen and his co-workers to make a transcriptomic cohort containing UV-responsive genes in human skin cells exposed the dysregulated genes present in squamous cell carcinomas of human keratinocytes. Base-pair mutations that accumulated in the case of melanomas illuminating an amazingly high rate of somatic mutation and lending support to the concept that point mutations constitute the major driver of melanoma progression [19]. A study by Berger and his co-workers indicated new paths for targeted discovery in melanoma, while also providing a prototype for large-scale transcriptome studies across many tumor types not only skin malignancy. A previous study by Berger also reveals that RNA-seq data has been used to characterize not only the entire melanoma transcriptome but also sequence mutations, gene expression levels, alternative splicing, and allele-specific expression. Thus the full spectrum of RNA-based alterations related to skin cancer is an emerging tool for integrative analysis.

The substantial connection between the UV signature and squamous cell carcinomas signature suggests that biomarker-based tests may also facilitate clinical diagnosis and early prediction of skin cancer risk in vulnerable persons due to UV induced skin damage. With the vertical reductions in the run times as well as costs of next-generation sequencing technologies, profiling an individual's transcriptome has become a possible clinical diagnosis. Thus one can expect that the UV biomarker panel, in combination with RNA-sequencing and bioinformatics tools, will develop the next-generation diagnostic tests to reduce the skin cancer cases by early detection of human skin malignancy.

8.2.4 Radiomics Approach in Skin Cancer Therapy

The term "radiomics" has developed in the imaging field as a novel area of study in the last few years. Radiomics is a recently evolving area of radiology capable of extracting and analyzing quantitative/measurable characteristics from biomedical/diagnostic images that could lead to the needs of precision medicine [20]. This novel concept obtaining image data from examinations such as computed tomography (CT), magnetic resonance imaging (MRI), single-photon emission computed tomography (SPECT), positron emission tomography (PET), etc. This conception has received considerable interest in clinical implementation; it could lead to strategies for medication selection and patient stratification. It can also assist in the invention of novel diagnostics, routine clinical practice, and chemotherapeutic treatments.

The workflow of radiomics can be (1) acquisition of diagnostic image data, (2) calibration and segmentation of tumor regions, (3) extraction and quantification of features, (4) image database establishment, (5) modeling and analysis, and (6) classification and prediction for treatment [21]. With the help of these workflow and acceptable algorithms, the harvested findings have wide applicability and capability for a significant positive impact in radiology. For instance, health professionals can assess the effectiveness of treatment, predict the position of tumor metastases, correlate findings with histopathological observations, or identify the type of cancer more accurately. Numerous studies have evaluated the radiometric characteristics of various forms of cancer based on different imaging modes [22–24]. Besides, some studies have examined the reproducibility and heterogeneity of radiomic features in various clinical settings [25–27], while others have documented important predictive and prognostic radiomic characteristics [28, 29]. Studies have observed that the correlation between radiomic features and tumor histology (stages/grades), metabolism, the survival of the patient, and several other clinical outcomes have also been documented [23, 30, 31]. Moreover, certain radiogenic studies have documented the relation between radiomic traits and basic patterns of gene expression [32, 33]. These reports suggest that radiomics could enhance selection and treatment follow-up. All radiomics process is faced with several challenges, but challenges also coexist with opportunities [34, 35].

Radiomics, which incorporates radiology, oncology, and machine learning methodologies, is still a newly proposed and rapidly evolving field. In the assessment of accurate diagnostics and oncology, it plays a highly significant role [36]. Further study can be focused on reproducibility and interpretability to make radiomics even more appropriate in this field.

8.2.5   Microbiomics Approach in Skin Cancer Therapy

Microbiomics is an evolving discipline that deals with microbes that live in and on the human body and play a vital role in human physiology and health. The human skin microbiome consists of numerous microbial populations [37, 38]. Several studies have indicated that these microbes play a key role in carcinogenesis and may also affect the response to cancer therapy [39, 40]. There has been a growing interest in human microbiomes and skin diseases in recent years.

Microbiome research is being used in numerous ways in the treatment of skin cancer such as the link between skin microbes in the process of inflammation and the association of commensal microbes with skin cancer [37, 38, 41]. Keratinized skin cells, immune cells, and microbes work together under homeostatic and stable conditions to create the physical and immune barriers of the skin [42]. Microbes can modify the physiological and immune functions by which the human body can change the microbiome. For instance, a study showed that cachectic cancer patients' skin microbiome is less diverse than healthy participants, suggesting an effect of cancer and cachexia on human skin microbial diversity [41, 43].

Furthermore, gut microbiome interactions have been shown with gastrointestinal cancer and skin cancer. The skin microbiome itself is as a complex group as the gut microbiome, but research is only beginning to unravel its impact on the host [41, 44]. The use of health beneficial microbiological strains in oral or topical probiotics can reduce the risk of skin cancer and possibly even increase the probability of treatment success ([44]; Górska et al. 2015; [40, 45]). Moreover, like as the bacterial flora is present in normal skin and mucous membranes, so viral flora is also existing, and some of them are correlated with skin cancers [46, 47]. Several efforts are currently being made to improve therapy by modulating the gut microbiota. For instance, (1) fecal microbiota transplantation, (2) microbiota mediated immune-based tactics [48, 49], (3) targeting and modulating the tumor microbiota [50, 51], (4) diet, prebiotics, and postbiotics [40, 52], (5) engineered live bacterial therapy [53]. However, various strategies will need to be developed to track and modulate these factors to optimize both the prognostic and therapeutic outlook [37]. Although there are significant differences in our research or understanding of the complex relationship between microbiome and skin cancer, particularly related to chemoprevention. Many questions remain unanswered about this relationship. Even more, studies are needed to establish new opportunities for possible skin cancer therapies. The application of microbiomes in skin cancer research appears to become a potential area and can help to provide new possibilities for the prevention and treatment of skin cancer by microbes.

8.3   Future of Multi-OMICS Studies in Skin Cancer Prevention

Recent advancements in high-throughput next-generation sequencing and mass spectrometric techniques have facilitated large-scale studies involving the whole cellular system analyses. The potent computational tools known to date have been able to recognize the link between genomic aberrations involving differentially expressed mRNAs, proteins, and concerned metabolites that may be associated with cancer driven cellular disturbance. The incorporation of multi-OMICS techniques gives a platform to relate the genomic or epigenomic modifications to interrelated proteome, transcriptome, and metabolome system. The future advances of research in systems biology will be based on models that can transact with multiple mRNA, protein, and metabolite alterations dynamically. The systems biology-based approach can develop efficient approaches to foster personalized cancer treatment [54]. The main aim of this approach is to build up extrapolative models that are advanced and constrained by experimental corroboration. These predictive model approaches or techniques will be predominantly helpful to select patients based on personalized multi-OMICS driven data and will be further grading the patients to conclude who is most likely to gain from targeted approach therapies [55]. In conclusion, the systems biology model approach determined by multi-OMICS data techniques may help in the future to augment the one-drug efficiency and surmount the developed resistant cancer cell phenotypes during chemotherapy or immunotherapy making them susceptible to targeted therapies and eventually for the betterment of patients' lives.

Acknowledgments Deepti Chopra thanks the Indian Council of Medical Research (ICMR), Delhi, India, for awarding Research Associateship (GAP-385) at CSIR-Indian Institute of Toxicology Research, Lucknow.

References

1. Hasin Y, Seldin M, Lusis A (2017) Multi-omics approaches to disease. Genome Biol 18 (1):1–15
2. Manzoni C, Kia DA, Vandrovcova J, Hardy J, Wood NW, Lewis PA, Ferrari R (2018) Genome, transcriptome and proteome: the rise of omics data and their integration in biomedical sciences. Brief Bioinform 19(2):286–302
3. Gallagher IJ, Jacobi C, Tardif N, Rooyackers O, Fearon K (2016, June) Omics/systems biology and cancer cachexia. In: Seminars in cell & developmental biology, vol 54. Academic Press, Cambridge, MA, pp 92–103
4. Yu KH, Snyder M (2016) Omics profiling in precision oncology. Mol Cell Proteomics 15 (8):2525–2536
5. Yan W, Xue W, Chen J, Hu G (2016) Biological networks for cancer candidate biomarkers discovery. Cancer Inform 15:S39458
6. Epstein RJ, Lin FP (2017) Cancer and the omics revolution. Aust Family Phys 46(4):189
7. Meyerson M, Gabriel S, Getz G (2010) Advances in understanding cancer genomes through second-generation sequencing. Nat Rev Genet 11:685–696
8. Rowley JD (1973) A new consistent chromosomal abnormality in chronic myelogenous leukaemia identified by quinacrine fluorescence and Giemsa staining. Nature 243:290–293
9. Network CGAR (2012) Comprehensive genomic characterization of squamous cell lung cancers. Nature 489:519
10. Kumar-Sinha C, Kalyana-Sundaram S, Chinnaiyan AM (2015) Landscape of gene fusions in epithelial cancers: seq and ye shall find. Genome Med 7:129
11. Tsai HY, Boonyapranai K, Sriyam S, Yu CJ, Wu SW, Khoo KH et al (2011) Glycoproteomics analysis to identify a glycoform on hapto-globin associated with lung cancer. Proteomics 11:2162–2170
12. Zhan X, Wang X, Desiderio DM (2013) Pituitary adenoma nitroproteomics: current status and perspectives. Oxidative Med Cell Longev 2013:580710
13. Guo T, Zhu Y, Gan CS, Lee SS, Zhu J, Wang H et al (2010) Quantitative proteomics discloses MET expression in mitochondria as a direct target of MET kinase inhibitor in cancer cells. Mol Cell Proteomics 9:2629–2641
14. Le Naour F, Brichory F, Misek DE, Brechot C, Hanash SM, Beretta L (2002) A distinct repertoire of autoantibodies in hepatocellular carcinoma identified by proteomic analysis. Mol Cell Proteomics 1:197–203
15. Pleasance ED, Cheetham RK, Stephens PJ, McBride DJ, Humphray SJ, Greenman CD et al (2010) A comprehensive catalogue of somatic mutations from a human cancer genome. Nature 463(7278):191–196. https://doi.org/10.1038/nature08658
16. Robinson JK (2005) Sun exposure, sun protection, and vitamin D. JAMA 294(12):1541–1543
17. Wu S, Han J, Laden F, Qureshi AA (2014) Long-term ultraviolet flux, other potential risk factors, and skin cancer risk: a cohort study. Cancer Epidemiol Biomark Prev 23(6):1080–1089. https://doi.org/10.1158/1055-9965.EPI-13-0821
18. Shen Y, Kim AL, Du R, Liu L (2016) Transcriptome analysis identifies the dysregulation of ultraviolet target genes in human skin cancers. PLoS One 11(9):e0163054. https://doi.org/10.1371/journal.pone.0163054
19. Berger MF, Levin JZ, Vijayendran K et al (2010) Integrative analysis of the melanoma transcriptome. Genome Res 20(4):413–427. https://doi.org/10.1101/gr.103697.109
20. Lambin P, Rios-Velazquez E, Leijenaar R, Carvalho S, Van Stiphout RG, Granton P, Zegers CM, Gillies R, Boellard R, Dekker A, Aerts HJ (2012) Radiomics: extracting more information from medical images using advanced feature analysis. Eur J Cancer 48(4):441–446
21. Lambin P, Leijenaar RT, Deist TM, Peerlings J, De Jong EE, Van Timmeren J, Sanduleanu S, Larue RT, Even AJ, Jochems A, van Wijk Y (2017) Radiomics: the bridge between medical imaging and personalized medicine. Nat Rev Clin Oncol 14(12):749–762

22. Aerts HJ, Velazquez ER, Leijenaar RT, Parmar C, Grossmann P, Carvalho S, Bussink J, Monshouwer R, Haibe-Kains B, Rietveld D, Hoebers F (2014) Decoding tumour phenotype by noninvasive imaging using a quantitative radiomics approach. Nat Commun 5(1):1–9

23. Chiesa-Estomba CM, Echaniz O, Larruscain E, Gonzalez-Garcia JA, Sistiaga-Suarez JA, Graña M (2019) Radiomics and texture analysis in laryngeal cancer. Looking for new frontiers in precision medicine through imaging analysis. Cancers 11(10):1409

24. Jain R, Poisson LM, Gutman D, Scarpace L, Hwang SN, Holder CA, Wintermark M, Rao A, Colen RR, Kirby J, Freymann J (2014) Outcome prediction in patients with glioblastoma by using imaging, clinical, and genomic biomarkers: focus on the nonenhancing component of the tumor. Radiology 272(2):484–493

25. Alic L, Niessen WJ, Veenland JF (2014) Quantification of heterogeneity as a biomarker in tumor imaging: a systematic review. PLoS One 9(10):e110300

26. Traverso A, Wee L, Dekker A, Gillies R (2018) Repeatability and reproducibility of radiomic features: a systematic review. Int J Rad Oncol Biol Phys 102(4):1143–1158

27. Yang F, Simpson G, Young L, Ford J, Dogan N, Wang L (2020) Impact of contouring variability on oncological PET radiomics features in the lung. Sci Rep 10(1):1

28. Fornacon-Wood I, Mistry H, Ackermann CJ, Blackhall F, McPartlin A, Faivre-Finn C, Price GJ, O'Connor JP (2020) Reliability and prognostic value of radiomic features are highly dependent on choice of feature extraction platform. Eur Radiol 30:6241–6250

29. Parmar C, Leijenaar RT, Grossmann P, Velazquez ER, Bussink J, Rietveld D, Rietbergen MM, Haibe-Kains B, Lambin P, Aerts HJ (2015) Radiomic feature clusters and prognostic signatures specific for lung and head & neck cancer. Sci Rep 5:11044

30. Mayerhoefer ME, Riedl CC, Kumar A, Gibbs P, Weber M, Tal I, Schilksy J, Schöder H (2019) Radiomic features of glucose metabolism enable prediction of outcome in mantle cell lymphoma. Eur J Nucl Med Mol Imaging 46(13):2760–2769

31. Sanduleanu S, Woodruff HC, De Jong EE, Van Timmeren JE, Jochems A, Dubois L, Lambin P (2018) Tracking tumor biology with radiomics: a systematic review utilizing a radiomics quality score. Radiother Oncol 127(3):349–360

32. Bodalal Z, Trebeschi S, Nguyen-Kim TD, Schats W, Beets-Tan R (2019) Radiogenomics: bridging imaging and genomics. Abdom Radiol 44(6):1960–1984

33. Segal E, Sirlin CB, Ooi C, Adler AS, Gollub J, Chen X, Chan BK, Matcuk GR, Barry CT, Chang HY, Kuo MD (2007) Decoding global gene expression programs in liver cancer by noninvasive imaging. Nat Biotechnol 25(6):675–680

34. Limkin EJ, Sun R, Dercle L, Zacharaki EI, Robert C, Reuzé S, Schernberg A, Paragios N, Deutsch E, Ferté C (2017) Promises and challenges for the implementation of computational medical imaging (radiomics) in oncology. Ann Oncol 28(6):1191–1206

35. Liu Z, Wang S, Di Dong JW, Fang C, Zhou X, Sun K, Li L, Li B, Wang M, Tian J (2019) The applications of radiomics in precision diagnosis and treatment of oncology: opportunities and challenges. Theranostics 9(5):1303

36. Guerrisi A, Loi E, Ungania S, Russillo M, Bruzzaniti V, Elia F, Desiderio F, Marconi R, Solivetti FM, Strigari L (2020) Novel cancer therapies for advanced cutaneous melanoma: the added value of radiomics in the decision making process–a systematic review. Cancer Med 9 (5):1603–1612

37. Byrd AL, Belkaid Y, Segre JA (2018) The human skin microbiome. Nat Rev Microbiol 16 (3):143

38. Parello CS (2020) Microbiomics. In: Translational systems medicine and Oral disease. Academic Press, Cambridge, MA, pp 137–162

39. Garrett WS (2015) Cancer and the microbiota. Science 348(6230):80–86

40. Helmink BA, Khan MW, Hermann A, Gopalakrishnan V, Wargo JA (2019) The microbiome, cancer, and cancer therapy. Nat Med 25(3):377–388

41. Sherwani MA, Tufail S, Muzaffar AF, Yusuf N (2018) The skin microbiome and immune system: potential target for chemoprevention? Photodermatol Photoimmunol Photomed 34 (1):25–34

42. Belkaid Y, Tamoutounour S (2016) The influence of skin microorganisms on cutaneous immunity. Nat Rev Immunol 16(6):353–366
43. Siegel R, Ma J, Zou Z, Jemal A (2014) Cancer statistics, 2014. CA Cancer J Clin 64:9–29
44. Yu Y, Champer J, Beynet D, Kim J, Friedman AJ (2015) The role of the cutaneous microbiome in skin cancer: lessons learned from the gut. J Drugs Dermatol 14(5):461–465
45. Górska A, Przystupski D, Niemczura MJ, Kulbacka J (2019) Probiotic bacteria: a promising tool in cancer prevention and therapy. Curr Microbiol 1:1–1
46. Foulongne V, Sauvage V, Hebert C, Dereure O, Cheval J, Gouilh MA, Pariente K, Segondy M, Burguière A, Manuguerra JC, Caro V (2012) Human skin microbiota: high diversity of DNA viruses identified on the human skin by high throughput sequencing. PLoS One 7(6):e38499
47. Harjes U (2020) Benevolent viruses in skin cancer. Nat Rev Cancer 20(1):2
48. Fessler J, Matson V, Gajewski TF (2019) Exploring the emerging role of the microbiome in cancer immunotherapy. J Immunother Cancer 7(1):108
49. Strickley JD, Messerschmidt JL, Awad ME, Li T, Hasegawa T, Ha DT, Nabeta HW, Bevins PA, Ngo KH, Asgari MM, Nazarian RM (2019) Immunity to commensal papillomaviruses protects against skin cancer. Nature 575(7783):519–522
50. Bashiardes S, Tuganbaev T, Federici S, Elinav E (2017) The microbiome in anti-cancer therapy. In: Seminars in immunology, vol 32. Academic Press, Cambridge, MA, pp 74–81
51. Raza MH, Gul K, Arshad A, Riaz N, Waheed U, Rauf A, Aldakheel F, Alduraywish S, Rehman MU, Abdullah M, Arshad M (2019) Microbiota in cancer development and treatment. J Cancer Res Clin Oncol 145(1):49–63
52. Ley RE, Hamady M, Lozupone C, Turnbaugh PJ, Ramey RR, Bircher JS, Schlegel ML, Tucker TA, Schrenzel MD, Knight R, Gordon JI (2008) Evolution of mammals and their gut microbes. Science 320(5883):1647–1651
53. Charbonneau MR, Isabella VM, Li N, Kurtz CB (2020) Developing a new class of engineered live bacterial therapeutics to treat human diseases. Nat Commun 11(1):1–1
54. Werner HM, Mills GB, Ram PT (2014) Cancer systems biology: a peek into the future of patient care? Nat Rev Clin Oncol 11(3):167
55. GuhaThakurta D, Sheikh NA, Meagher TC, Letarte S, Trager JB (2013) Applications of systems biology in cancer immunotherapy: from target discovery to biomarkers of clinical outcome. Expert Rev Clin Pharmacol 6(4):387–401

Artificial Intelligence in Skin Cancer: Diagnosis and Therapy

9

Trishala Das, Vijay Kumar, Amresh Prakash, and Andrew M. Lynn

Abstract

Skin cancer is one of the major public health problems worldwide. Its early diagnosis and timely therapy are immensely important in improving patient health. Thus, the improved and accessible diagnostic systems for skin cancer are the most potent determinant of getting the right treatment at the right time. The last two decades have seen unprecedented growth in the application of artificial intelligence (AI) for skin cancer research. Recent advancement in the computational power, digitization of medical imaging, rise of -omics data have accumulated a new opportunity. The ability of AI methods to detect hidden or unknown patterns from such complex datasets reveals their importance. The AI approach in skin cancer has helped to improve the diagnostic and therapeutic strategies, from risk assessment using genomic sequences, accessible smartphone-based "apps" for diagnosis to predict the likelihood of therapy response amidst others. This technology holds a promising potential to automate and assist primary clinicians in improving patient health outcomes through effective diagnostic and therapy strategies using the complex healthcare data paving in the way for precision medicine.

T. Das · A. M. Lynn
School of Computational & Integrative Sciences, Jawaharlal Nehru University, New Delhi, India

V. Kumar
Amity Institute of Neuropsychology & Neurosciences (AINN), Amity University, Noida, Uttar Pradesh, India

A. Prakash (✉)
Amity Institute of Integrative Sciences and Health, Amity University Haryana, Gurgaon, India
e-mail: aprakash@ggn.amity.edu; amreshprakash@jnu.ac.in

A. Dwivedi et al. (eds.), *Skin Cancer: Pathogenesis and Diagnosis*,
https://doi.org/10.1007/978-981-16-0364-8_9

143

Keywords

Skin cancer · Melanoma · Non-melanoma · Artificial intelligence · Machine learning · Deep learning · Convolutional neural network · Image analysis · Targeted therapy

Abbreviations

2-D	Two-dimensional
3-D	Three-dimensional
AI	Artificial intelligence
AK	Actinic keratosis
ANN	Artificial neural network
apps	Applications
ATAC-seq	Assay for transposase-accessible chromatin using sequencing
AUC	Area under the curve
BCC	Basal cell carcinoma
CADe	Computer-aided detection
CADx	Computer-aided diagnosis
cDNA	Complementary DNA
ChIPseq	Chromatin immunoprecipitation
CNN	Convolutional neural network
CT	Computed tomography
CTCs	Circulating tumor cells
CUPs	Cancer of unknown primary
DL	Deep learning
DNA	Deoxyribonucleic acid
DNN	Deep neural network
DTRs	Dynamic treatment regimes
EHRs	Electronic health records
EMRs	Electronic medical records
FDA	Food and drug administration
GANs	Generative adversarial networks
GATK	Genome analysis toolkit
GDL	Genome deep learning
GWAS	Genome-wide association studies
H&E	Hematoxylin and Eosin
HAM10000	Human Against Machine with 10,000 training images
HLA	Human leukocyte antigen
IHC	Immunohistochemistry
ISIC	International Skin Imaging Collaboration
ISRO	Indian Space Research Organization
KSC	Keratinocyte skin cancer
MCC	Merkel cell carcinoma

MHC	Major histocompatibility complex
ML	Machine learning
MRI	Magnetic resonance imaging
mRNA	Messenger RNA
MSC	Melanoma skin cancer
NGS	Next-generation sequencing
NLP	Natural language processing
NMSC	Non-melanoma skin cancer
NNs	Neural networks
OTR	Organ transplant recipients
PCA/DA	Principal component analysis discriminant analysis
PET	Positron emission tomography
PLS/DA	Partial least squares discriminant analysis
PPIs	Protein–protein interactions
PRS	Polygenic risk score
RNA	Ribonucleic acid
ROIs	Region of interests
SCC	Squamous cell carcinoma
scRNAseq	Single-cell RNA sequencing
SKCM	Skin cutaneous melanoma
SNPs	Single nucleotide polymorphisms
SVMs	Support vector machines
TA	Texture analysis
TCGA	The cancer genome atlas
TD	Teledermatology
TDD	Teledermoscopy
TF	Transcription factor
TMB	Tumor mutational burden
T-VEC	Talimogene laherparepvec
UM	University of Michigan
US	Ultrasound
UV	Ultraviolet
WES	Whole exome sequencing
WHO	World Health Organization

9.1 Introduction

The highest reported cancer globally is the occurrence of skin cancer. And, the most common types are melanoma and keratinocyte skin cancer (KSC), particularly characterized by light pigmented skin populations. This rising incidence of skin cancer is mainly attributed by the increased exposure to ultraviolet (UV) radiation. Stabilization of mortality rates of melanoma in the USA, Australia, and in European countries probably reflects the success of the new systemic treatments [1]. The ongoing trends towards thinner melanoma are mainly attributed to earlier diagnosis [1, 2]. This gives motivation for developing methods relevant from diagnosis to therapy. Generally, skin cancer diagnoses are mainly determined visually which involves clinical screening, dermoscopic analysis, biopsy test, and histopathological examination [3].

In recent years, the applications of artificial intelligence (AI) have been shown their efficacy to accurately differentiate skin lesions in the diagnosis of skin cancer. Many studies suggest that the medical applications of AI can perform better for the automated classification of skin lesions in diagnosing the disease [1, 3, 4]. Although the images processing is a challenging task to characterize and detect the fine-grained variability. To improve the classification accuracy of skin lesions, the potential ability of deep convolutional neural networks (CNNs) can be exploited for general classification to highly variable tasks, categorizing for the fine-grained objects [1, 3]. Thus, the potential of AI to analyze the complex abundant data to find relevant hidden features is preferentially being used as an opportunity in diagnosing the skin lesions to overcome the standard practices [5–7]. However, the robustness of AI on the clinical diagnosis of diseases relies on the ability of scalability, accuracy, and the integration of clinical augments for the potential impact in medical diagnostic scenarios [8–10].

The domain of AI makes machine-based inferences using statistical and machine learning algorithms. The subdomain of AI, machine learning (ML) uses algorithms for recognizing relationships and patterns from available training data for clustering or classifying new data samples [3, 11, 12]. A recently introduced branch of ML, deep learning (DL), has been shown for effectively identifying such patterns in skin cancer research. These algorithms have led to the development of computer-aided diagnostics, prognostic models, monitoring drug efficacies, and predicting treatment response. The underlying biology of this cancer has also been studied using -omics data. AI models have been widely used and accepted for detecting malignancy in images. Thus, this technology holds the promising potential to provide information to primary clinicians and patients which can effectively guide diagnosis, reduce delays in diagnosis and the improvement of therapeutic strategies in the clinical treatment of skin cancer [3, 6, 12–14].

9.1.1 Overview of Skin Cancer

The report of World Health Organization (WHO) approximates that one in every three cases of cancer is being diagnosed as skin cancer, globally each year (https://www.who.int/news-room/q-a-detail/ultraviolet-(uv)-radiation-and-skin-cancer). It is an uncontrollable growth of abnormal skin cells caused by unrepaired DNA damage that triggers mutations. These mutations generally develop in areas exposed to UV radiation. However, they can also be found in body parts unexposed to sunlight. The white-skinned populations generally have a much higher risk of developing skin cancers than colored populations due to their relative lack of skin pigment, the melanin [15–17]. In addition to lightly pigmented skin, chronic exposure to UV radiation, light-colored hair, blue, green, or hazel eyes, deep tanning, i.e., tendency to burn rather than a suntan, family or personal history, genetics, smoking are other risk factors [18, 19]. Individual risk factors for developing skin cancer are abnormal sized moles, precancerous skin lesions, exposure to carcinogenic substances, immunomodulation, and immunosuppression, and transplant patients have also been shown to predispose to the development of skin cancer [20–22].

Skin cancer is primarily divided into Non-Melanoma Skin Cancer (NMSC) and Melanoma Skin Cancer (MSC).Non-melanoma skin cancer (NMSC) represents a major skin cancer occurrence, particularly in the white-skinned population. Also known as keratinocyte skin cancer (KSC) they account for 1/third of all reported cancers in the USA with over 600,000 new cases a year [23]. The occurrence of NMSC is attributed to the combination of genetic, environmental, and phenotypic factors. Exposure to UV light and genetic mutations are important cofactors [24]. Usually, the organ transplant recipients (OTR) and immunosuppressed patients are strongly susceptible to NMSC [24]. The head and neck regions are the most frequent sites for NMSC. The most common forms of NMSC are basal cell carcinoma (BCC) and squamous cell carcinoma (SCC). Among them, BCC is the most common cancer accounts for the growing public health care problem. Though the metastasis is reported extremely rare in the case of BCC, but the high risk of metastasis in SCC turns to be lethal [24, 25].

BCC originates in certain cells from the basal layer of the epidermis and its appendages, which are the most commonly on sun-exposed areas, e.g., face, nose, ears, and the backs of hands, but it may spread anywhere on the body. Although BCC is a slow-growing cancer, rarely metastasizes. Thus, the life-threatening risk is low, but may cause significant morbidity due to local invasion. However, a slight increase in this risk has been found with more aggressive BCC subtypes for which the surgery remains the mainstay of treatment [19, 23, 26]. Based on the distinct characteristics and histologic findings, typically three subtypes of BCC, superficial, nodular, and infiltrative (morphea form) have been reported [27–29]. The nodular BCC is the most common subtype followed by superficial BCC and infiltrative subtype. Of these three, infiltrative BCC is generally thought to be the most aggressive. It displays a high risk for local destruction, thus requiring timely management [23].

The SCC originates from the epidermal keratinocytes, and is the most lethal due to metastatic property [23]. This cancer type is further divided into invasive, clear-cell, spindle cell, verrucous, and sarcomatoid SCC. Besides, the multiple precursor lesions such as actinic keratosis (AK) and Bowen's disease also fall under the umbrella of SCC. Thus, the risk factors for the recurrence of cutaneous SCC must be taken into account [17, 27, 29].

Other rare pathologies of NMSC also exist which include cutaneous lymphoma, Kaposi's sarcoma, Merkel cell carcinoma (MCC), and angiosarcomas [27, 30]. Among them, MCC is the high-risk form of NMSC, considering the rising incidence and poor prognosis [31]. Recent studies on MCC suggest that existence of nodal metastasis in 26% of cases with distant metastasis in 8%cases. They also observed a significant correlation between the extent of disease and five-year survival which recommend the prompt diagnosis of MCC in the clinical management of NMSC [32].

Melanoma skin cancer originates from the pigment-producing skin cells (melanocytes). Although it is less common but has high metastatic properties. The prognostic approach of cutaneous melanoma involves the depth and location of primary tumor, and the absence or presence of localized and distant metastasis [27]. It is suggested that early diagnosis may result in at least 5 years survival in up to 95% cases [33]. The most common subtype of melanoma cancer is superficial spreading melanoma. Present as a mole, a pigmented skin lesion that changes size, shape, or color. Other subtypes of melanoma include nodular melanoma, lentigo maligna, and acral lentiginous melanoma. Based on the genomic alterations, large-scale of RNA sequencing efforts results in the classification of four major subtypes of melanoma, which are (1) BRAF-mutant, (2) NRAS-mutant, (3) NF1-deficient, and (4) triple wild-type [30, 34]. Furthermore, these studies also suggest that the occurrence of mutation in melanoma genomes is higher as compared to other forms of cancers which result in high neoantigen load [35]. People with pigmented or Asian skin are more susceptible to acral lentiginous melanoma than the Caucasian population [36, 37]. Over the last 30 years, the incidences of melanoma have quadrupled in the Caucasian population and are also assumed to increase incidence over the next 20 years [22]. This makes early detection and improved treatment vital for improving patient survival.

With the evident of global rise in skin cancer cases, early diagnosis and effective therapy are gaining considerable attention. Much progress has been made for metastatic melanoma, evident in the literature. Traditionally, the skin cancer diagnosis involves dermatologists screening the suspicious skin lesions using their experience. They also include clinical information of the patient, like their age, location of the lesion among others. This is followed by biopsy and histopathology for confirmation. Although both of them are standard methods for definitive diagnosis, a biopsy is an invasive procedure with limitations [38, 39]. Histopathology, on the other hand, is time-consuming, often delaying diagnosis and management of the skin lesions [40]. Several non-invasive imaging technologies have emerged in recent years to overcome these diagnostic challenges. Techniques like coherence tomography microscopic imaging, confocal microscopy, dermoscopy, fluorescence, reflectance, and Raman spectroscopy showed promising results in diagnosis [41]. Recent development in dermoscopic techniques has been greatly improving the diagnostic accuracy of both pigmented and non-pigmented lesions [42]. The advantages of dermoscopy involve its ease of operating, shorten observation times, and allow better visualization of skin subsurface structures revealing lesion details [43]. However, this tool is an operator-dependent test, requiring training and experience in "pattern analysis" which refers to concurrent assessment of the diagnostic features of lesions [44]. Furthermore, the strong lack of efficient dermatologists and the availability of advanced dermatoscopes in the developing countries [38, 39, 42]. In the previous two decades, the computer-based systems, computer-aided detection (CADe), and computer-aided diagnosis (CADx) have been widely explored for assisting the doctors in making clinical decisions [45, 46], comprised of multiple approaches, AI, ML, computer vision, and medical image processing [47]. Thus, there is the great need of computer-based systems for the diagnosis of skin cancer which can be easy and efficiently distinguished the skin lesions.

9.1.2 Artificial Intelligence (AI) and Its Applications in Healthcare

The ability of AI to extract analytical information from the complex images and sophisticated medical reports, both structured and unstructured data, decisive for the clinical decisions makes it a widely accepted technique in the improvement of healthcare management systems [5, 9, 48, 49]. The advantages of this technology have been extensively discussed in the medical literature for better prevention, detection, diagnosis, and treatment of disease [48, 49]. The structured data can be stored in computer and able to display in a consistent and organized manners, which include numerical values, e.g., height, weight, and blood pressure, categorical values, e.g., blood types, and the ordinal values defining the stages of disease diagnosis. Whereas the unstructured data residing in the electronic medical records (EMRs) and electronic health records (EHRs) which lacks the organization and structural precision. One of the biggest problems associated with healthcare system is that the inaccessibility of large amount of medical data (approximately 80%) which remains unstructured and untapped, during the clinical diagnostic and treatments (e.g., text, image, signal, etc.) [38, 40]. With the advancement in healthcare organizations, have started to leverage the implication of AI for the access of plethora of unstructured data from patients which may include images and videos, bio-signal data of patients that are been displayed on the screen of monitoring systems with wearable health monitoring devices, and the audio data that are verbally or nonverbally created from the patient's pathophysiologically, in operating rooms or intensive care units [38–40]. Thus, the ability to extract information from a large set of data of patient's population makes AI crucial for real-time inferences of clinical health management systems.

Based on strength, breadth, and applicability, AI can further be classified into Narrow or Weak AI, Generalized or Strong AI, and Conscious or Super AI. In the current scenario, we have only gained access to narrow AI, where a machine learns to complete a single goal. The application of AI in medicine involves major two branches, virtual and physical. The inference of ML and algorithms for diagnosis, sorting, and treatment define under the virtual component, whereas physical components include the extrapolation of data from the medical devices and the delivering care through robots [41].

The field of AI encompasses machine learning or ML uses mathematical and statistical approaches to enhance the performance of computers [42]. It is the scientific discipline that utilizes computer algorithms to learn from data, identify patterns to make predictions. Identifying such patterns from data has provided an unprecedented opportunity for the discovery of biomarkers. A biomarker is defined as a feature that is indicative of a disease state, response to therapy, or another relevant biological state [43]. ML uses two types of data: "labeled" and "unlabeled data" for making models. Labeled data has an associated tag or an outcome assigned to it. Unlabeled data has no such assigned labels to it. The learning of machines can be supervised learning, unsupervised learning, and semi-supervised. Unsupervised learning is a well-known approach for the extraction of features, whereas the supervised learning approach is suitable for the development of predictive models which involves the building of relationships between the inputs as patient traits and outcomes (output) in terms of defined interest. In the recent years, the hybrid technique of supervised and unsupervised which also known as semi-supervised learning is observed as a suitable method for scenarios where the outcome is missing for certain subjects. Relevant techniques used in supervised machine learning include rigorous regression analyses, naive bayes classifiers, nearest neighbor, decision tree, random forest, discriminant analysis, support vector machine (SVM), and neural network (NN). Whereas the unsupervised learning includes clustering and principal component analysis (PCA) as the two major components. For the supervised learning, algorithm is developed by supplying the labeled data which define as learning process for desired output. Thus, for the classification of images as diseased or non-diseased, the classification algorithm is supplied with images, as features and the categorical data labeled as diseased or non-diseased. In unsupervised learning, unlabeled data is used for the learning algorithm, to identify patterns from input data. The other technique, reinforcement learning which is a hybrid method, learns by interacting with the environment trial and error search receiving feedback from its actions. This learning has been utilized to automate the discovery and generation of optimal DTRs (Dynamic Treatment Regimes) in a variety of chronic diseases including cancer [40, 50]. In 2017, Fei Jiang and colleagues surveyed the machine learning algorithms used in the medical literature in PubMed [13, 44]. This search suggests that SVM and neural networks are the popular choices of modeling; however, SVMs are preferred as they can achieve considerable generalizability and are reliable for the classification of new samples. Useful in dichotomous classification, this algorithm performs optimally as it maps the input vector onto a feature space of higher dimensionality. It then finds the best hyperplane separating the data points in two clusters. This visualization ease of boundary decision along with producing higher accuracy makes it favorable. On the other hand, neural network (NNs) which work on the principle of linear regression can be used to estimate the complex non-linear relationships between the input and output variables. And the multiple hidden layers with the amalgamations of prespecified functionals are used to depict the functionalities between the input and outcome variables. Neural networks can be "shallow" or "deep" depending on the number of hidden layers as shown in Fig. 9.1.

Deep learning (DL), which is also define as the modern extension of classical NNmethod, and acts as subfield of ML, is characterized by the operation of multi-layered artificial neural networks [38, 39, 41, 50]. The rapid advancement in the modern computing system enables the development NN system having many hidden layers, serving the feasibility of DL which enables to explore more complex data, having non-linear patterns. In the clinical applications, the more commonly used DL

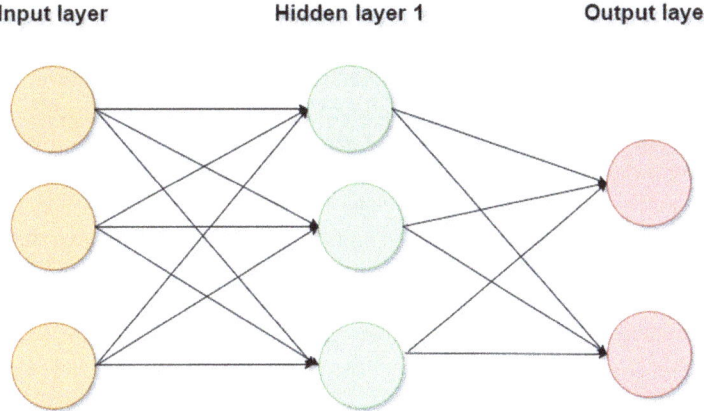

Fig. 9.1 Diagrammatic illustration of neural networks with a shallow structure. Here, the shallow neural network is represented by one hidden layer. It is the basic neural network though deep neural networks can have up to "nth" hidden layers, located in between the input and output. In this algorithm, the weighted functions assigned to the inputs in this hidden layer which directs the output happens through the activation function

algorithms for handling the medical data include convolutional neural network (CNN), recurrent neural network (RRN), deep neural network machine learning (DNN-ML), and deep belief network (DBN) algorithms.

Considering the accelerating growth in the healthcare sector, AI has been the key driver in (generation) of novel diagnostics, risk assessment, and therapeutic interventions. Globally, there are considerable efforts ongoing in the development and application of standard and novel artificial intelligence methods towards biomarker discovery pattern recognition from different-different sources, e.g., omics data, medical images, and hospital records.

9.2   Application of AI in the Early Detection of Skin Cancer

The rising incidence of skin cancer cases has burdened the patient care health management system to opt for the new strategies for improvising the fast and accurate diagnosis outcomes. This trend can be counteracted using primary prevention (avoidance of risk factors) and secondary prevention (secondary prevention) [16]. However, the overall survival rate depends on the type and stage of skin cancer. According to the melanoma research alliance (MRA), the five-year survival rate for melanoma stages 0, 1, and 2 is 98.4% and for stage 3 melanoma and stage 4 is 63.6% and 22.5%. For basal cell carcinoma, the survival rate is five-years for almost 100% cases, whereas the survival rate for squamous cell carcinoma is predicted as 5 years in the 95% cases, according to the Canadian Cancer Society.

Thus, for the early detection of skin cancer, necessarily required the identification of people who are prone to develop skin cancer. Environmental risk factors and personal or family history, skin type, and the number of melanocytic nevi are used as risk (group) markers for primary prevention. Apart from risk (group) markers, different classes of biomarkers have already been used in skin cancer research. They are classified as exposure markers, internal dose markers, biologically effective dose and altered structure markers, markers of susceptibility, markers for diagnostics, prognosis, progression, and metastasis [46, 47]. The field of AI has increased specificity and sensitivity of the biomarker identification and has made previously unknown revelations. AI in skin cancer diagnosis involves discovering information from medical images and array-based techniques fueling efficient and new studies in the field. Traditional diagnosis of skin cancer was dependent on the accessibility and experience of the primary clinicians. AI has led to improvement of traditional diagnostic systems to non-invasive and accessible CAD systems.

9.2.1 Image-Based Detection

An innovation of AI was the development of CADx systems for skin cancer detection using medical image analysis. It is a fundamental method for recognizing, differentiating, and quantifying diverse types of images [48, 49]. The typical steps involve in a CADx using images for skin cancer are summarized in Fig. 9.2.

The typical steps for the diagnosis of skin cancer from the image of skin lesions:

Step 1. *Image Acquisition for Screening Skin Lesions*: The input image is given to the system for unaided visual inspection of the skin.

Step 2. *Preprocessing*: This step involves a comprehensive examination of pigmented skin lesion which discriminate the lesion from a healthy skin. This step also includes the improvisation of the image data by enhancing the image quality while suppressing unwanted distortions. Preprocessing of images comprised of image resizing, contrast, and brightness adjustment. However, the dermoscopy images are often comprise with several artifacts which are noted as uneven illumination, black frames, dermoscopic gel, ink markings, rulers, intrinsic cutaneous features, and air bubbles, that are broadly affected the detection efficiency to differentiate between the blood vessels, skin lines and texture, and hairs [51, 52].

Step 3. *Segmentation*: This step is very crucial step for the scrutiny of skin lesion images which is done by removing the healthy and normal skin from the obtained image to differentiate the regions containing skin lesion. Segmentation divides an input image into regions or segments and defining the boundary for object detection as due to complexity of biological images, obtaining good segmentation is one of a difficult task [53]. Several segmentation techniques have been developed over the years, and also allowing its improvement in skin cancer image analysis [52, 54–56].

Step 4. *Feature Extraction*: Feature extraction involves measuring of certain properties or features that can reduce the original data from set, help to differentiate the input pattern from one and another. It includes the measurements of pixels which signify as the segmented object that allow the computing of several topographical features. Such features are also termed as "imaging biomarkers." An imaging biomarker for melanoma is defined as a quantitative metric extracted from a

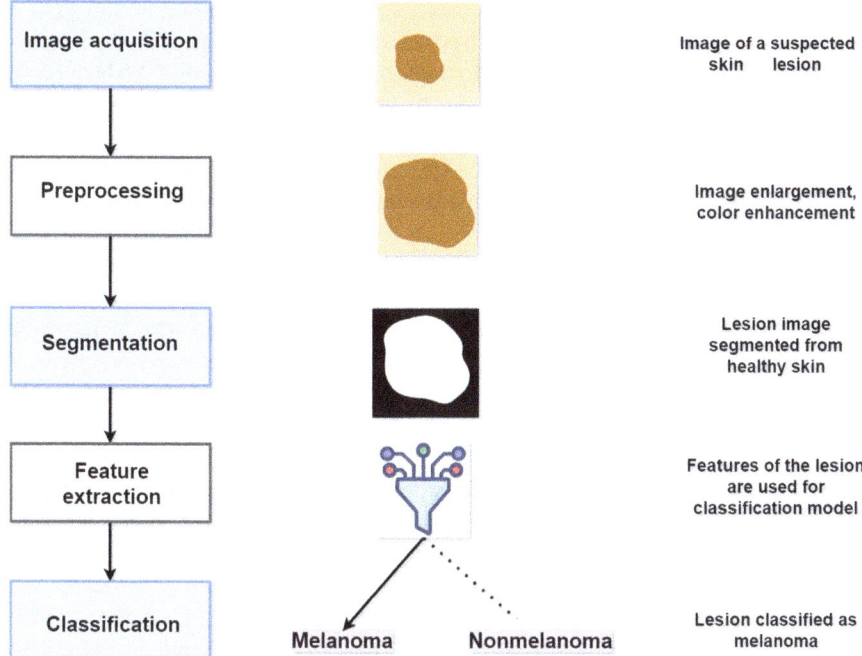

Fig. 9.2 A typical workflow for a CADx image analysis. This workflow shows an example of a suspected skin lesion for image analysis which involves five steps: the image acquisition, preprocessing, segmentation, feature extraction, and classification. Class labels are provided. Here, a suspected skin lesion is provided. Following image processing and segmentation, the extracted features and the model would classify the image into "melanoma" or "nonmelanoma." Here, the image has been classified as "melanoma." In machine learning models, features are either manually provided by the user or feature selection methods are used. Relevant features are automatically "learned" in the case of deep learning models

dermoscopy image using computer algorithms that is stated as 1 and 0 representing high for melanoma and low for a nevus, respectively [57]. Dimensions of imaging biomarkers are used to define the features which are associated with normal and pathological features. These features include symmetry of biomarkers images, number of colors, border, brightness, organization of pigmented network pattern, etc. [57]. Different feature extraction methods have been reported in the literature including the ABCD-E system, 7-point checklist, 3-point checklist, pattern analysis, and Menzies method to extract texture based features of the lesion which offers greater advantage [58]. Two methods are exclusively applied for feature extraction, ML and DL. ML models require manual extraction of features by the user, whereas DL models have the ability of automatic extraction of features.

Step 5. *Classification*: The classification phase is the most important step in developing a reliable diagnostic system. Hence, the above steps must be dealt with precisely or near to produce unbiased results. For the classification of images, two different approaches have been explored which includes (1) the dichotomous classification for assigning "class" labels to the data item, in terms of "0" or "1", (2) and the second model assigns a "class" label along with the probability of class membership. SVMs are used for dichotomous classification problems. ANN, logistic regression, nearest neighbors, and decision trees are the algorithms used in the second approach [41, 58].

9.2.1.1 Dermatoscopic Images and Datasets for the Development of AI-Based Model

Dermatoscopic (dermoscopic) images are commonly acquired using a dermatoscope (dermoscope), help to visualize structures of melanocytic skin lesions, diagnosis of benign nevi, and malignant melanoma and non-melanoma lesions. For dermoscopic observations of melanocytic lesions, the important features are colored structures of globules, pigment network, dots, and streaks which are used for non-melanoma skin cancer diagnosis [59]. However, for the development of efficient neural network based automated diagnostic model a large set of training and test set data are required which is now available as HAM10000 ("Human Against Machine with 10000 training images") and ISIC2020 (https://challenge2020.isic-archive.com/), preferentially can be explored for featurization of skin lesions as melanoma and non-melanoma skin cancer. The pioneer works on CADx systems reported the use of low-level handcrafted features for classifying melanoma and non-melanoma skin cancer [60, 61]. With time different computational approaches were developed for selecting features using ABCD(E) rule, pattern analysis, and 7-point checklist and feeding them to a classifier [54, 62, 63]. However, these approaches are associated with two major drawbacks: (1) they are applicable for pigmented lesions, only and (2) it could not help to differentiate BCC or SCC and further lacks for the generalization of extracted features [64].

In recent years, the developments of AI-based approach which includes DL and CNN models are gaining popularity in developing CADx. In 2018, Brinker et al. [65] had performed the systematic review of skin cancer using CNN to classify the skin lesions and detecting melanoma from image data. The well-known CNN architectures used for image classification are AlexNet [66], VGG [67], GoogLeNet [68], and ResNet [69] which can be used for learning from the scratch. Another study on the skin cancer detection using DL and sound analysis algorithms for the classification of dermal cell images helps researchers and practitioners in building DL models without any programming [70, 71]. Similarly, studies focused on wavelet-based logistic discriminator of melanoma images and multiclass skin cancer classification using five pre-trained CNNs, and the ensemble of four models, suggest maximum 93.20% accuracy for individual models and among the model sets and maximum 92.83% accuracy was obtained for ensemble models [72].

A major breakthrough was achieved in 2017, Esteva et al. [3, 50] used a pre-trained CNN architecture (GoogleNet Inception v3) to train over 129,450 mobile photographic images and applied binary classification for achieving dermatologist-level diagnostic classification of benign nevi versus malignant melanomas. Similarly, DL and Google's Inception v4 CNN models were developed to classify dermoscopic melanoma images which can accurately diagnose melanoma, having accuracy >0.87 [73, 74]. Remarkably, the recent advancement in AI models for the skin lesions diagnosis successfully demonstrated higher accuracy in skin tumor diagnosis [75–77]. This may lead to the conclusion that CNN based diagnostic systems may help dermatologists, irrespective of their experience. Other effort methods of DL such as feature aggregation of different models, an ensemble of models, among others have been implemented.

Another implication of AI has been seen in diagnosing melanoma from two-dimensional (2-D) and three-dimensional (3-D) skin lesions. Recent studies highlighted the importance of "depth" for melanoma as it is "skin deep." This 3-D reconstruction technique is used to estimate the depth of dermoscopic images which provide the basis for features extraction along with regular color, texture, and 2-D shape features [78–80]. Apart from melanoma, in-situ melanoma, the proposed system also can apply to diagnose BCC, dermatofibroma, blue nevus, seborrheic keratosis, hemangioma, and normal mole lesions. Most of the above studies used dermoscopic images as their training dataset. This may perhaps be due to the less availability of mobile photographic images. Recent efforts have been made for providing datasets composed of such images for skin cancer diagnosis. Pacheco et al.[81] introduced a new skin cancer dataset, PAD-UFES-20 dataset [82] which is composed by the images taken from patients using smartphones, and related clinical data. They developed an application that also allowed tracking of patient lesions followed by its evolution. These results suggest that the substantial clinical features are required for the improvement of CNN models performance. However, the classification of SCC and BCC remained challenging as they almost share the same clinical features. One of the major constraints associated with computer-aided diagnostic techniques for the classification of skin lesion is the scarcity of labeled data and imbalance class dataset. To improve the performance of classification model, Qin et al. proposed skin lesion style-based GANs that can produce high-quality skin lesion imaging [83], thus helping dermatologists in more accurate diagnostic decisions. The CADx systems work on the dermoscopic images, however, the availability of dermatoscope in most of the developing countries is very limited, which constrains the use of these systems.

Now, the many AI-based tools and methods have also been developed for finding hidden patterns or features. The majority of the NGS analysis tools are based on algorithms. GATK is one such example. Apart from GATK, Cerebro, Genome Deep Learning, CancerSPP, finding potential neoepitopes has been developed to drive skin cancer research. Most of them have supervised deep learning methods at their backends, mostly convolution neural networks. The transcriptional and epigenome machinery has also been investigated for its role. The mRNA expression levels and the chromatin state have been found as important predictors of the mutational landscape in cancer cells. Integrated analysis of RNAseq data, ChIPseq, and scRNAseq data to understand melanoma progression has been studied. The resulting combination of TF networks and PPIs has been said as potential drug targets in melanoma. This ability of AI to work with multi-modal data has powered precision medicine. The precision medicine approach takes individual variability in genes, environment, and lifestyle into account for prediction of prevention and treatment

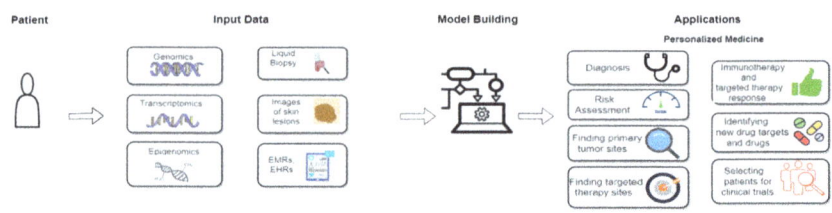

Fig. 9.3 An overview of the input datasets for skin cancer and the applications of AI in skin cancer research. Genomics, epigenomics, transcriptomics, liquid biopsy, images of lesions and patient healthcare records, EHRs, and EMRs are taken as "input data." These data are then used as input data for model building using artificial intelligence-based algorithms. These models then generate intelligence insights into the system and generate output. These "output data" pave the way from diagnosis to improvements in therapy and management for skin cancer patients

strategies may provide the best strength for the care of individual patient, as represented schematically in Fig. 9.3.

However, this impressive pace of AI in skin cancer diagnosis and therapy has certain drawbacks as most of the studies have used dermoscopic images. These images are enlarged and enhanced, under controlled lighting conditions. More diagnostic applications using clinical images are slowly showing up. This popularity of dermoscopy in literature can be attributed to its publicly available image datasets. Clinical(non-dermoscopic) image datasets are fewer in number compared to dermatoscopic images. Most of the available datasets are imbalanced (ISIC dataset, PAD-UFES-20 dataset). Therefore, effective methods for dealing with imbalanced datasets must be taken into account, like GAN based methods for synthetic image generation for the diagnostic accuracy of AI.

9.2.1.2 Mobile Applications in the Personal Monitoring of Skin Cancer

Bridging this gap, the CAD systems embedded in smartphones gained limelight offering accessibility and low cost for general users. With modern smartphones, the capturing of high-quality images is possible which provide a wealth for the development mobile apps, "skin," a chance for the better care of skin cancer patients [84]. Between the years 2014–17, approximately 235 new dermatology smartphone applications (apps) have been identified which uses an inbuilt AI algorithm that classifies lesion images in the range of low to high risk for the prevention and diagnosis of skin cancer, more precisely the melanoma skin cancer [85, 86]. These mobile apps can be explored as resource for the collection of information to assist the monitoring and self-examination of skin conditions, lesions as well as for providing the advice or guidance in the case of required medical attentions. These apps having "inbuilt algorithms" which can work as classified medical devices and able make medical decisions considering the claims and conditions of patients. However, these apps are required for regulatory approval which also comes under the authority of FDA, https://ec.europa.eu/docsroom/documents/17921). Similarly, the smartphone apps for mobile medical applications approved by EU Medical Device Directive come under "class 1 devices." The potential ability of theses apps for the earlier diagnosis and treatment of skin lesions may influence the survival of patients. Apps like Miiskin(https://miiskin.com/), UMSkinCheck (http://myhealthapps.net/app/details/123/umskincheck), MoleScope(www.molescope.com), SkinVision (https://www.skinvision.com/about), among others are available for personalized diagnosis. Miiskin able to capture the hi-resolution digital images, used for mole mapping to analyze the skin conditions. UMSkinCheck developed at the School of Medicine, University of Michigan (UM) allows users, full-body self-assessment of skin cancer, as well as the tracking of moles history, their growths, and lesions. The app, MoleScope installed on smartphone is devised to capture and share photos with dermatologist, thus facilitate the online checkup of patients. SkinVision claims to aid early detection of melanoma. In 2019, Freeman and colleagues carried out a systematic review on the diagnostic accuracy studies of algorithm-based smartphone-based apps [86] which suggest the higher diagnostic accuracy of SkinVision as compared to SkinScan (https://teleskin.org/skinscan.html). Thus, these AI-based technologies are promising and helpful to bridge the gap where some patients are not provided with quality dermatological care facilitating personal monitoring.

9.2.1.3 Teledermatology and Teledermoscopy in the Detection of Skin Cancer

Dermatology, the field of medicine dealing with skin is particularly well-suited for telemedicine. Ubiquitous access to information and communication technologies provides ease in virtual conversations. Teledermatology (TD), on the other hand, is a subspecialty of dermatology that uses these technologies, facilitating the diagnosis, monitoring, treatment, preventions, collection of data for research, as well as to educate people over a distance which makes easier accessibility for the patients care [87, 88]. However, it has both pros and cons to it as it depends on good quality patient images to make inferences [87]. To facilitate the growth of telemedicine, Indian Space Research Organization (ISRO) has taken initiatives and pilot projects have been launched in 2001, aiming the needs of rural India for delivering dermatology care which can help diagnose many cases that otherwise would have left unattended.

For the sequential monitoring of skin lesions, especially in Brazil and many Asian and African countries, where the access to dermatologists is limited, teledermoscopy (TDD) plays important role which involve the AI-based image analysis method for acquisition and storage of digital dermoscopic images [89]. For automating such a situation, a mobile application system has been developed which employs internet cloud computing to access image-based diagnostic databases and delivers possibilities of diagnosis and differential classification of lesions which also provide assistance to the non-dermatologist physician. Recently TDD has been gaining attention for its efficiency. It was found comparable to a human expert in the field of medical management and diagnosis of hospitalized patients beside the skin conditions [90]. Hence, these techniques provide a suitable alternative for the care patients in absence of a dermatologist or can be associated with assisting the clinicians. It has also been used for the diagnosis of pigmented skin lesions [91].

9.2.2 Clinical Data-Based Skin Cancer Detection

After virtual screening of skin lesions by the dermatologist, pathological examinations remain the gold standard for the final diagnosis which is primarily carried out using a tissue biopsy. In a tissue biopsy diagnosis, the fine slices from tissue specimen are used to prepare the slides, and the slides staining with Hematoxylin and Eosin (H&E) dye are used to study under the microscope by the certified histopathologist. If the pathologist observed suspicious lesion of melanoma, then the immunohistochemistry method is applied for further confirmation of cancerous lesions [92]. These examinations are however time-consuming and tedious. Efficient automated techniques have been developed for the diagnosis of skin whole-slide images, which consist of the modules of five techniques: (1) epidermis segmentation, (2) keratinocytes segmentation, (3) melanocytes detection, (4) feature construction, and (5) classification [93]. Based on the pathological examination of segmented epidermis, keratinocytes and melanocytes, pathologists can determine the regions of interest(ROIs), which helps to define the morphological features and spatial distribution of lesions. These specified features are used as classifier for SVM, resulting in approximately 90% accuracy, thus such high-performance classification provides remarkable assistance to pathologist in the histopathological diagnosis and analysis of skin tissue. Another study using histopathological classification of melanoma images with DNN, when trained with 595 histopathologic images of melanomas and nevi suggested that images from digital whole-slide images were cropped randomly [94]. Such information can be explored for the comparative classification of human pathological examination, using machine learning. Thus, on-par performance explains the ability of AI to mine "subvisual" image features that have been never observed by dermatologist using the naked eye [95, 96].

In clinical practice, the dermatologists along with the screening skin lesion also used clinical data of the patient. The electronic medical record (EMR) was initially introduced as a health tool for improving patient health. According to the National Cancer Institute, an EMR is a collection of medical information about a person that is stored on a computer (https://www.cancer.gov/publications/dictionaries/cancer-terms/def/electronic-medical-record). This information is generally found in a provider's paper chart: diagnoses, medical history, allergies, medications, immunizations, lab results, and doctor's notes. This digitized version has both structured and unstructured formats. The structured data consist of laboratory tests, diagnosis codes, drug orders, and medications, whereas the text-based radiology reports, pathology findings, and clinical progress notes are stored as unstructured data [97]. The digitized records of EMRs combined with the longitudinal overview of a specific patient are referred to as an EHR (Electronic health records), which are used for tracking the health progression of patients over time [98]. With the advent of widespread connectivity and remote server accessibility, skin cancer research has benefited from the use of EMRs. Recently, this digitized version of information has been deciphered using Natural Language Processing (NLP), the technique used to identify the target texts and transform into machine-readable structured data, which can be assessed by applying ML approach [44]. This device of AI is used to extract findings from the clinical unstructured data, clinical notes, and medical journals, as supplementary data for the enrichment of existing structured medical data. This pipeline involves text processing using NLP which identifies the user provided keywords from the supplied medical records and clinical notes available in the databases and the classification [44, 99]. For the evaluation of classification, a subset of the keywords is selected and applied on normal and disease cases to examine their effects. After that, the validated keywords used to enter and enrich the structured data to support clinical decision making. Thus, the availability of patient clinical data is equally important to tune the AI models for the substantial improvement in the prediction accuracy [81, 100].

9.3 Artificial Intelligence in Skin Cancer Therapy

The conventional approach of skin cancer therapy involves skin biopsy and the removal of precancerous skin lesions (actinic keratoses) which depends on the type, size, location, and depth of the lesions. Additional treatment includes cryosurgery, excisional surgery, Mohs surgery, curettage and electrodesiccation radiation therapy, chemotherapy, biological therapy along with site-directed therapy and immunotherapy. Understanding the cancer landscape can only facilitate the development of new effective therapy. This is due to the high complexity and heterogeneity of cancer, characterized by a series of genetic, metabolic, and functional changes at the cellular and tissue level. Now, the existence of computational or mathematical models assisted melanoma diagnosis can give better emphasis on the complex interaction of molecular network, suggesting the novel strategies for individualized patient treatment, decisions about the novel molecular drug targets, optimization of immunotherapies, and personalized medicine trials [101, 102]. This may give a direction that cancer needs to be understood from a holistic perspective of the integration of images and omics data.

To unravel the complexity of the disease, next-generation sequencing (NGS) is one of the other advance techniques which can tackle the high dimensional -omics data to enable a deeper understanding of the disease complexity. There are three major areas where AI can be used within -omics data analysis. The first involves obtaining optimal coverage across the genome or region (that is, the gene of interest) followed by mapping or assembly of the reads to the genome. Another prominent application of AI includes the identification of variants. Several AI-based tools including the Genome Analysis Toolkit (GATK) (https://gatk.broadinstitute.org/hc/en-us) have been developed for identifying SNPs and small insertions and deletions (indels) in germline DNA and RNA Seq data. Once variants are called, the next step is to determine which variants are statistically or clinically relevant. Here, AI can be used to detect patterns of variants (mutations) within healthy or diseased patients, for instance, to determine which variants are relevant. These steps are labor-intensive. Hence, AI has drastically reduced the time and effort in finding key clinical drivers. These genome sequences and variants have also made big revelations in cancer diagnosis and therapy. One of the important aspects of cancer therapy is determining the staging of the patient and stratifying patients into low or high risk.

9.3.1 Risk Assessment Models

The conventional approach of skin cancer therapy involves skin biopsy and the removal of precancerous skin lesions (actinic keratoses) which depends on the type, size, location, and depth of the lesions. Additional treatment includes cryosurgery, Mohs surgery, excisional surgery, curettage, chemotherapy, electrodesiccation radiation therapy, biological therapy along with site-directed therapy and immunotherapy. Understanding the cancer landscape can only facilitate the development of new effective therapy. This is due to the high complexity and heterogeneity of cancer, identified by several changes at the molecular, cellular, and tissue level. Now, the existence of computational or mathematical models assisted melanoma diagnosis can give better emphasis on the complex interaction of molecular network, suggesting the novel strategies for individualized patient treatment, decisions about the novel molecular drug targets, optimization of immunotherapies, and personalized medicine trials [101, 102]. This may give a direction that cancer needs to be understood from a holistic perspective of the integration of images and omics data.

To unravel the complexity of the disease, next-generation sequencing (NGS) is one of the other advance techniques which can tackle the high dimensional -omics data to enable a deeper understanding of the disease complexity. The three central areas where application of AI can be used for -omics data analysis involve obtaining optimal genome coverage or a specific gene followed by mapping or assembly of the reads to the genome. Another prominent application of AI includes the identification of variants. Several AI-based tools including the Genome Analysis Toolkit (GATK) (https://gatk.broadinstitute.org/hc/en-us) have been developed for identifying variants (mutations) in germline DNA and RNA-Seq data. Once the variants are being called, finding which of these are statistically or clinically relevant is the next step. Here, AI can be used to distinguish variant patterns from healthy and diseased patients for determining relevant variants. These steps are labor-intensive. Hence, AI has drastically reduced the time and effort in finding key clinical drivers. These genome sequences and variants have also made big revelations in cancer diagnosis and therapy. One of the important aspects of cancer therapy is determining the staging of the patient and stratifying patients into low or high risk.

9.3.2 Risk Assessment Models

The staging of cancer is crucial for planning the course of therapy for the patient. Staging describes the growth and the possibility of metastatic spread. Basal and squamous cell carcinoma rarely metastasizes as compared to malignant melanoma. Hence, early diagnosis and prognosis of cancer are important as they can be used to inform patients and guide therapeutic management [103, 104]. Physical tests like imaging (CT scans, PET scans, X-rays, and ultrasound), biopsies of the suspected skin lesion, and blood test reports may also help in finding the stage of the cancer cells. Collectively the amalgamation of information from gene sequences, EMRs, images is essential for enrichment of AI-model to make it capable to predict the disease state accurately.

In 2019, Hsiao-Han Wang et al. used CNN to develop a novel prediction model for NMSC incidence accurately identifying individuals at high risk which was based on non-imaging and multidimensional medical information [105]. The EMR of every patient was transformed into an image-like matrix with longitudinal medical events. Several promising factors for prognosis like the history with precancerous lesions, usage of a-few photosensitizing medications were recognized. Another study associates important genomic level features that may play a role in contributing to the melanoma oncogenesis along with novel putative markers for cutaneous melanoma metastasis using genomic profiles of patients. This study was able to successfully classify metastatic melanoma from the primary tumors. The team has also put forward a web server, CancerSPP to predict metastatic and primary tumor samples of SKCM (metastatic Skin Cutaneous Melanoma) [106].

Diagnostic models evaluate the possibility of an individual being diseased, whereas prognostic models predict the risk of a person experiencing a particular outcome in the future [104]. The use of univariate and multivariate models has also been explored in predicting survival and recurrence of melanoma and non-melanoma in patients [107, 108]. Examples of models include the logistic regression model, cox regression, partial least squares discriminant analysis (PLS-DA), principal component analysis discriminant analysis (PCA-DA). Univariate models use one predictor for modeling its outcome. Multivariate data analysis on the other hand requires multiple predictors for its model. Features such as patient's age, sex, severity, test results which are assumed or known to be contributing to the disease outcome may be considered as a predictor.

9.3.3 Genome Variants for Skin Cancer Therapy

Apart from diagnostic and predictive models, variants identified using AI-based tools have been studied for investigating its role in cancer therapy. The key driver genes in early tumorigenesis are single-nucleotide alterations and small insertions or deletions. Over time, additional mutations and cancers accumulate influencing the underlying biology of the tumor cell. This represents new opportunities for therapeutic interventions. With the extensive exon and genome-sequencing studies, it is established that major types of tumor harbor different patterns of somatic mutation [109–111]. This availability of big data has paved way for classifying cancer using ML by identifying alterations at the genetic level and make necessary arrangements for patients regarding their therapy and management. AI has also been successfully used in delivering tools in identifying somatic mutations. Wood et al. developed a ML tool called Cerebro for calling validated somatic mutations in tumor samples from cancer patients with increased accuracy [112]. This tool was able to surpass six other mutation detection methods by better differentiating technical artifacts in the sequencing data. A study of melanoma and non-small cell lung cancer patient samples found Cerebro in precisely classifying patients according to their immunotherapy response, indicating that the authors' mutation calling method could positively direct patient care. Sun et al.[113] used a method called GDL (genome deep learning) based on deep neural networks (DNN) using genomic information for identifying cancer. They used WES (Whole Exome Sequencing) variation data of 12 types of cancer, including Skin Cutaneous Melanoma available at TCGA (The Cancer Genome Atlas) for their models. Accuracy, specificity, and sensitivity of the total-specific model were 94.70%, 85.54%, and 97.30%, respectively, GDL also introduces a novel methodology to determine cancer risk before diagnosis, leaving enough time for treatment. The use of Genome-Wide Association Studies and Polygenic Risk Score (PRS) has also been studied in skin cancer. A PRS compares a person's risk to others with a different genetic constitution. A review of available work for melanoma, basal cell carcinoma (BCC), and cutaneous squamous cell carcinoma (cSCC) using GWAS and PRS is done in this study and potential clinical utility is discussed [114]. Another potential of AI has been reported in site directed, immunotherapy, and combination therapy for determining the origin of a metastatic tumor [115, 116].

9.3.4   Transcriptomics and Epigenomics in Skin Cancer Therapy

When cancer immunotherapy succeeds, the effect can be transformative for the patients while some either develop resistance or the patient shows no response at all to the treatment. These clinical concerns have strengthened the discovery of new drugs and their targets. The main purpose is to aid patients who have either intrinsic or acquired resistance to the treatment options. For the treatment of metastatic melanoma, many studies have utilized the basic transcriptional machinery as a target for cancer therapy. One of the key features of all cancer cells is the deregulation of expression at mRNA level. A recent study involving chromatin immunoprecipitation (ChIP) seq, RNAseq, and single-cell (sc) RNAseq data of melanoma was done to decipher the cancer progression. Several other networks AP1, Elk1, and E12 TF were identified indicating them to aid in progression of melanoma. Moreover, in invasive melanoma the sumoylation-associated interactome seems to be upregulated. Altogether, this bioinformatics analysis for melanoma suggests a combination of protein–protein interactions (PPIs) and TF networks in disease progression. However, its confirmation in experimental conditions needs to be verified before they are used as targets for drug intervention in melanoma [117]. Another key predictor in the mutational landscape of cancer is the chromatin state. Studies show using the assay for transposase-accessible chromatin with high-throughput sequencing (ATAC-seq) data for analyzing chromatin accessibility for melanoma using ChromHMM, a multivariate HMM (hidden Markov model) [118, 119].

9.3.5 Imaging for Skin Cancer Therapy

AI has also been assisting in selecting patients for adjuvant immunotherapy and accelerating clinical trial design. Adjuvant therapy is often used after primary treatments, such as surgery, to lessen the chances of cancer recurrence. While effective adjuvant therapies are available, these therapies are on the costlier side and often incur significant toxicity. Precise biomarkers would therefore allow clinicians to identify and treat the high-risk patients, sparing lowest-risk patients with cost and toxicities of treatment. A deep neural network architecture for identifying patients at risk for visceral recurrence and death using digital images of slides stained with H&E dye or primary melanoma tumors was found in the literature. This study eliminates the need for sample shipment, manipulation, and shows an applied advance over current genetic and immunohistochemistry (IHC) based methods [120]. AI has also been investigated to identify targeted therapy sites and for anticancer treatment. Targeted therapy is a branch of cancer therapy that aims to target a specific site, leaving the surroundings unaffected. Anticancer treatment on the other hand involves methods to stop or prevent cancer. A synergistic result was observed on combining immunotherapy and targeted therapy in the preclinical studies and clinical trials for metastatic melanoma treatment. Recently, a study reported four machine learning models (linear model, random forest, XGBoost, and LightGBM) to predict the response to immunotherapy and targeted therapy in stage IIIc or IV melanoma patients. They considered age, sex, Breslow, melanoma type, ulceration, spontaneous regression, mitotic index, number of invaded lymph nodes, extracapsular extension, mutational status, melanoma stage, number of metastasis sites, lines of treatments, and time between first melanoma excision and metastatic relapse for their models. This field of radiomics is a newly emerging field in radiology which has the ability to utilize biomedical images and abstract features that might provide a direction in responding to precision medicine needs [121].

9.3.6 Liquid Biopsy in Skin Cancer Therapy

The clinical relevance of liquid biopsy in melanoma studies has already been established for early diagnosis, prognosis, and follow-up of the cancer. Liquid biopsy is a non-invasive blood-based test to look for cell-free DNA, extracellular vesicles, and cells from the tumor that might be circulating in the blood. A study presented by Magali Boyer et al. suggested the implication of liquid biopsy in melanoma for studying biomarkers (e.g., ctDNA, CTCs, and exosomes), with its clinical relevance presently in the investigation of clinical trials [122]. They also pointed out that in MCC, the research is still in the early stages and has few published articles. Furthermore, no clinical trial evaluating liquid biopsy for MCC has been reported so far. Thus, the wide acquisition of artificial intelligence in skin cancer therapy shows encouraging results. However, timely diagnosis holds key to improved therapy and management. Several biomarkers/features including mutations, genes show the capability of AI to mine hidden patterns in big data.

9.4   Conclusion

Over the past two decades, an enormous rise in the applications of artificial intelligence (AI) in skin cancer research has been reported which suggest the emerging role of AI for diagnosis, modeling prognosis, mining information from patient healthcare, i.e. EMRs and EHRs, and improving the patient health care data. Moreover, it plays a decisive role for identifying the novel therapeutics. Previously, the diagnosis of skin cancers relied on different traditional techniques which were of invasive nature. However, with the evolution of AI, many progresses have been towards developing non-invasive tools and methods for diagnostics and therapy of skin cancer. Now the digitization of images, imaging modalities for diagnostics, and monitoring of diseases have been user friendly. In clinical diagnostics, AI-based algorithms used for classifying *skin cancer images with an accuracy that complements or even may surpass primary care clinicians, radiologists, pathologists.* These developments in AI hold the potential for assisting clinicians in prioritizing suspicious skin lesions. Furthermore, AI has also leveraged the uses of advancing communication and high-speed internet facilities which make easy accessibility of consultations with clinicians using smartphone-based apps like SkinVision and teledermatology, teledermoscopy have been made possible. On the other hand, AI-based non-invasive computer-aided systems incorporating patient clinical data are now established with promising accuracy. Risk assessment methods using genomic sequences, EMRs, and image data provide a great benefit in stratification and the development of diagnostic and prognostic models which can be easily applied to investigate and access the risk, staging, survival, and the recurrence in skin cancer. These models have greatly benefitted clinical decision making by providing immediate care for high risk and reducing avoidable excisions for low-risk patients. The role of AI has also been seen at the -omics level. Identifying the variants and genes of interest for associating genotype to phenotype has provided deep insights into the underlying mechanism. The availability of big data has provided a great opportunity to investigate cancer classification using AI and make decisions regarding patient therapy and management. From identifying the somatic and passenger mutations for the primary tumor. Using the AI, the passenger mutation patterns can be easily predicted for the successful classification of primary and metastatic skin cancer. Predicting primary tumor sites for CUPS and identifying cancer risk even before the diagnosis might help in saving time and cost for treatment. Its ability to further classify patients according to their immunotherapy response has significantly improved health outcomes. The role of TMB, tumor mutational burden, and durable response to immunotherapy has been considered. Other applications of AI have been seen in identifying potential neoepitopes for vaccine development, finding targeted therapy sites, predicting patient response to immunotherapy, selecting patients for adjuvant immunotherapy and targeted therapy which are essential for accelerating the clinical trials.

Acknowledgement TD is thankful to UGC (University Grants Commission) for providing fellowship. Authors gratefully acknowledge the computational facility funded by Science and Engineering Research Board (SERB), Government of India (Ref. No.: YSS/2015/000228/LS).

Conflict of Interest The author declares no conflict of interest.

References

1. Leiter U, Keim U, Garbe C (2020) Epidemiology of skin Cancer: update 2019. Adv Exp Med Biol 1268:123–139. https://doi.org/10.1007/978-3-030-46227-7_6
2. Sacchetto L, Zanetti R, Comber H, Bouchardy C, Brewster DH, Broganelli P et al (2018) Trends in incidence of thick, thin and in situ melanoma in Europe. Eur J Cancer 92:108–118. https://doi.org/10.1016/j.ejca.2017.12.024
3. Esteva A, Kuprel B, Novoa RA, Ko J, Swetter SM, Blau HM et al (2017) Dermatologist-level classification of skin cancer with deep neural networks. Nature 542(7639):115–118. https://doi.org/10.1038/nature21056
4. Narla A, Kuprel B, Sarin K, Novoa R, Ko J (2018) Automated classification of skin lesions: from pixels to practice. J Invest Dermatol 138(10):2108–2110. https://doi.org/10.1016/j.jid.2018.06.175
5. Brinker TJ, Schlager G, French LE, Jutzi T, Kittler H (2020) Computer-assisted skin cancer diagnosis: is it time for artificial intelligence in clinical practice? Hautarzt 71(9):669–676. https://doi.org/10.1007/s00105-020-04662-8
6. Hogarty DT, Su JC, Phan K, Attia M, Hossny M, Nahavandi S et al (2020) Artificial intelligence in dermatology-where we are and the way to the future: a review. Am J Clin Dermatol 21(1):41–47. https://doi.org/10.1007/s40257-019-00462-6
7. Jutzi TB, Krieghoff-Henning EI, Holland-Letz T, Utikal JS, Hauschild A, Schadendorf D et al (2020) Artificial intelligence in skin cancer diagnostics: the patients' perspective. Front Med 7:233. https://doi.org/10.3389/fmed.2020.00233
8. Hosny A, Parmar C, Quackenbush J, Schwartz LH, Aerts H (2018) Artificial intelligence in radiology. Nat Rev Cancer 18(8):500–510. https://doi.org/10.1038/s41568-018-0016-5
9. Currie G, Hawk KE, Rohren E, Vial A, Klein R (2019) Machine learning and deep learning in medical imaging: intelligent imaging. J Med Imaging Radiat Sci 50(4):477–487. https://doi.org/10.1016/j.jmir.2019.09.005
10. Pouly M, Koller T, Gottfrois P, Lionetti S (2020) Artificial intelligence in image analysis-fundamentals and new developments. Hautarzt 71(9):660–668. https://doi.org/10.1007/s00105-020-04663-7
11. Wang S, Summers RM (2012) Machine learning and radiology. Med Image Anal 16(5):933–951. https://doi.org/10.1016/j.media.2012.02.005
12. Tran WT, Jerzak K, Lu FI, Klein J, Tabbarah S, Lagree A et al (2019) Personalized breast Cancer treatments using artificial intelligence in Radiomics and Pathomics. J Med Imaging Radiat Sci 50(4 Suppl 2):S32–S41. https://doi.org/10.1016/j.jmir.2019.07.010
13. Rajkomar A, Dean J, Kohane I (2019) Machine learning in medicine. N Engl J Med 380(14):1347–1358. https://doi.org/10.1056/NEJMra1814259
14. Lim BCW, Flaherty G (2019) Artificial intelligence in dermatology: are we there yet? Br J Dermatol 181(1):190–191. https://doi.org/10.1111/bjd.17899
15. Beleza S, Santos AM, McEvoy B, Alves I, Martinho C, Cameron E et al (2013) The timing of pigmentation lightening in Europeans. Mol Biol Evol 30(1):24–35. https://doi.org/10.1093/molbev/mss207
16. Leiter U, Eigentler T, Garbe C (2014) Epidemiology of skin cancer. Adv Exp Med Biol 810:120–140. https://doi.org/10.1007/978-1-4939-0437-2_7

17. Perez MI (2019) Skin cancer in hispanics in the United States. J Drugs Dermatol 18(3):s117–s120
18. Armstrong BK, Cust AE (2017) Sun exposure and skin cancer, and the puzzle of cutaneous melanoma: a perspective on fears et al. mathematical models of age and ultraviolet effects on the incidence of skin cancer among whites in the United States. American journal of epidemiology 1977; 105: 420-427. Cancer Epidemiol 48:147–156. https://doi.org/10.1016/j.canep.2017.04.004
19. Willemze R, Cerroni L, Kempf W, Berti E, Facchetti F, Swerdlow SH et al (2019) The 2018 update of the WHO-EORTC classification for primary cutaneous lymphomas. Blood 133 (16):1703–1714. https://doi.org/10.1182/blood-2018-11-881268
20. Bradford PT (2009) Skin cancer in skin of color. Dermatol Nurs 21(4):170–177
21. Suppa M, Gandini S, Njimi H, Bulliard JL, Correia O, Duarte AF et al (2019) Association of sunbed use with skin cancer risk factors in Europe: an investigation within the Euromelanoma skin cancer prevention campaign. J Eur Acad Dermatol Venereol 33(Suppl 2):76–88. https://doi.org/10.1111/jdv.15307
22. Jones OT, Ranmuthu CKI, Hall PN, Funston G, Walter FM (2020) Recognising skin Cancer in primary care. Adv Ther 37(1):603–616. https://doi.org/10.1007/s12325-019-01130-1
23. Kansara S, Bell D, Weber R (2020) Surgical management of non-melanoma skin cancer of the head and neck. Oral Oncol 100:104485. https://doi.org/10.1016/j.oraloncology.2019.104485
24. Samarasinghe V, Madan V (2012) Nonmelanoma skin cancer. J Cutan Aesthet Surg 5 (1):3–10. https://doi.org/10.4103/0974-2077.94323
25. Brantsch KD, Meisner C, Schonfisch B, Trilling B, Wehner-Caroli J, Rocken M et al (2008) Analysis of risk factors determining prognosis of cutaneous squamous-cell carcinoma: a prospective study. Lancet Oncol 9(8):713–720. https://doi.org/10.1016/S1470-2045(08)70178-5
26. Malone JP, Fedok FG, Belchis DA, Maloney ME (2000) Basal cell carcinoma metastatic to the parotid: report of a new case and review of the literature. Ear Nose Throat J 79(7):511–515
27. Linares MA, Zakaria A, Nizran P (2015) Skin cancer. Prim Care 42(4):645–659. https://doi.org/10.1016/j.pop.2015.07.006
28. Karagas MR, Stukel TA, Greenberg ER, Baron JA, Mott LA, Stern RS (1992) Risk of subsequent basal cell carcinoma and squamous cell carcinoma of the skin among patients with prior skin Cancer. JAMA 267(24):3305–3310. https://doi.org/10.1001/jama.1992.03480240067036
29. Siegel R, Ma J, Zou Z, Jemal A (2014) Cancer statistics, 2014. CA Cancer J Clin 64(1):9–29. https://doi.org/10.3322/caac.21208
30. Yanofsky VR, Mercer SE, Phelps RG (2011) Histopathological variants of cutaneous squamous cell carcinoma: a review. J Skin Cancer 2011:210813. https://doi.org/10.1155/2011/210813
31. Ramahi E, Choi J, Fuller CD, Eng TY (2013) Merkel cell carcinoma. Am J Clin Oncol 36 (3):299–309. https://doi.org/10.1097/COC.0b013e318210f83c
32. Harms KL, Healy MA, Nghiem P, Sober AJ, Johnson TM, Bichakjian CK et al (2016) Analysis of prognostic factors from 9387 Merkel cell carcinoma cases forms the basis for the new 8th edition AJCC staging system. Ann Surg Oncol 23(11):3564–3571. https://doi.org/10.1245/s10434-016-5266-4
33. Leonardi GC, Falzone L, Salemi R, Zanghi A, Spandidos DA, McCubrey JA et al (2018) Cutaneous melanoma: from pathogenesis to therapy (review). Int J Oncol 52(4):1071–1080. https://doi.org/10.3892/ijo.2018.4287
34. Yeh I, Jorgenson E, Shen L, Xu M, North JP, Shain AH et al (2019) Targeted genomic profiling of Acral melanoma. J Natl Cancer Inst 111(10):1068–1077. https://doi.org/10.1093/jnci/djz005
35. Gupta R, Janostiak R, Wajapeyee N (2020) Transcriptional regulators and alterations that drive melanoma initiation and progression. Oncogene 39:7093–7105. https://doi.org/10.1038/s41388-020-01490-x

36. Bellew S, Del Rosso JQ, Kim GK (2009) Skin cancer in asians: part 2: melanoma. J Clin Aesthet Dermatol 2(10):34–36
37. Gupta AK, Bharadwaj M, Mehrotra R (2016) Skin cancer concerns in people of color: risk factors and prevention. Asian Pac J Cancer Prev 17(12):5257–5264. https://doi.org/10.22034/APJCP.2016.17.12.5257
38. Kong HJ (2019) Managing unstructured big data in healthcare system. Healthc Inform Res 25 (1):1–2. https://doi.org/10.4258/hir.2019.25.1.1
39. Househ MS, Aldosari B, Alanazi A, Kushniruk AW, Borycki EM (2017) Big data, big problems: a healthcare perspective. Stud Health Technol Inform 238:36–39
40. Belle A, Thiagarajan R, Soroushmehr SM, Navidi F, Beard DA, Najarian K (2015) Big data analytics in healthcare. Biomed Res Int 2015:370194. https://doi.org/10.1155/2015/370194
41. Londhe VY, Bhasin B (2019) Artificial intelligence and its potential in oncology. Drug Discov Today 24(1):228–232. https://doi.org/10.1016/j.drudis.2018.10.005
42. Nguyen G, Dlugolinsky S, Bobák M, Tran V, López García Á, Heredia I et al (2019) Machine learning and deep learning frameworks and libraries for large-scale data mining: a survey. Artif Intell Rev 52(1):77–124. https://doi.org/10.1007/s10462-018-09679-z
43. McDermott JE, Wang J, Mitchell H, Webb-Robertson BJ, Hafen R, Ramey J et al (2013) Challenges in biomarker discovery: combining expert insights with statistical analysis of complex omics data. Expert Opin Med Diagn 7(1):37–51. https://doi.org/10.1517/17530059.2012.718329
44. Jiang F, Jiang Y, Zhi H, Dong Y, Li H, Ma S et al (2017) Artificial intelligence in healthcare: past, present and future. Stroke Vasc Neurol 2(4):230–243. https://doi.org/10.1136/svn-2017-000101
45. Biomarkers Definitions Working Group (2001) Biomarkers and surrogate endpoints: preferred definitions and conceptual framework. Clin Pharmacol Ther 69(3):89–95. https://doi.org/10.1067/mcp.2001.113989
46. Greinert R (2009) Skin cancer: new markers for better prevention. Pathobiology 76(2):64–81. https://doi.org/10.1159/000201675
47. Torres R, Lang UE, Hejna M, Shelton SJ, Joseph NM, Shain AH et al (2020) MicroRNA ratios distinguish melanomas from nevi. J Invest Dermatol 140(1):164–173. https://doi.org/10.1016/j.jid.2019.06.126
48. Leon R, Martinez-Vega B, Fabelo H, Ortega S, Melian V, Castano I et al (2020) Non-invasive skin cancer diagnosis using hyperspectral imaging for in-situ clinical support. J Clin Med 9 (6):1662. https://doi.org/10.3390/jcm9061662
49. Rey-Barroso L, Burgos-Fernandez FJ, Delpueyo X, Ares M, Royo S, Malvehy J et al (2018) Visible and extended near-infrared multispectral imaging for skin cancer diagnosis. Sensors 18 (5):1441. https://doi.org/10.3390/s18051441
50. Esteva A, Robicquet A, Ramsundar B, Kuleshov V, DePristo M, Chou K et al (2019) A guide to deep learning in healthcare. Nat Med 25(1):24–29. https://doi.org/10.1038/s41591-018-0316-z
51. Hoshyar AN, Al-Jumaily A, Hoshyar AN (2014) The beneficial techniques in preprocessing step of skin cancer detection system comparing. Procedia Comput Sci 42:25 31. https://doi.org/10.1016/j.procs.2014.11.029
52. Guerra-Rosas E, Alvarez-Borrego J (2015) Methodology for diagnosing of skin cancer on images of dermatologic spots by spectral analysis. Biomed Opt Express 6(10):3876–3891. https://doi.org/10.1364/BOE.6.003876
53. Uchida S (2013) Image processing and recognition for biological images. Develop Growth Differ 55(4):523–549. https://doi.org/10.1111/dgd.12054
54. Celebi ME, Kingravi HA, Uddin B, Iyatomi H, Aslandogan YA, Stoecker WV et al (2007) A methodological approach to the classification of dermoscopy images. Comput Med Imaging Graph 31(6):362–373. https://doi.org/10.1016/j.compmedimag.2007.01.003

55. Abbas Q, Fondon I, Rashid M (2011) Unsupervised skin lesions border detection via two-dimensional image analysis. Comput Methods Prog Biomed 104(3):e1–e15. https://doi.org/10.1016/j.cmpb.2010.06.016

56. Ozturk S, Ozkaya U (2020) Skin lesion segmentation with improved convolutional neural network. J Digit Imaging 33(4):958–970. https://doi.org/10.1007/s10278-020-00343-z

57. Hosking AM, Coakley BJ, Chang D, Talebi-Liasi F, Lish S, Lee SW et al (2019) Hyperspectral imaging in automated digital dermoscopy screening for melanoma. Lasers Surg Med 51(3):214–222. https://doi.org/10.1002/lsm.23055

58. Masood A, Al-Jumaily AA (2013) Computer aided diagnostic support system for skin cancer: a review of techniques and algorithms. Int J Biomed Imaging 2013:323268. https://doi.org/10.1155/2013/323268

59. Fargnoli MC, Kostaki D, Piccioni A, Micantonio T, Peris K (2012) Dermoscopy in the diagnosis and management of non-melanoma skin cancers. Eur J Dermatol 22(4):456–463. https://doi.org/10.1684/ejd.2012.1727

60. Umbaugh SE, Moss RH, Stoecker WV, Hance GA (1993) Automatic color segmentation algorithms-with application to skin tumor feature identification. IEEE Eng Med Biol Mag 12(3):75–82. https://doi.org/10.1109/51.232346

61. Green A, Martin N, Pfitzner J, O'Rourke M, Knight N (1994) Computer image analysis in the diagnosis of melanoma. J Am Acad Dermatol 31(6):958–964. https://doi.org/10.1016/s0190-9622(94)70264-0

62. Oliveira RB, Papa JP, Pereira AS, Tavares JMRS (2018) Computational methods for pigmented skin lesion classification in images: review and future trends. Neural Comput Applic 29(3):613–636. https://doi.org/10.1007/s00521-016-2482-6

63. Barata C, Celebi ME, Marques JS (2015) Improving Dermoscopy image classification using color Constancy. IEEE J Biomed Health Inform 19(3):1146–1152. https://doi.org/10.1109/jbhi.2014.2336473

64. Yu L, Chen H, Dou Q, Qin J, Heng P (2017) Automated melanoma recognition in Dermoscopy images via very deep residual networks. IEEE Trans Med Imaging 36(4):994–1004. https://doi.org/10.1109/tmi.2016.2642839

65. Brinker TJ, Hekler A, Utikal JS, Grabe N, Schadendorf D, Klode J et al (2018) Skin Cancer classification using convolutional neural networks: systematic review. J Med Internet Res 20(10):e11936. https://doi.org/10.2196/11936

66. Hosny KM, Kassem MA, Fouad MM (2020) Classification of skin lesions into seven classes using transfer learning with AlexNet. J Digit Imaging 33(5):1325–1334. https://doi.org/10.1007/s10278-020-00371-9

67. Liu S, Deng W (2015) Very deep convolutional neural network based image classification using small training sample size. 2015 3rd IAPR Asian Conference on Pattern Recognition (ACPR). pp. 730–734

68. Hirano G, Nemoto M, Kimura Y, Kiyohara Y, Koga H, Yamazaki N et al (2020) Automatic diagnosis of melanoma using hyperspectral data and GoogLeNet. Skin Res Technol 26:891–897. https://doi.org/10.1111/srt.12891

69. Al-Masni MA, Kim DH, Kim TS (2020) Multiple skin lesions diagnostics via integrated deep convolutional networks for segmentation and classification. Comput Methods Prog Biomed 190:105351. https://doi.org/10.1016/j.cmpb.2020.105351

70. Dascalu A, David EO (2019) Skin cancer detection by deep learning and sound analysis algorithms: a prospective clinical study of an elementary dermoscope. EBioMedicine 43:107–113. https://doi.org/10.1016/j.ebiom.2019.04.055

71. Toraman S, Alakus TB, Turkoglu I (2020) Convolutional capsnet: a novel artificial neural network approach to detect COVID-19 disease from X-ray images using capsule networks. Chaos Solitons Fractals 140:110122. https://doi.org/10.1016/j.chaos.2020.110122

72. Surówka G, Ogorzalek M (2020) Wavelet-based logistic discriminator of dermoscopy images. Expert Syst Appl 2020:113760. https://doi.org/10.1016/j.eswa.2020.113760

73. Marchetti MA, Codella NCF, Dusza SW, Gutman DA, Helba B, Kalloo A et al (2018) Results of the 2016 international skin imaging collaboration international symposium on biomedical imaging challenge: comparison of the accuracy of computer algorithms to dermatologists for the diagnosis of melanoma from dermoscopic images. J Am Acad Dermatol 78(2):270–277. https://doi.org/10.1016/j.jaad.2017.08.016

74. Haenssle HA, Fink C, Schneiderbauer R, Toberer F, Buhl T, Blum A et al (2018) Man against machine: diagnostic performance of a deep learning convolutional neural network for dermoscopic melanoma recognition in comparison to 58 dermatologists. Ann Oncol 29 (8):1836–1842. https://doi.org/10.1093/annonc/mdy166

75. Fujisawa Y, Otomo Y, Ogata Y, Nakamura Y, Fujita R, Ishitsuka Y et al (2019) Deep-learning-based, computer-aided classifier developed with a small dataset of clinical images surpasses board-certified dermatologists in skin tumour diagnosis. Br J Dermatol 180 (2):373–381. https://doi.org/10.1111/bjd.16924

76. Maron RC, Weichenthal M, Utikal JS, Hekler A, Berking C, Hauschild A et al (2019) Systematic outperformance of 112 dermatologists in multiclass skin cancer image classification by convolutional neural networks. Eur J Cancer 119:57–65. https://doi.org/10.1016/j.ejca. 2019.06.013

77. Brinker TJ, Hekler A, Enk AH, Klode J, Hauschild A, Berking C et al (2019) Deep learning outperformed 136 of 157 dermatologists in a head-to-head dermoscopic melanoma image classification task. Eur J Cancer 113:47–54. https://doi.org/10.1016/j.ejca.2019.04.001

78. Satheesha TY, Satyanarayana D, Prasad MNG, Dhruve KD (2017) Melanoma is skin deep: a 3D reconstruction technique for computerized Dermoscopic skin lesion classification. IEEE J Transl Eng Health Med 5:4300117. https://doi.org/10.1109/JTEHM.2017.2648797

79. Muller I, Kulms D (2018) A 3D Organotypic melanoma spheroid skin model. J Vis Exp 135:57500. https://doi.org/10.3791/57500

80. Kaur A, Ecker BL, Douglass SM, Kugel CH 3rd, Webster MR, Almeida FV et al (2019) Remodeling of the collagen matrix in aging skin promotes melanoma metastasis and affects immune cell motility. Cancer Discov 9(1):64–81. https://doi.org/10.1158/2159-8290.CD-18-0193

81. Pacheco AGC, Krohling RA (2020) The impact of patient clinical information on automated skin cancer detection. Comput Biol Med 116:103545. https://doi.org/10.1016/j.compbiomed. 2019.103545

82. Pacheco AGC, Lima GR, Salomao AS, Krohling B, Biral IP, de Angelo GG et al (2020) PAD-UFES-20: a skin lesion dataset composed of patient data and clinical images collected from smartphones. Data Brief 32:106221. https://doi.org/10.1016/j.dib.2020.106221

83. Qin Z, Liu Z, Zhu P, Xue Y (2020) A GAN-based image synthesis method for skin lesion classification. Comput Methods Prog Biomed 195:105568. https://doi.org/10.1016/j.cmpb. 2020.105568

84. Buechi R, Faes L, Bachmann LM, Thiel MA, Bodmer NS, Schmid MK et al (2017) Evidence assessing the diagnostic performance of medical smartphone apps: a systematic review and exploratory meta-analysis. BMJ Open 7(12):e018280. https://doi.org/10.1136/bmjopen-2017-018280

85. Flaten HK, St Claire C, Schlager E, Dunnick CA, Dellavalle RP (2018) Growth of mobile applications in dermatology - 2017 update. Dermatol Online J 24(2):13030

86. Freeman K, Dinnes J, Chuchu N, Takwoingi Y, Bayliss SE, Matin RN et al (2020) Algorithm based smartphone apps to assess risk of skin cancer in adults: systematic review of diagnostic accuracy studies. BMJ 368:m127. https://doi.org/10.1136/bmj.m127

87. Pasquali P, Sonthalia S, Moreno-Ramirez D, Sharma P, Agrawal M, Gupta S et al (2020) Teledermatology and its current perspective. Indian Dermatol Online J 11(1):12–20. https://doi.org/10.4103/idoj.IDOJ_241_19

88. Chuchu N, Dinnes J, Takwoingi Y, Matin RN, Bayliss SE, Davenport C et al (2018) Teledermatology for diagnosing skin cancer in adults. Cochrane Database Syst Rev 12: CD013193. https://doi.org/10.1002/14651858.CD013193

89. Bleicher B, Levine A, Markowitz O (2018) Going digital with dermoscopy. Cutis 102 (2):102–105

90. Keller JJ, Johnson JP, Latour E (2020) Inpatient teledermatology: diagnostic and therapeutic concordance among a hospitalist, dermatologist, and teledermatologist using store-and-forward teledermatology. J Am Acad Dermatol 82(5):1262–1267. https://doi.org/10.1016/j.jaad. 2020.01.030

91. Barcaui CB, Lima PMO (2018) Application of Teledermoscopy in the diagnosis of pigmented lesions. Int J Telemed Appl 2018:1624073. https://doi.org/10.1155/2018/1624073

92. Hekler A, Utikal JS, Enk AH, Berking C, Klode J, Schadendorf D et al (2019) Pathologist-level classification of histopathological melanoma images with deep neural networks. Eur J Cancer 115:79–83. https://doi.org/10.1016/j.ejca.2019.04.021

93. Lu C, Mandal M (2015) Automated analysis and diagnosis of skin melanoma on whole slide histopathological images. Pattern Recogn 48(8):2738–2750. https://doi.org/10.1016/j.patcog. 2015.02.023

94. Madabhushi A, Lee G (2016) Image analysis and machine learning in digital pathology: challenges and opportunities. Med Image Anal 33:170–175. https://doi.org/10.1016/j.media. 2016.06.037

95. Lodha S, Saggar S, Celebi JT, Silvers DN (2008) Discordance in the histopathologic diagnosis of difficult melanocytic neoplasms in the clinical setting. J Cutan Pathol 35(4):349–352. https://doi.org/10.1111/j.1600-0560.2007.00970.x

96. Corona R, Mele A, Amini M, De Rosa G, Coppola G, Piccardi P et al (1996) Interobserver variability on the histopathologic diagnosis of cutaneous melanoma and other pigmented skin lesions. J Clin Oncol 14(4):1218–1223. https://doi.org/10.1200/JCO.1996.14.4.1218

97. Sharma H, Mao C, Zhang Y, Vatani H, Yao L, Zhong Y et al (2019) Developing a portable natural language processing based phenotyping system. BMC Med Inform Decis Mak 19 (Suppl 3):78. https://doi.org/10.1186/s12911-019-0786-z

98. Hubbard RA, Huang J, Harton J, Oganisian A, Choi G, Utidjian L et al (2019) A Bayesian latent class approach for EHR-based phenotyping. Stat Med 38(1):74–87. https://doi.org/10. 1002/sim.7953

99. Afzal N, Sohn S, Abram S, Scott CG, Chaudhry R, Liu H et al (2017) Mining peripheral arterial disease cases from narrative clinical notes using natural language processing. J Vasc Surg 65(6):1753–1761. https://doi.org/10.1016/j.jvs.2016.11.031

100. Kharazmi P, Kalia S, Lui H, Wang ZJ, Lee TK (2018) A feature fusion system for basal cell carcinoma detection through data-driven feature learning and patient profile. Skin Res Technol 24(2):256–264. https://doi.org/10.1111/srt.12422

101. Albrecht M, Lucarelli P, Kulms D, Sauter T (2020) Computational models of melanoma. Theor Biol Med Model 17(1):8. https://doi.org/10.1186/s12976-020-00126-7

102. Pennisi M, Russo G, Di Salvatore V, Candido S, Libra M, Pappalardo F (2016) Computational modeling in melanoma for novel drug discovery. Expert Opin Drug Discov 11(6):609–621. https://doi.org/10.1080/17460441.2016.1174688

103. Kourou K, Exarchos TP, Exarchos KP, Karamouzis MV, Fotiadis DI (2015) Machine learning applications in cancer prognosis and prediction. Comput Struct Biotechnol J 13:8–17. https:// doi.org/10.1016/j.csbj.2014.11.005

104. Hendriksen JMT, Geersing GJ, Moons KGM, de Groot JAH (2013) Diagnostic and prognostic prediction models. J Thromb Haemost 11(s1):129–141. https://doi.org/10.1111/jth.12262

105. Wang HH, Wang YH, Liang CW, Li YC (2019) Assessment of deep learning using nonimaging information and sequential medical records to develop a prediction model for nonmelanoma skin Cancer. JAMA Dermatol 155(11):1277–1283. https://doi.org/10.1001/ jamadermatol.2019.2335

106. Bhalla S, Kaur H, Dhall A, Raghava GPS (2019) Prediction and analysis of skin Cancer progression using genomics profiles of patients. Sci Rep 9(1):15790. https://doi.org/10.1038/ s41598-019-52134-4

107. Ferrone CR, Panageas KS, Busam K, Brady MS, Coit DG (2002) Multivariate prognostic model for patients with thick cutaneous melanoma: importance of sentinel lymph node status. Ann Surg Oncol 9(7):637–645. https://doi.org/10.1007/BF02574479
108. Silveira FL, Pacheco MT, Bodanese B, Pasqualucci CA, Zangaro RA, Silveira L Jr (2015) Discrimination of non-melanoma skin lesions from non-tumor human skin tissues in vivo using Raman spectroscopy and multivariate statistics. Lasers Surg Med 47(1):6–16. https://doi.org/10.1002/lsm.22318
109. Jiao W, Atwal G, Polak P, Karlic R, Cuppen E, Danyi A et al (2020) A deep learning system accurately classifies primary and metastatic cancers using passenger mutation patterns. Nat Commun 11(1):728. https://doi.org/10.1038/s41467-019-13825-8
110. Kandoth C, McLellan MD, Vandin F, Ye K, Niu B, Lu C et al (2013) Mutational landscape and significance across 12 major cancer types. Nature 502(7471):333–339. https://doi.org/10.1038/nature12634
111. Lawrence MS, Stojanov P, Polak P, Kryukov GV, Cibulskis K, Sivachenko A et al (2013) Mutational heterogeneity in cancer and the search for new cancer-associated genes. Nature 499 (7457):214–218. https://doi.org/10.1038/nature12213
112. Wood DE, White JR, Georgiadis A, Van Emburgh B, Parpart-Li S, Mitchell J et al (2018) A machine learning approach for somatic mutation discovery. Sci Transl Med 10(457):eaar7939. https://doi.org/10.1126/scitranslmed.aar7939
113. Sun Y, Zhu S, Ma K, Liu W, Yue Y, Hu G et al (2019) Identification of 12 cancer types through genome deep learning. Sci Rep 9(1):17256. https://doi.org/10.1038/s41598-019-53989-3
114. Roberts MR, Asgari MM, Toland AE (2019) Genome-wide association studies and polygenic risk scores for skin cancer: clinically useful yet? Br J Dermatol 181(6):1146–1155. https://doi.org/10.1111/bjd.17917
115. Bochtler T, Kramer A (2019) Does Cancer of unknown primary (CUP) truly exist as a distinct Cancer entity? Front Oncol 9:402. https://doi.org/10.3389/fonc.2019.00402
116. Chen Y, Sun J, Huang LC, Xu H, Zhao Z (2015) Classification of Cancer primary sites using machine learning and somatic mutations. Biomed Res Int 2015:491502. https://doi.org/10.1155/2015/491502
117. Singh K, Baird M, Fischer R, Chaitankar V, Seifuddin F, Chen YC et al (2020) Misregulation of ELK1, AP1, and E12 transcription factor networks is associated with melanoma progression. Cancers 12(2):458. https://doi.org/10.3390/cancers12020458
118. Ernst J, Kellis M (2017) Chromatin-state discovery and genome annotation with ChromHMM. Nat Protoc 12(12):2478–2492. https://doi.org/10.1038/nprot.2017.124
119. Lindberg M, Bostrom M, Elliott K, Larsson E (2019) Intragenomic variability and extended sequence patterns in the mutational signature of ultraviolet light. Proc Natl Acad Sci U S A 116 (41):20411–20417. https://doi.org/10.1073/pnas.1909021116
120. Shah M, Wedam S, Cheng J, Fiero MH, Xia H, Li F et al (2020) FDA approval summary: tucatinib for the treatment of patients with advanced or metastatic HER2-positive breast cancer. Clin Cancer Res 27(5):1220–1226. https://doi.org/10.1158/1078-0432.ccr-20-2701
121. Guerrisi A, Loi E, Ungania S, Russillo M, Bruzzaniti V, Elia F et al (2020) Novel cancer therapies for advanced cutaneous melanoma: the added value of radiomics in the decision making process-a systematic review. Cancer Med 9(5):1603–1612. https://doi.org/10.1002/cam4.2709
122. Boyer M, Cayrefourcq L, Dereure O, Meunier L, Becquart O, Alix-Panabieres C (2020) Clinical relevance of liquid biopsy in melanoma and merkel cell carcinoma. Cancers 12 (4):960. https://doi.org/10.3390/cancers12040960

Biomedical Engineering in Cancer Diagnosis and Therapy

10

Jovel Varghese Jose and Rashmi Prem Prakash Maurya

Abstract

This chapter crosses the divide between bioengineering and cancer biology. It relies on a "bottom-up" view of the connections between molecules, cells, tissues, organs, animals, and health and functions—all within the framework of bioengineering. The chapters cover the key approaches, innovations, and devices that could better detect cancer faster and more helpful therapies. The chapter adopts an interdisciplinary approach that is suitable for those who need knowledge on design strategies and devices that assist with their care.

Keywords

Cancer · Bioengineering · Diagnosis · Treatment

10.1 Introduction

Cancer is caused due to the unrestricted growth of cells and is also one of the main causes of deaths. As per World Health Organization cancer is the second largest death cause disease globally which is also responsible for an approximate 9.6 million deaths in the year 2018. The death rate is as high as 1 in 6 deaths due to cancer. By 2030, the cancer-related deaths are expected to rise to 13.1 million. Cancer is an assembly of diseases with every organ and system developing a particular set of diseases. Cancer is caused due to modifications of genes inherited from parents and environmental factors such as smoking, sunlight exposure, unbalanced diet, and alcohol consumption. In addition with continuous cell growth cancer outspreads whole over the human body, while the normal cells become insensitive to the

J. V. Jose (✉) · R. P. P. Maurya
Amity University Mumbai, Mumbai, India

© The Author(s), under exclusive license to Springer Nature Singapore Pte Ltd. 2021
A. Dwivedi et al. (eds.), *Skin Cancer: Pathogenesis and Diagnosis*,
https://doi.org/10.1007/978-981-16-0364-8_10

immune-checkpoint receptors such as PD1 and CTLA4 guiding to growth of tumors and metastasis of cells. The proliferation of uncontrolled growth of cells forms malignant tumor and invades the nearby parts of body. Till date there are over 200 different kinds of cancer which are identified that can affect whole over the human body. The most cancer types include blood, skin, prostate, stomach, ovary, lung, breast, liver, and colon cancer. To identify and cure cancer diagnosis, imaging and therapy steps are necessary for killing of cancerous cells.

Biomedical engineering (BME) has advent in the field of medical science by integrating various fields of biology, medicine, physics, and chemistry along with principles of engineering to evolve new devices and procedures to solve health-related and medical issues in the current world. Biomedical engineering uses chemical, optical, electrical, engineering, and mechanical principles to control, modify, and understand biological systems. BME can be also known as biological engineering or bioengineering. BME has been an emerging field in clinical application which has been constantly evolving through research of engineering medicine and biology integrating various algorithms and processes by developing new devices which have large scope in medical practice and healthcare distribution. BME is involved in diagnosis and treatment of various diseases to treat sick individuals and provide effective treatment in early stage with reduced costs. BME treatments are based on stem-cell technologies, surgical tools, new drugs, and new drug delivery methods to treat and diagnose various diseases including cancer. With the help of BME diagnosis of most health issues through devices, software, and instruments health care system can be improved globally. BME has been also involved in treatment of diseases and can be more accurately monitored depending on patients who are acutely or chronically diseased in low costs.

There are various bioengineering strategies to diagnose and treat cancer. The goal of bioengineering strategy can used to deliver high dosage of anticancer drug to cancer cells, enhance drug uptake by tumor cells, and also can help in minimization of drug uptake in normal cells. The main approach to target the cancer cells is to design drug delivery system. Advancements in micro and nanotechnology have led to development of particles such as micelles and liposomes that encapsulate the drugs and target cancer cells. Chemotherapy and radiation are the current way of treating cancer, but such traditional methods have many limitations. Radiation therapy is mainly focused on targeting cancer tumor, but can cause negative effects to non-malignant tissues surrounding the cancerous cells. Radiation also has limited effectiveness in treating metastasized cancers because it requires the detection and treatment of each tumor. Chemotherapy is mainly a systemic treatment that mostly targets highly proliferative cancerous cells but faces disadvantages as it exposes all the cells to the drugs. Chemotherapy lacks specificity and also damages non-malignant cells such as gonads, bone marrow, hair follicles, and gastrointestinal mucosa which results in systemic toxicity and acute complications. To achieve fully treatment efficacy the drug should be delivered to the target cancerous cells. Integrated treatment of chemotherapy and radiation to cancer cells can cure cancer and will increase treatment efficacy and also reduce side effects causing to normal cells. Still there is an urgent need to find an effective diagnostic methods and more targeted approach to kill cancer cells. In this book chapter we review the recent biomedical strategies and various applications to identify, diagnose, imaging and treatment of cancerous cells.

10.2   Types of Biosensors for Cancer Diagnostics

10.2.1 Piezoelectric Biosensors

Some experiments have been documented on piezoelectric biosensors for the identification of biomarker cancer. A piezoelectric immune sensor to detect AFP using AuNPs coated nano-sized hydroxyapatite [1]. Piezoelectric crystals are covered with this hybrid nanomaterial in which anti-AFP antibodies are immobilized to make the sensor. These piezoelectric crystals are well immersed in a reaction where an AFP-containing sample solution is added. Frequency variations detected during immune responses between the AFP and the piezoelectric probes are measured, accompanied by electrochemical measurements. This immune sensor is capable of detecting AFP in the range of 15.3–600.0 ng mL^{-1}. The addition of AuNPs has been shown to improve the reusability of the immunosensor, developed a quartz crystal microbalance (QCM) immune sensor for a tumor marker, human ferritin [2]. Human ferritin antibodies are immobilized on the QCM gold disk in this immune tracker by adsorption and chemical therapy methods. These antibodies interact with ferritin in the samples. Ferritin is evaluated in mouse serum and buffersamples in a 0.1--100 ng mL^{-1} concentration range. Another label-free piezoelectric biosensor for the detection of PSA and AFP [3] where in this case, immobilized AFP and PSA antibodies are on lead titanate zirconate (PZT) ceramic resonator transducers. The samples are applied to the PZT ceramic surface, and the antigen/antibody reactions sensor AFP and PSA are derived from the frequency differences in the two ceramic resonator surfaces.

10.2.2 Colorimetric Biosensors

Colorimetric biosensors used to detect exosomes are of great value for realistic r point-of-care (POC) applications due to their simple operation and convenient readability. Colorimetric biosensors could be detached into two formats: solution-based and paper-based. Paper-based colorimetric biosensors use paper as a substrate and are needed for field-based application due to those alleviate utilization and limited sample volume. Lateral flow biosensors (LFBs) are considered classified among much promise emerging technologies due to their low cost, rapid analysis, simplicity, and high specificity and sensitivity. LFBs consist of four components: a conjugate pad, a sample pad, a control and test line absorbent pad, and nitrocellulose membrane. The sample solution migrates through capillary movement and flows through both of these sheets. The capture factor catches targeting exosomes fixed on the test line. The detection elements labeled with nanoparticles are then added to the exosomes to form sandwich complexes resulting in a color shift that can be visualized due to the aggregation of nanoparticles over this test line. A combination of anti-CD81 and anti-CD9 as a catch antibody and anti-CD63 branded with gold nanoparticles as a detection antibody. Different exosomal antigens for LFB production have shown that using CD9 and exosomal MICA as targets is more appropriate [4]. Solution-based colorimetric biosensors that use nanomaterials or enzymes as signal tags to produce color shift can be beneficial for fast and easy detection by using relatively large sample volumes. It uses gold nanoparticles that show red color as a colorimetric signal. A biosensor platform uses aptamers to shield gold nanoparticles from aggregation in a high-salt solution [5]. A bivalent-cholesterol (BChol)-labeled DNA anchor was injected into the exosome membrane to facilitate a blue-colored hybridization chain reaction to HRP. The natural enzyme as a signal tag contributes to certain drawbacks of HRP, such as the need for a complicated purification procedure and careful storage conditions. Nanozymes with the inherent properties of mimicking natural enzyme behavior have gained extensive attention for biosensor construction due to their benefits, for instance, low cost, bulk preparation capacity, high pH tolerance, and temperature changes. Therefore, those simple strategies have a great potential to become standard.

10.2.3 Fluorescent Biosensors

Appropriate to elevated sensitivity, fluorescent biosensors designed for detecting exosomes demonstrate essential advantages. Usually, fluorescent signal production relies on fluorescent dyes, fluorophores, fluorescent proteins, or fluorescent nanoparticles being used. Three device formats can be categorized into fluorescent biosensors: micro-platform, solution-based, and paper-based. Paper-based fluorescent biosensors, which are paper-based analytical instruments, can also be designed as an essential analytical tool (PADs). Creation of fluorescent PAD to detect exosomes derived from hepatocellular carcinoma (HepG2) cells using conversion nanoparticles (UCNPs) and gold nanorods (AuNRs) as fluorescence quenching nanopairs [6].

Interestingly, to grab exosomes and form a sandwich structure, the CD63 aptamer sequence has been broken into two different pieces. To produce green luminescence, UCNPs and CP were preloaded onto the sodium periodate-oxidized filtrate. DP-modified AuNRs were combined about exosomes and aliquoted on the paper to reduce the gap between UCNPs and AuNRs by the sandwich shape, which quenched the green luminescence by the transfer of energy through luminescence resonance centered on fluorescent copper nanoparticles (CuNPs) [7]. A cost-effective and straightforward fluorescent biosensor was developed for exosome detection. Via the acidolysis of the transformation of CuO NP into copper (II) ions ($Cu2+$) and the reduction of $Cu2+$ into fluorescent CuNPs by sodium ascorbate in the presence of poly (thymine), fluorescence was achieved [8]. The detection period in their architecture is accomplished by the enzyme DNase I as it digests aptamers and releases fluorophores, the available exosomes undergo a new detection cycle to produce an improved fluorescence signal. Micro platform-based fluorescent biosensors can be useful for exosome identification because they can boost analytical efficiency by system manufacture and provide digital output through random delivery [9].

10.2.4 Gold Nanoparticle (AuNP)-Based Sensors

AuNP-based fluorescent sensors generally carry benefit of the excellent fluorescence quenching potential, that occurs after the discharge of a fluorescent molecule convergence with the plasmon band of nanoparticles. Interestingly, AuNPs will quench chromophores' fluorescence 100-fold in excess of molecular quenchers and current greater quenching performance still in near-infrared dyes. In addition to its extraordinary quenching properties, fluorescent oligonucleotide probes' ability to identify single-base mutations is nearly eight-fold greater when using AuNPs as quenchers relative to traditional molecular quenchers. Therefore, replacement of the molecular quencher with AuNP results in a more alert oligonucleotide probe and thus increases its selectivity. Nanoflares have also been developed to reflect an alternative to MBs [10]. They comprise functionalized AuNPs with a fragment of dsDNA. The target sequence is complemented by one strand, and the rest is a small fluorescently tagged reporter sequence. In the lack of a nucleic acid biomarker, the fluorophore is retained close to the AuNP quencher, and no fluorescence is released. In the existence of the only biomarker of interest, the report sequence is transferred from the AuNP, and the characteristic fluorescence signal will continue to be released. It is also interesting that many AuNPs functionalized with oligonucleotides can be quickly internalized into cells without the need for transfecting agents, making them useful sensors to identify intracellular nucleic acid cancer biomarkers [11]. AuNP-based oligonucleotide sensors may also be developed to enable colorimetric detection.

10.3 Imaging Methods for Cancer Detection

The imaging method produces visual depiction in the form of images of the body's interior to reveal the human body organs function, structure, and pathology for cancer diagnosis and treatment. Several imaging techniques view the human body's interior structure; each type gives different information about the human organ being treated or studied for effective medical diagnosis and treatment. There are some imaging techniques available for cancer diagnosis and treatment of human cancer, which are x-ray, ultrasound (US), computed tomography (CT), positron emission tomography (PET), magnetic resonance imaging (MRI), single-photon emission computed tomography (SPECT), and optical imaging. There is diverse imaging usage as per cancer is interested; similarly, screening of cancer is where imaging is employed to review abnormalities that could be cancerous. In diagnosis, images could be utilized to determine cancer location and how much it has spread. Guiding cancer Treatment: imaging can focus on cancer's exact location during treatment and determine whether treatment is working or not. The cancer imaging should image or detect the minimum conceivable number of tumor cells, preferably earlier the angiogenic switch. The detection and imaging are arbitrary and the size of the imaging modality used and the threshold for detection remains of paramount significance [12, 13].

10.3.1 Ultrasound (US)

The majority of widespread imaging modalities are Ultrasound (US), which uses 1–10 MHz sound waves for the human body analysis. In real-time, internal organs of the human body are analyzed, such as reproductive system imaging, malfunctions of cardiac valve assessment, and liver perfusion throughout abdominal tumors identification. There are two distinct categories of US, which are diagnostic and therapeutic US. The ultrasonography is a known diagnostic US for anatomical images to produce information maps [10]. The evaluation and action following the evident differences in the structure or function of organs using these information maps. This technique is inexpensive, versatile, multifunctional, and portable compared with computed tomography and magnetic resonance. Soundwaves are highly scattered and have imaging depth approximate 10 cm in many parts of the body example, bones. They have a high resolution with a 0.25–1 μm in diameter exogenous difference in microbubbles diameter to generate a signal. Ultrasound employs purpose is to interact with body tissues, leading to their modification or destruction. US-induced fragmentation of kidney stones and blood clots, thermal destruction of tumors that are malignant in nature, and site-specific drug delivery mediation in the body are reached using very-intensity sound beams that are nonionizing, thus preventing the high risk of tissue damage [11].

10.3.2 X-Ray and Computed Tomography (CT).

In 1895, the progress in health sciences led to the development of X-ray. Plain films and CT follow the x-ray beam's principle reflecting through the body and measuring its attenuation. The CT around the patient rotated the source and detector's pair, so the data acquired can be reconstructed into a 3-D image. This medical tool imaging technique has various procedures. It also uses electromagnetic radiation to produce images on the radiograph [14]. This X-ray is passed through the human body to show images of tumors, bones, and dense matter. The produced rays are sometimes absorbed and attenuated. Mainly dense tissue is more attenuated, producing a white color image; meanwhile, darker x-ray images are caused by the less dense tissues because of the less attenuation. Now X-rays are used for cancer diagnosis and staging and guiding treatment. In radiation therapy, X-rays were used to destroy cancer cells. The exogenous contrast agents need high concentrations and a high atomic number to x-ray attenuation. In clinical, the exogenous agents used were injected to become invisible, having molar concentrations following merely a some-fold dilution in the blood [15]. Bone x-ray and chest x-ray are some of the different types of x-rays helping the doctors diagnose cancer and comparing the tumor size before and after treatment.

10.3.3 Magnetic Resonance Imaging (MRI)

Magnetic resonance imaging chiefly images the limited abundance in the Boltzmann distribution of spins through the magnetic field. Since hydrogen nuclei (protons) are approximately 1.5 T, this excess is the maximum parts per million (ppm) of the total number of hydrogen nuclei indicated. Since most tissue has a total proton concentration of about 80 M, the MRI signal originates from 80μmol/L of the protons present. Improving the signal interference ratio by increasing the magnetic field intensity from 1.5 T to 3 T and beyond is a significant MRI trend. Since the signal interference ratio scales linearly with field power, an increase from 1.5 T to 7 T results in an improvement of approximately 4.7 times, importantly, however, other issues, such as increased tissue heating and standing wave patterns present at higher radio wave frequencies, can arise from high field power [16]. When intravenously administered gadolinium (Gd^{3+})-based contrast agents are used, $Gd3^+$ is not seen, but instead, the influence of $Gd3^+$ on the magnetic resonance relaxation properties of the protons present in the tissue. This relaxation effect is only detectable at $Gd3^+$ concentrations greater than approximately 50μmol/L, making it challenging to produce targeted agents. MRI has been fascinating for a variety of reasons. Next, MRI does not use radiation exposure and is usually non-invasive. Imaging depends on a large universal polarizing magnetic field, weaker "gradient" magnetic fields, and radiofrequency magnetic fields, neither of which affects the body's tissues [17].

10.3.4 Single-Photon Emission Computed Tomography (SPECT)

An important technique for quantifying the distribution of radioactive compounds in humans is Single-Photon Emission Computed Tomography (SPECT). It also uses toxic compounds that are pumped into veins in the body. One or more gamma rays, containing unique energies, are emitted in random directions by SPECT radioisotope decay. Considering that photons with high energy cannot be concentrated using traditional lenses, collimators' use restricts the angle of emitted photons that enter the detector. To capture the flow of blood and chemical reactions in the body, the SPECT scanner is used to render computerized 2D and 3D images. These radioactive substances bind to tumor cells, which can be identified by the SPECT scanner for cancer diagnosis. In alleviating the photon energies of SPECT isotopes, living tissue is entirely effective. In image processing algorithms and hardware technology, SPECT is a strong field that has changed a lot over the last few years. The SPECT elements used, including photon transducers and scintillators, have been improved. The latest development in SPECT involves hybrid SPECT/CT systems and cardiac

SPECT systems with high count sensitivity. Advances in algorithms reduce the time of image processing while preserving diagnostic efficiency [15, 18].

10.3.5 Positron Emission Tomography (PET)

PET positrons are discharged out of proton-rich nuclei that was antimatter which is equal in mass nevertheless opposite in charge of an electron. Positrons travel an average length before interacting with an electron, depending on their energy. But not generally apprehended, the density of electrons in the tissue would severely impact dissolution distance. Less dense tissues have a longer dissolution distance, resulting in lower inherent resolution, for example, the lungs [19]. Matter and antimatter are annihilating each other and creating two antiparallel photons of 511-keV. In a stationary ring, detector crystals are placed, and only specific 511-keV photons simultaneously entering opposing crystals are counted. The body also attenuates 511-keV photons with just 10% left after passage within 25 cm of solid tissue, including SPECT isotopes. PET detects around 1/2000th of the photons emitted at the cancer site during factorization of the susceptibility and tissue attenuation. Since the cumulative effects of tissue attenuation and noise attenuation, current PET technology can only detect solid tumors $\geq 10^9$ cells in size. Glucose-mimetic 2-deoxy-2-[^{18}F] fluoro-D-glucose ([17] FDG) is the most widely used PET drug since it is recovered by metabolically active cells, is not metabolized, and is trapped intracellularly after hexokinase phosphorylation. It is not a perfect PET radiotracer for cancer imaging and has a reasonably high penetration in numerous normal tissues and organs [20].

10.3.6 Optical Imaging (OI)

Since starting medicine, optical imaging has shaped the primary support for disease diagnosis and treatment. When living tissue is interreacted with a photon of light, it can be absorbed or scattered. Therefore absorption-based and scattering-based are the two significant types of OI. The majority of optical methods use comparatively simple instrumentation to image-reflected fluorescence emission light, or excitation light, with a surface. OI has begun to make more broadly used to detect and inspect cancer outside of simple detection through the naked eye. That was permitted by identifying the surgical field with a color camera system specifically either mounted on the near end of an endoscope or in more contemporary times downsized and located at the tip. Tissue reflectivity imaging is high resolution and fast. The 1/e optical penetrance limits sensitivity since the multiple light dispersion and contrast are acquired mainly from superficial structures, typically up to about 3 mm in depth. Tomographic optical spectroscopy and imaging deed multiple light scattering and utilize computational models to rebuild absorbing and scattering structures in thick tissues [21]. The color retaliation of the red-green-blue image data is finely balanced to the human eye. It can be provided on a color display to the surgeon in the operating theater for straightforward visual guidance of the interference. Imaging the white-light characteristics of the tissue reflected is a purely conventional procedure on supplying a visually perceivable picture of the tissue to the surgeon and lacks the possibility of light to disclose contrary hidden tissue information. It is possible that biophotonic techniques can lead to diagnosis and therapies [21].

10.4 Cancer Therapy

There are two fundamental therapeutic methodologies in treating disease: [22] killing previous tumors or mass of cancerous cells and [23] controlling further metastasis of cancerous cells. For individuals in the late-stage malignant growth, it might not be conceivable to take out tumor tissue, and rather the attention lies on managing additional the disease to mitigate side effects and increase the survival years. Clinicians commonly combine therapies to deal with target malignant cancerous cells. These therapies maybe generally assembled into radiotherapy to kill cancerous cells and reduce tumor size, immunotherapy to actuate the body's immune system to battle disease, drug delivery, and medical surgeries to extract cancerous tissue. The kind of malignant growth treatment a patient gets relies upon various components, including tumor type, area, seriousness of sickness, and any previous conditions.

All the treatments are discussed one by one.

10.4.1 Drug Delivery

Tumors are strange developments of cancer cells, encircled by a microenvironment of tumor. The microenvironment normally comprises tumor cells, immune cells, healthy cells, and blood vessels to supply oxygen and nutrition to the cells [22]. To treat the tumor, clinicians can utilize medications to target biological processes in the tumor. These medication based treatments plan to establish an antagonistic climate to restrict cancer cell endurance and tumor development. For instance, chemotherapeutic medications can be utilized to forestall the fast division of cells, causing death of cancer cells [23].

Cancerous cells release vascular (blood vessels forming) development factors (i.e., PDGF and VEGF) that contribute to vessel development in the microenvironment of tumor. Newly formed vessels in the vicinity of the tumor increase the stream of blood to the tumor. This assists with satisfying the metabolic needs of developing cancer cells and furthermore gives the disease local vasculature that encourages its migration and metastasis. Obstructing this neovascularization and forestalling stabilization of leaking vessels are accordingly a promising methodology to restrict cancer development. Angiogenic inhibitors, for example, Bevacizumab are sedates ordinarily administered in a combination with chemotherapeutics to kill tumor cells and limit vessel development.

Some cancerous tumors are hormone sensitive like those from gynecology or orthology. Tumors from these cancers very often have hormone receptors on their cell surface and the cell growth is affected by the degree of hormone in the microenvironment of tumor [24, 25]. When the amount of hormone in the microenvironment of tumor increases, then they can bind to hormone receptors on the cell surface for rapid proliferation of the cancer cells. Hormone levels are kept low throughout the body by clinicians, in cancer patients to prevent the interaction of hormone with hormone receptors and slow down cancer proliferation.

The most popular class of medications to treat cancer are chemotherapeutic agents. Cytotoxic chemotherapeutic medications intrude the cell cycle by focusing on particular cell measures happening in every one of the periods of division of cell. Alkylating agents, antimetabolites, enzyme inhibitors, antitumor antibiotics, and antimicrotubule agents are the five primary types of chemotherapeutic drugs. DNA replication is intruded by a considerable lot of these chemotherapeutic drugs. Carboplatin is one case of this class and is regularly the primary line chemotherapeutic used to treat numerous types of cancer, exhibiting the broad utilization of this technique.

Other chemotherapy methodologies centred around repressing the synthesis of new DNA utilizing antimetabolites. Antimetabolites are atoms that are fundamentally the same as substances used to construct DNA, regularly found in the cell. Be that as it may, they are somewhat unique to endogenous substances and keep the nucleic acid, DNA from being utilized appropriately, causing cell death. At last, alkaloids removed from plants can be successful at forestalling division of cells by disturbing microtubules formation in the cell. These tubules are required to adjust the recently formed DNA prior to division; forestalling microtubule formation assisting with easing back cancer development.

Albeit practically all cells progress through this cycle, cancer growth happens at a lot quicker pace compared to ordinary cells. By spacing chemotherapeutic medicines properly, oncologists attempt to guarantee that chemotherapeutic medications intrude on cell division just in rapidly dividing cells, leaving most of ordinary cells safe. Shockingly, this frequently implies that healthy cells that grow quickly (i.e., hair, nails, and white blood cells) are additionally influenced, prompting undesirable results, for example, low white blood cell count and balding. To decrease these unwanted side effects, bioengineers can design better delivery systems to guarantee the correct medication arrives at the correct target.

10.4.2 Immunotherapy

A large number of recent cancer treatments center around diverting the patient's own immune system to better identify and target cancerous tissue. Techniques incorporate conveying small particle agents that can actuate neighborhood immune cells or antibodies that can impede the cell surface receptors that cancer cells commonly use to dodge the immune system [26, 27]. Cancer vaccines can likewise be used to prepare the immune system to perceive and react to cancer cell epitopes [28]. In the most recent treatments a patient's own immune cells can be extricated from tissue biopsy, searched for the most potent anticancer cells, expanded, and reinfused. On the other hand, a patient's T cells can be taken out and genetically engineered to express a chimeric antigen receptor, which can assist cells with distinguishing and targeting harmful cancerous cells.

Several methodologies have been developed to improve patient-expected cytotoxic T lymphogen reaction by genetic modification ex vivo from anti-cancers targeting dendritic cells [29–31] to resistant control point blockages [32, 33] restoring and improving the T cell function, to chimeric antigen receptor [34, 35] cell treatments. The use of anticancer vaccines containing antigenic materials, such as TAA or immune boosting adjuvants, has been investigated for quite a few years, among these. In general, the restorative benefits that anticancer antibodies can deliver in clinical settings are not at all like efficient traditional vaccines targeting foreign bodies, challenges in selecting the correct antigenic content and the powerless selection of the vaccines in lymphatic systems. Checkpoint obstructions, such as CTLA-4 and PD-1 antibodies, are the most commonly successful immunotherapies to date and have shown phenomenal clinical reactions in melanoma, cellular lung cancer of non-small cells, head and neck cancer, renal cancer, Hodgkin's lymphoma, and many others [36]. Unfortunately, problems such as extreme side effects and limited response rates still exist [37–40]. All in all, non-specific immune system activation is responsible for the adverse side effects observed in patients. Subsequently, the main test is to achieve selective activation of the right immune cells in order to enhance tumor-specific immune reactions and reduce systemic exposure to potent therapeutic agents.

10.4.3 Radiotherapy

Radiation therapy (also called radiotherapy) is a cancer therapy that uses high doses of radiation to kill cancer cells and reduce tumor size. At low doses, radiation is used in x-rays to be seen inside the body, similar to x-rays in your teeth or broken bones. Radiation treatment kills cancer cells at high doses or reduces their development by damaging their DNA. Cancer cells, the DNA of which is damaged far beyond repair, stop cell division or die. At the point when cancer cells die, they are separated and eliminated by the body. Radiation treatment does not immediately kill cancer cells. After that, cancerous cells continue to die for weeks after radiation treatment completes.

Two fundamental kinds of radiation treatment exist, namely, external beam and internal beam.

Many components can be used to treat radiation, including cancer, tumor proportions, the position of the tumor in the body and the closeness to which the tumor is with healthy tissues that are sensitive to radiation and the general well-being and clinical history of the patient. External beam radiation therapy is given by a machine which points to cancer radiation. The machine is massive and may be bullish. It does not touch the individual, but from several directions it may travel around and radiation is sent to a region of the body. External beam radiation is a local treatment that involves treating a specific region of the body. For example, if you have a chance of having cancer cells in your lung, they will radiate only to your chest, not the whole body. Internal radiation therapy is a therapy where the body has a source of radiation. Solid or liquid can be the source of the radiation. Radiation therapy is called brachytherapy if it is done with a solid source. In this treatment, inside or near the tumor; seeds, ribbons, or capsules that contain a source of radiation are kept. Local treatment, like external beam radiation treatment, also involves external therapy and treats only a certain part of the body. The radiation source will give radiation out of the body for some time after this therapy. If the internal radiation treatment is performed using a liquid source, then the treatment is called systemic therapy. This means that cancer cells can be found and killed from blood to tissues around the body. This therapy is performed through swallowing, a vein or an injection via an IV line. With this therapy, body fluids, such as urine, sweat, and saliva, have been emit radiation for a while.

10.4.4 Robotic Assisted Laproscopic Surgeries

The term MIS is used to refer to any single procedure and intercession based on reducing trauma to healthy or vital tissues. While MIS is the most common type of laparoscopic surgery (and in some cases used as a similar word), versatile endoscopy, neurosurgery, and percutaneous interventions are included in the more detailed idea of MIS, together with non-contained therapeutic procedures, including energy emissions. Diminishing healing time, pain, analgesics, or postoperative drawbacks has extraordinary advantages for surgical procedures.

Robotic technology has the ability to demonstrate its empowering nature at any point it may exhibit. The vast majority of these procedures are performed using the Da Vinci Surgical System by Intuitive Surgical Inc., the market leader in automated procedures, with 4986 surgical systems being used far and wide [41] and more than six million procedures being performed towards the end of 2018. The patient cart contains numerous articulated arms for the control of the laparoscope and a few laparoscopic instruments. These are handled in a master-slave style by the surgeon, who sits at a vivid reassure with 3D HD perception and ergonomic handles.

On the one side sits the surgeon, who clearly has ergonomic developments for robots, for example, greater control over the surgical equipment, a superior view of the surgical site, and a more convenient workspace. The primary stakeholder is then again: the patient. Urologic procedures to eliminate prostate cancer have shown that robotic methodologies can provide more completed cancer expulsion and less side effects from conventional laparoscopic prostatectomy [42] but with a substantial vulnerability.

10.5 In Vitro Models of Cancer

In Latin, in vitro, means "in the glass." Hence, experiments in vitro are conducted on or in the glass. This refers to the cycle by which cells are removed from living tissues onto a plate to examine them beyond their normal environment. Glass slides were originally used as a cell culture support to justify the use of the word "in vitro." There are nowadays different forms of supported materials that are used for cell culture, not really glass [43]. The term in vitro is in any case commonly used to mean, for the most part, that cells in a research laboratory outside their normal natural environments are investigated. In vitro research today has grown to be its own field in biomedical testing.

10.5.1 Why In Vitro Models?

Before we discuss the subtleties of in vitro cancer research models, we shall understand why research has been central and why prospective biomedical researchers deserve exceptional attention. In vitro models initially significantly contribute to the understanding of the biological mechanisms behind normal and pathological processes. By cultivating and studying "on dishes," researchers are able to plan easy yet unbelievable experiments, which will help them learn more about how cells function in vivo. Second, drug development is used in in vitro models. This can be achieved using in vitro models as methods to track the pharmacological target via medicines libraries. Parallel to these in vitro models, basic parameters, such as the dosage of the medication are to be tested, examined, and rationalized in order to predict its suitability or toxicity in people. The cells in 3D tended to respond to drugs uniquely as opposed to 2D cells, and the finding that drugs tested in 3D cells gave results similar to those in vivo, perhaps, was more important than that.

10.5.2 Existing 3D Models of Essential and Metastatic Malignancy

There are different 3D in vitro models, many of which are used for research on cancer. They all allow cancer cells to grow in 3D but differ in configuration or technology on which they depend [44]. We speak here of the most commonly used portion of organizations today: spheroids, scaffolds, microfluid, and bioreactors. Be aware that scaffolds can be mixed, for example, often put within microfluidic systems, or inside scaffolds, spheroids can be placed.

10.5.2.1 Spheroids
Spheroids are self-organized cell clusters, including tumor cells, which can be formed with different cell types. A spheroid tumor, itself a lump of tumor cells, reiterates large portions of the tumor. Cells can be conglomerated into spheroids through different well-established protocols that minimize their adherence to the well. Tumor spheroids may either be formed by the use of non-adherent surfaces,

suspension in a drop of fluid hanging from an upside-down well plate or by agitating cells with spinning fluids or rotating systems. Tumor cells discharge their own extracellular matrix within spheroids. In the light of the decreased spread of supplements and oxygen, as is seen in large tumors in vivo the middle of the spheroids has become hypoxic and necrotic [45]. This equally leads to areas of the rates of cell division that are more relaxed than the cells at the central point of the spheroid.

The absence of vascularization is a current weakness of spheroids grown in vitro. Spheroids therefore are not relevant to the consideration of vascularized tumors and are used to impersonate primary avascular tumors, some micrometastases or avascular tumor microregions [45]. Note that spheroids are model primary tumor, but they do not represent a broad array of formations of metastatic tumors. Spheroids have some benefits which have made them a significant 3D cell culture model for discovery of pharmaceuticals. They are generally easy to shape, use, and ideal for screening drugs [46], since individual spheroids can be shaped and studied independently within plates that contain various wells. The imaging by fluorescence of fluorescent tumor cells is particularly unbelievable in the analysis of spheroids because fluorescent scenes can give estimates of the size, multiplication, or reaction of the spheroids.

10.5.2.2 Scaffolds

Scaffolds are 3D in vitro research structures used to provide three-dimensional biochemical and mechanical anchorage [47]. It can be made with natural or synthetic material. Natural scaffolds are proteins which constitute the extracellular matrix of tissues, such as collagen, fibrin, or hyaluronic acid, or other biomaterials naturally present, such as gelatine. These biomaterials provide different sites for adhesion between proteins. The merit of biomaterials obtained naturally is that they are in vivo and are therefore physiologically essential. In addition, in any instance their specific components are not clearly specified and biodegradable. Biodegradability is powerful and essential in studies where scaffolds are embedded in the body. However, this biodegradability for in vitro studies can restrict the study length and cause unintended uncontrolled effects due to scaffold degradation by-products.

Scaffolds can also include plastic biomaterials made of polymers, ceramic material like bioactive glasses, or self-assembled peptides. They are synthetic. They also have established chemical composition, are inert, do not biodegrade, ensure a more viable and less toxic effect, and are free of components from animals, in contrast to natural biomaterials, which appear to be derived from certain animal tissue and can cause interspecies differences in use with human cells. An emerging method for creating tissue decellularization of ECMs by naturally derived scaffolds. This method eliminates cellular tissue elements, but retains the ECM. It preserves the tissue's native microarchitecture and eliminates the allogenic or xenogenic cellular antigens from the tissues as they are the origins of immunogenicity after implantation. The ECM is preserved between species and is thus immunologically tolerated well. However, seeds of cells inside of the scaffold can be hard and inhomogeneous.

10.5.2.3 Microfluidic Devices

In the previous decade, microfluidic models were developed as important devices for investigating in vitro cancer. Tiny channels from tens to several micrometers high or wide for small liquid volumes are found in microfluidic systems [48]. Microfluidic studies are usually advance physiologically in comparison to other in vitro models as they take specific cellular, physical, and biochemical microenvironment regulation into account [49]. They can be planned easily according to experimental requirements and have different channels and compartments. Each microfluidic compartment includes separately, a specific population of cells that allows well specified cultures.

This partitioning allows large-scale spatial regulation of the physiological cell distribution. The existence of microfluidic channels allows precise flux regulation, allowing for the study of many essential biomechanical processes, such as shear pressure. The channels also allow for the regulated transmission of cells or nanoparticles. Also, direct and control flow valves can be added. These canals may also be used to properly create physical (for example, interstitial pressure) or chemical (for example, cytokines) gradients in a more precise and sustained way in microfluid testing than in in vitro macroscale systems [50]. The channels permit local control by associating the microchannels to gas or vacuum cell sources of other natural environmental elements, such as pressure or strain or hypoxia. For example, it was designed to mimic the alveolar capillary interface in the lung [51] by means of a microfluidic system consisting of a permeable membrane cellulose between two applied microchannels. A vacuum pump that puts cyclical pressure on the main canal containing the permeable membrane, cyclically stretches cells, as in the case of traditional relaxation, was connected with two major flanking canals. Cells grown in 2D or in 3D, embedded in hydrogels, can be in microfluidical instruments. Since they are small, they need only a small number of often expensive, rare, or difficult to obtain cells and reagents. More importantly, it is easier to imagine high resolution cells in comparison to large traditional in vitro 3D models [52] from the biological samples on the device to the microscope lens objective.

10.5.2.4 Bioreactors

Closed systems that regulate local factors such as perfusion, temperature, humidity, and gas exchange are bioreactors [53]. A bioreactor normally includes a centralized chamber (which contains cells), segments of actuators, sensors, and test software. In order to facilitate 3D cell culture, cells can be put in 3D cells within those bioreactors. Bioreactors allow for close control of the conditions of culture and enable the tissue to physically imitate the forces of cells in the body. Sensors help create computer models and get accurate test data [53]. In some interesting ways, bioreactors were used in cancer studies [54]. Bioreactors were first used for cell expansion. Second, they were used to promote the consistent colonization of scaffolds through cells, particularly when the cells were dropped onto the scaffold under the dynamic flow conditions within a bioreactor. Third, bioreactors have been used to monitor important environmental factors, such as hypoxia and tissue strain, in the production of cancer [54]. Perfusion in bioreactors, especially in thick 3D scaffolds, promotes long-term survival of cells by continuously providing new media and by promoting the removal of the cell's metabolic products. Interestingly, ordinary in vitro experiments are subject to the discerning daily replacement of the media, which only hit the limited area in the 3D scaffold.

Different kinds of bioreactors are available, for example, rotary, stirring, perfusion, or hollow-fiber bioreactors to ensure that the necessary cells are exchanged inside the scaffolds [54]. Different bioreactors are available to monitor and study the effects of tumor cells on pressure or stress. For example, a bioreactor experiment used to exercise pressure by using 3D in vitro rollers on 295 tumor-celled gels that demonstrate modified gene expression and a metastatic potential. These are fascinating factors for the development of cancer which show that non-physiological mechanical stimuli typically occur in tumors. This showed the key models in vitro for cancer research and also how each can advance our understanding of the disease in their own way. Most of the 3D cell culture designs mentioned are used routinely and can be difficult to distinguish. Without a doubt, new tactics would add aspects to the advantages that we have presented from current techniques.

10.6   Conclusion

Despite a steady increase worldwide in global cancer prevalence, over the last decade Europe and the United States have seen a 1 percent reduction in age-standardized death rates associated with the disease (ASMR) [55, 56]. In the United Kingdom between 2014 and 2035 the combined cancer mortality rate is predicted to decrease by 15% to 280 deaths per 100,000 by 2035 [57]. That has been at least partly made possible by constant developments in the diagnosis and treatment of cancer patients, using groundbreaking bioengineering innovations, medicines, and instruments. Bioengineers will provide doctors and specialists with creative tools and solutions that meet important yet unsatisfied medical needs for their users and patients at the receptive end, with the aid of potential end-users and direct experience in cancer patients and their families. Public screening diagnosis offers the best chance before initial clinical symptoms begin to be diagnosed with early cancer, when patients are more likely to undergo therapy. Imaging methods such as magnetic resonance imaging, digital imaging, and ultrasound imaging often provide new knowledge which diagnostic studies typically fail to provide. This includes details on the size and location of the tumor which also is critical for the consultation of the clinician before or after a targeted biopsy or tumor excision. Technological developments in this area have led to substantial increases in image resolution, which allow early cancer detection simulations of smaller tumors. Although early diagnosis usually involves higher survival rates, cancer mortality minimizes cancer patients, be it chemotherapy, immunotherapy, radiotherapy, or surgery, or some combination of these, requires the most effective treatment. The development of experimental drugs, their optimizing direct delivery at a tumor site in order to minimize secondary effectiveness, and the supply of modern robotic techniques in order to enhance accuracy play an important role in each of these areas. But both scientific advances also provide a detailed understanding of the development, growth, and reaction of cancer cells. This can best be tested by providing detailed 2- or 3-dimensional in vitro models to the scientific community [58, 59]. Cancer research is a prime example of a sector in which new technologies, by means of industrial research, greatly influence the diagnosis, management, and treatment of this disease. Although survival of cancer has doubled over the last 40 years, progress for all kinds of diseases has not been achieved consistently. The powerful effects of the access of modern technology have been demonstrated by major regional inequalities.

References

1. Ding L, Bond AM, Zhai J, Zhang J (2013) Utilization of nanoparticle labels for signal amplification in ultrasensitive electrochemical affinity biosensors: a review. Anal Chim Acta 797:1–12
2. Chou SF, Hsu WL, Hwang JM, Chen CY (2002) Development of an immunosensor for human ferritin, a nonspecific tumor marker, based on a quartz crystal microbalance. Anal Chim Acta 453(2):181–189
3. Su L, Zou L, Fong CC, Wong WL, Wei F, Wong KY et al (2013) Detection of cancer biomarkers by piezoelectric biosensor using PZT ceramic resonator as the transducer. Biosens Bioelectron 46:155–161
4. López-Cobo S, Campos-Silva C, Moyano A, Oliveira-Rodríguez M, Paschen A, Yáñez-Mó M et al (2018) Immunoassays for scarce tumour-antigens in exosomes: detection of the human NKG2D-ligand, MICA, in tetraspanin-containing nanovesicles from melanoma. J Nanobiotechnol 16(1):47
5. Jiang Y, Shi M, Liu Y, Wan S, Cui C, Zhang L, Tan W (2017) Aptamer/AuNP biosensor for colorimetric profiling of exosomal proteins. Angew Chem Int Ed 56(39):11916–11920
6. Chen X, Lan J, Liu Y, Li L, Yan L, Xia Y et al (2018) A paper-supported aptasensor based on upconversion luminescence resonance energy transfer for the accessible determination of exosomes. Biosens Bioelectron 102:582–588
7. He F, Wang J, Yin BC, Ye BC (2018) Quantification of exosome based on a copper-mediated signal amplification strategy. Anal Chem 90(13):8072–8079
8. Wang H, Chen H, Huang Z, Li T, Deng A, Kong J (2018) DNase I enzyme-aided fluorescence signal amplification based on graphene oxide-DNA aptamer interactions for colorectal cancer exosome detection. Talanta 184:219–226
9. Zhang P, He M, Zeng Y (2016) Ultrasensitive microfluidic analysis of circulating exosomes using a nanostructured graphene oxide/polydopamine coating. Lab Chip 16(16):3033–3042
10. Coutinho C, Somoza Á (2019) MicroRNA sensors based on gold nanoparticles. Anal Bioanal Chem 411(9):1807–1824
11. Heuer-Jungemann A, Harimech PK, Brown T, Kanaras AG (2013) Gold nanoparticles and fluorescently labelled DNA as a platform for biological sensing. Nanoscale 5(20):9503–9510
12. Groebe K, Mueller-Klieser W (1996) On the relation between size of necrosis and diameter of tumor spheroids. Int J Radiat Oncol Biol Phys 34(2):395–401
13. Naumov GN, Akslen LA, Folkman J (2006) Role of angiogenesis in human tumor dormancy: animal models of the angiogenic switch. Cell Cycle 5(16):1779–1787
14. Meneses CT, Flores WH, Sotero AP, Tamura E, Garcia F, Sasaki JM (2006) In situ system for X-ray absorption spectroscopy experiments to investigate nanoparticle crystallization. J Synchrotron Radiat 13(6):468–470

15. Hsiang D, Shah N, Yu N, Su MY, Cerussi A, Butler J et al (2005) Coregistration of dynamic contrast enhanced MRI and broadband diffuse optical spectroscopy for characterizing breast cancer. Technol Cancer Res Treat 4(5):549–558
16. Zhang S, Merritt M, Woessner DE, Lenkinski RE, Sherry AD (2003) PARACEST agents: modulating MRI contrast via water proton exchange. Acc Chem Res 36(10):783–790
17. Nioka S, Miwa M, Orel S, Shnall M, Haida M, Zhao S, Chance B (1994) Optical imaging of human breast cancer. In: Oxygen transport to tissue XVI. Springer, Boston, MA, pp 171–179
18. Kelloff GJ, Hoffman JM, Johnson B, Scher HI, Siegel BA, Cheng EY et al (2005) Progress and promise of FDG-PET imaging for cancer patient management and oncologic drug development. Clin Cancer Res 11(8):2785–2808
19. Kumar R, Chauhan A, Zhuang H, Chandra P, Schnall M, Alavi A (2006) Standardized uptake values of normal breast tissue with 2-deoxy-2-[F-18] fluoro-D-glucose positron emission tomography: variations with age, breast density, and menopausal status. Mol Imaging Biol 8 (6):355–362
20. Choy G, Choyke P, Libutti SK (2003) Current advances in molecular imaging: noninvasive in vivo bioluminescent and fluorescent optical imaging in cancer research. Mol Imaging 2 (4):15353500200303142
21. Ke S, Wen X, Gurfinkel M, Charnsangavej C, Wallace S, Sevick-Muraca EM, Li C (2003) Near-infrared optical imaging of epidermal growth factor receptor in breast cancer xenografts. Cancer Res 63(22):7870–7875
22. Matsumura Y, Maeda H (1986) A new concept for macromolecular therapeutics in cancer-chemotherapy— mechanism of tumoritropic accumulation of proteins and the antitumor agent SMANCS. Cancer Res 46(12 Part 1):6387–6392
23. Parmar H et al (1988) Response to D-TRP-6-Luteinising hormone-releasing hormone (decapeptyl) microcapsules in advanced ovarian-cancer. Br Med J 296(6631):1229
24. Small EJ et al (2000) Immunotherapy of hormone-refractory prostate cancer with antigen-loaded dendritic cells. J Clin Oncol 18(23):3894–3903
25. Maher J, Davies ET (2004) Targeting cytotoxic T lymphocytes for cancer immunotherapy. Br J Cancer 91(5):817–821
26. Capitini CM, Mackall CL, Wayne AS (2010) Immune-based therapeutics for pediatric cancer. Exp Opin Biol Ther 10(2):163–178
27. Huye LE, Dotti G (2010) Designing T cells for cancer immunotherapy. Discov Med 9 (47):297–303
28. Chekmasova AA, Brentjens RJ (2010) Adoptive T cell immunotherapy strategies for the treatment of patients with ovarian cancer. Discov Med 9(44):62–70
29. Jena B, Dotti G, Cooper LJ (2010) Redirecting T-cell specificity by introducing a tumor-specific chimeric antigen receptor. Blood 116(7):1035–1044
30. Li WA, Mooney DJ (2013) Materials based tumor immunotherapy vaccines. Curr Opin Immunol 25(2):238–245
31. Guo C et al (2013) Therapeutic cancer vaccines: past, present, and future. Adv Cancer Res 119:421–475
32. Hu Z, Ott PA, Wu CJ (2018) Towards personalized, tumour-specific, therapeutic vaccines for cancer. Nat Rev Immunol 18:168
33. Melero I et al (2014) Therapeutic vaccines for cancer: an overview of clinical trials. Nat Rev Clin Oncol 11:509
34. Leach DR, Krummel MF, Allison JP (1996) Enhancement of antitumor immunity by CTLA-4 blockade. Science 271:1734–1736
35. Tumeh PC et al (2014) PD-1 blockade induces responses by inhibiting adaptive immune resistance. Nature 515:568
36. Davila ML et al (2014) Efficacy and toxicity management of 19-28z CAR T cell therapy in B cell acute lymphoblastic leukemia. Sci Transl Med 6:224ra225

37. Ma L et al (2019) Enhanced CAR-T cell activity against solid tumors by vaccine boosting through the chimeric receptor. Science 365(6449):162–168. https://doi.org/10.1126/science. aav8692
38. Teng F, Meng X, Kong L, Yu J (2018) Progress and challenges of predictive biomarkers of anti PD-1/PDL1 immunotherapy: a systematic review. Cancer Lett 414:166–173
39. Hodi FS et al (2010) Improved survival with ipilimumab in patients with metastatic melanoma. N Engl J Med 363:711–723
40. Larkin J et al (2015) Combined nivolumab and ipilimumab or monotherapy in untreated melanoma. N Engl J Med 373:23–34
41. Topalian SL et al (2012) Safety, activity, and immune correlates of anti–PD-1 antibody in cancer. N Engl J Med 366:2443–2454
42. Zou W, Wolchok JD, Chen L (2016) PD-L1 (B7-H1) and PD-1 pathway blockade for cancer therapy: mechanisms, response biomarkers, and combinations. Sci Transl Med 8:328rv324
43. Intuitive Surgical Inc (2018) Q4 2018 preliminary financial data tables, Available from: https:// isrg.gcsweb.com/static-files/3a12c816-6637-4a3a-bfef-247a60c1fbd7
44. Ramsay C, Pickard R, Robertson C, Close A, Vale L, Armstrong N et al (2012) Systematic review and economic modelling of the relative clinical benefit and cost-effectiveness of laparoscopic surgery and robotic surgery for removal of the prostate in men with localised prostate cancer. Health Technol Assess 16:1–313
45. Estabridis HM, Jana A, Nain A, Odde DJ (2018) Cell migration in 1D and 2D nanofiber microenvironments. Ann Biomed Eng 46:392–403
46. Tung Y-C et al (2011) High-throughput 3D spheroid culture and drug testing using a 384 hanging drop array. Analyst 136:473–478
47. Knight E, Przyborski S (2015) Advances in 3D cell culture technologies enabling tissue-like structures to be created in vitro. J Anat 227:746–756
48. Whitesides GM (2006) The origins and the future of microfluidics. Nature 442:368–373
49. Polacheck WJ, Li R, Uzel SGM, Kamm RD (2013) Microfluidic platforms for mechanobiology. Lab Chip 13:2252–2267
50. Kim S, Kim HJ, Jeon NL (2010) Biological applications of microfluidic gradient devices. Integr Biol 2:584
51. Huh D et al (2010) Reconstituting organ-level lung functions on a chip. Science 328:1662–1668
52. Boussommier-calleja A, Li R, Chen MB, Wong SC, Kamm RD (2016) Microfluidics: a new tool for modeling cancer-immune interactions. Trends Cancer 2:6–19
53. Wendt D, Riboldi SA, Cioffi M, Martin I (2009) Potential and bottlenecks of bioreactors in 3D cell culture and tissue manufacturing. Adv Mater 21:3352–3367
54. Guller AE, Grebenyuk PN, Shekhter AB, Zvyagin AV, Deyev SM (2016) Bioreactor-based tumor tissue engineering. Acta Nat 8:44–58
55. La Vecchia C, Rota M, Malvezzi M, Negri E (2015) Potential for improvement in cancer management: reducing mortality in the European Union. Oncologist 20(5):495
56. Siegel RL, Fedewa SA, Miller KD, Goding-Sauer A, Pinheiro PS, Martinez-Tyson D, Jemal A (2015) Cancer statistics for hispanics/latinos, 2015. CA Cancer J Clin 65(6):457–480
57. Smittenaar CR, Petersen KA, Stewart K, Moitt N (2016) Cancer incidence and mortality projections in the UK until 2035. Br J Cancer 115(9):1147–1155
58. Malik SH, Lone TA, Quadri SM (2016) Imaging techniques for cancer diagnosis and scope for enhancement. Int J Image Graphics Signal Process 8(5):83
59. Pradhan S et al (2017) A three-dimensional spheroidal cancer model based on PEG-fibrinogen hydrogel microspheres. Biomaterials 115:141–154

Skin Cancer Treatment with Emphasis on Nanotechnology

Baranya Murugan

Abstract

Cancer is the illness that proves to be a great challenge, despite current trends and modern improvements in medicine. Among the different cancer types, skin cancer is the most common cancer and has manifest vast growth in 5 years worldwide. No less than one in five Americans have skin cancer. Nanomedicine is used as a hub for diagnosis and therapy by developing different nanoparticles as a delivery carrier. The delivery nanocarrier can be nanocapsules, nanorods, nanotubes, nanoshells, and nanocages. The structure and properties of these nanoparticles prevent the drug from the degradation and enhance its stability. Synthesis and characterization of the nanoparticles like polymeric nanoparticles, polymeric micelles, liposomes, nanohydrogel, dendrimers, inorganic nanoparticles delivers the divergent anticancer agents. Functionalization of the nanoparticles gives rise to smart delivery systems through surface modifying agents and techniques used. The use of nanotechnology-based techniques improves a systematic delivery to the target cells. Skin cancer experiences many issues in detecting early forms of cancer for many years, and slower growth rate. This chapter describes on novel therapeutic approaches for skin cancer with emphasis on nanotechnology.

Keywords

Skin cancer · Nanotechnology · Cancer biology · Target cells · Therapeutics · Skin type · UV exposure

B. Murugan (✉)
Centre for Nanotechnology and Advanced Biomaterials, SASTRA University, Thanjavur, Tamil Nadu, India

© The Author(s), under exclusive license to Springer Nature Singapore Pte Ltd. 2021
A. Dwivedi et al. (eds.), *Skin Cancer: Pathogenesis and Diagnosis*,
https://doi.org/10.1007/978-981-16-0364-8_11

11.1 Introduction

11.1.1 Background

Skin, the biggest organ in the body, which has a surface area of about 1.8 m^2 and occupies 8% of the total body mass of an adult. Skin cancer is the second most common cancer worldwide [1, 2]. Millions of new cases occur every year all over the world. Various types of cancer are differentiated based on the origination and behaviour of the cell [3–5]. The most prominent types of cancers are basal cell carcinoma (BCC), squamous cell carcinoma (SCC), together known as nonmelanocytic skin cancer (NMSC) and malignant melanoma (MM) [6]. Basal and squamous cell carcinomas in the United States are around six million new cases of annually and approximately 77,000 new cases of malignant melanoma occur each year. The increase in number of cases bothers for patients as well as the health care departments [7–10]. The cost for the treatment of skin cancer is about 10 billion dollar every year in the United States. The prevalence of skin cancer occurs globally and most popularly happens in divergent populations, involving women and other Hispanic individuals [11–14]. A clear idea about the rate of incidence, varying risk factors, and genetic modifications of this deadly disease is of very crucial and significant to initiate a national and international public awareness of different populations [15].

11.1.2 Types of Skin Cancer

11.1.2.1 Malignant Melanoma

Melanoma is a type of skin cancer, occurs from continuous events of ultraviolet exposure causes the burning of the skin. Melanoma is said to be a more aggressive skin cancer and widely known to be multi drug resistance [16]. In Europe the occurrence of type of skin cancer is 10–20 cases among 100,000 inhabitants, whereas USA be at 20–30 among 100,000 cases. Slovenian occurrence, in the year 2012, been 23, 1 out of 100,000 in the male candidates and 23, 8 out of 100,000 in the female candidates. Therefore, the prevalence rate of the new diagnosis per year for Slovenia is around seven hundred new cases [17–19]. The malignant melanoma is more familiar in males as compared with females [20]. Melanoma constitutes a small portion of skin cancer occurrence, but it lasts for most of the skin cancer deaths. Melanoma can be treated, when it is diagnosed at an initial stage, which can be removed through surgery, with a survival rate of 99%. In contrast, in a metastasized condition, it leads to the death of 80% of patients right after the five years from the diagnosis [20, 21]. These melanoma types of skin cancer entirely depend on skin type and exposure to ultraviolet rays [22].

11.1.2.2 Nonmelanocytic Skin Cancer

NMSC is the malignancy that occurs in humans. Every year around four million cases account worldwide. In the USA alone, nonmelanocytic skin cancer is very common, and the incidence rate is approximately 1–3 million new patients [23]. While in Europe, Canada, and Australia, the occurrence rate is increasing by 9% every year, and it is expected to be double in the next few years [24]. The risk factors include ultraviolet rays, ionizing radiation, and chemical carcinogens [25]. The alarming increase in the number of skin cancer across the world has been attributed to age, gender, immunosuppression, UV exposure, skin type, sun radiation, and family history. The most common gold standard treatment for localized tumours is excision for these localized diseases without damaging normalized tissue [26].

It is possible to make an important influence on medicine by providing alterations in disease diagnosis and therapy. According to the federal US research and development programme agency, the National Nanotechnology Initiative (NNI), nanotechnology incorporates the progress of carrier's devices or systems sized in 1–100 nm range. At the same time, it can be widened up to 1000 nm. The unique factor, such as high surface-to-volume ratio and the feasible of tuning their properties, have gained significant interest and biomedical applications in imaging, diagnosis, and therapy [27, 28]. In the current health care domain, making use of nanotechnology can develop new efficient treatments, in a way to reduce the adverse effects and cost of the treatment both to governments and to the patients. In the current scenario, most of the researchers or scientists have been working on the development of new ways to release the drug to patients using nanoparticles as a nanocarrier without side effects and preventing damage to neighbouring cells [29]. Melanoma has been treated with conventional therapies through nanoscience and technology. The efficiency of the treatment via nano-drug delivery systems for chemotherapy, immunotherapy, targeted therapy, and photodynamic therapy has been developed to a great extent [30–32]. These nanoparticles can also address the water-soluble drugs, modify pharmacokinetics, enhance drug half-life by diminishing immunogenicity, bioavailability, and reducing the drug metabolism. Nanoparticles also play around in release of drugs, i.e. delivering two or more drugs at a time in terms of combination therapy. [33, 34]. Engineered nanocarriers also used as a combination of chemo and phototherapy to evaluate the treatment scenario in real-time, for synergistic and anticancer therapy [35]. This chapter summarizes the types of skin cancer and treatment with an emphasis on nanotechnology.

11.2   Pathology and Conventional Therapies of Skin Cancer

The treatment method depends on the tumour location; cell type, location, and depth; the cosmetic desires of the patient; the history of previous treatment; whether the tumour is invasive, and whether metastatic nodes are present.

11.2.1 Malignant Melanoma Skin Cancer (MSC)

Melanoma emerges from melanocytes, the cells which produce the melanin. In the pathological procedure, different mutations can occur, predominantly located in the epidermis, at the basal layer [35, 36]. The risk factors including for malignant melanoma are ultraviolet light exposure; it causes the mutations in melanocytes that results in the invasive metastatic characteristics [37]. The characteristics mutations involved in the malignant melanoma are BRAF/NRAS/MAPK/MEK pathways; these signalling pathways are mainly operated on the malignant melanoma, without causing mutations. Hence, these are repetitive targets to involve in the treatment of melanoma [38]. The treatment strategy is chosen based on the stage of cancer, and available conventional therapies include surgery. Radiation therapy and other inventive therapies include targeted therapy, immunotherapy, and a mixture of systemic, topical, and transdermal treatments [39]. Melanoma can cure about 90% in the patients with absence of metastatic ability; on the other hand, the survival rate of the patients with metastasis is nearly only ten% [40]. Surgery is preferred for the patients with lesions of well-defined borders, and only at an early stage. The complications behind the surgical excision involve lymph node and metastases [41]. The location and depth of the melanoma is decided based on the Breslow's tumour thickness, which is shown in Table 11.1 below

Radiation therapy has been used as an initial treatment for patients with a clear diagnosis and well-defined and clear bordered lesions. Radiation therapy has very good tumour reduction rates, and it is well tolerated with patients [42]. Along with this, radiation therapy can be given to patients with an advanced stage, provided with other interventional therapies such as immunotherapy. The mechanism behind melanocytic skin cancer has not been identified yet, and therefore treating the patients with the disease is a challenge. To defeat this challenge ahead, need innovative therapies with mainly focused on drug delivery systems with a focus on nanotechnology [43].

11.2.2 Non-Melanoma Skin Cancer (NMSC)

Non-melanoma skin cancer is not more aggressive and less invasive potential, and therefore the therapeutic strategies are more potential in non-melanoma skin cancer. Non-melanoma skin cancer is combined with good prognosis and survival rate than a more aggressive form of malignant melanoma skin cancer [44].

Table 11.1 Breslow's tumour thickness

Stage	Depth of the tumour
I	Tumour with <1.0 mm
IIA	1.01–2.0 mm
IIB	2.01–4.0 mm
III	4.0 mm < tumour depth

Squamous cell carcinoma (SCC) and basal cell carcinoma (BCC) emerge in keratinocytes and called keratinocyte carcinomas. BCC is familiar than SCC, reports about 70% of the cases, in contrast with 25% of SCC and more pronounced among all other types of cancer. Both BCC and SCC do not contribute to death. Still, these types of cancer are considered as public health issues, on behalf of high incidence rate [45]. There are plentiful risk factors which known to cause this type of neoplasia, including in terms of genetics, such as age, ultraviolet rays, ionizing radiation, immunosuppressors, and few of the medications are TNF-α inhibitors, tobacco use, severe skin and bone infections, and inflammatory conditions [46]. Nonmalignant skin cancer can be treated through surgical excision confined on the size and locations of the lesions. The non-surgical treatment also suggested for lesions with clear cut pictures with confined regions. The non-surgical treatments include are curettage, electrodesiccation, topical drug administration, cryosurgery, and radiation and photodynamic therapies. The choice of the treatment may differ based upon the lesion size and location, and also the cell signalling pathways [47]. Different types of nanoparticles have been used to treat nonmalignant skin cancer owing to the efficient in delivering drugs, via the signalling pathways, along with the administration route to make it low invasive [48–50].

11.3 Challenges to Skin Cancer Treatment

11.3.1 Biological Barriers

In the present scenario, nanoparticles encapsulated with anticancer molecule are administered via intratumourally, transdermal, intravenous, or via a mixture of these. For elderly patients, topical or transdermal applications are preferred due to its noninvasive, self-administered and for patients who are not ideally preferred for surgical excision. The routes of administration have been advantageous for premalignant lesions, superficial skin cancer, like noninvasive SCC; and BCC and melanoma in the early stages [48] the superficial layer is the epidermis, consists of stratum corneum, which is the main cutaneous barrier and enhance the intake of anticancer drugs to the targeted tissues. Stratum corneum is made up of 15–20 corneocyte cell layers, with a thickness of 10–20 μm. These layers are constituents of long epidermal maturation, differentiation, and keratinization processes [51] along with, different types of lipids are envelop corneocytes, like ceramides, triglycerides, cholesterols, and free fatty acids, to conceive multiple network of lipids and corneocytes which can absorb can consume water and influence the penetration of macromolecules and micro molecules over the skin [52].

The second viable epidermis is localized underneath the stratum corneum and extends the dermal–epidermal junction fabricate by the thin basal layer. The alike dermis, viable epidermis is consisting of keratinocytes at divergent stages of maturation and occupied by melanocytes, Langerhans cells, and Merkel cells and area with the depth of 50–100 μm. The viable epidermis receives nutritional support from the dermis. The dermis consisting of lymphatic vessels, sebaceous glands, collagen, elastin, sensory nerves, and hair follicles are and localized with the thickness of 0.1–0.4 cm thick [53].

There are different types of skin cancer with an increased quantity of keratin, causes diffusion-resistant tissue and leads to the significant barrier to the passive transport and holding of nanoparticles in the target cells [54]. Actinic keratosis secretes a large amount of keratin, creating the stratum corneum thicker and leads to difficulty in penetration and therefore use of nanoparticles towards the treatment of actinic keratosis had to be constructed to penetrate into the stratum corneum and enters to the deep layer of the epidermis, to enhance the immune response through the Langerhans cells [55].

The other biological barrier involving the intestinal tumour space consisting of collagen, proteins, elastic fibres, and glycosaminoglycans. Due to the increase in the intestinal fluid pressure, the drugs transported to the interior are disturbed. Moreover, the extracellular matrix present in the tumour microenvironment is inflexible and increased collagen acts as a barrier to the nanoparticles to pass through the cancer cells [56]. The physio and chemical properties of the nanoparticles have significance on interaction with tumour cells, relation to the cancer cells and also the physiological properties of the cells. The important interactions between cancer cells and nanoparticles are adsorption, cellular uptake, endocytosis, endosomal escape, metabolism, and degradation [57]. Few of the authors also discussed on the cell uptake pathways, trafficking, and kinetics, may also be disturbed through the factors of the nanoparticles.

In general, the plasma membrane is the barrier for the uptake of nanoparticles because of it is negatively charged and leads to selective permeability to drugs and nanoparticles depending on the size and location. A cellular barrier may be defeated through different routes and mechanism as follows, the entry of the nanoparticles directly to the cell or endocytosis mechanism. The other way, these systems transported through the cell membrane via lipid bilayer, other nanoparticles enter to the cytoplasm, hence, to get over the endosomal entrance through energy-dependent transport mechanism. The entry of the nanoparticles through endocytosis pathways is trapped inside the intracellular vesicles once they get into the cytoplasm [58].

There are different mechanisms for entry of nanoparticles via endocytosis, such as micropinocytosis, phagocytosis, caveolin-independent endocytosis, caveolin-dependent endocytosis, clathrin-independent endocytosis [59]. Once endosomes entrap the nanoparticle, nanoparticles are performed to exit and ready to act at the targeting site. Intratumoural injection is more advantageous as compared to other administration routes, nanoparticles can be injected intratumourally, and at high concentrations, minimally invasive and low doses can be preferred, painless than subcutaneous injection. The intratumoural injection is a potential site of vaccination through direct intratumoural injection or immunization, improves the magnitude, and improves the control of metastasis [60].

11.3.2 Multidrug Resistance (MDR)

Multidrug resistance is the mechanism where cancer drugs develop resistance to chemotherapy, which is the major issue for the failure of many forms of chemotherapy towards different cancers. Nanoscience and technology is an upcoming field to defeat the multidrug resistance. So, using nanotechnology other than the conventional method of treatment is to use a very low concentration of drugs with lesser adverse effects [61]. Nanocarrier is used effectively with various chemotherapeutic agents and combinational therapies and molecules for achieving effective and acts synergistically against cancer cells that are shown resistance to conventional treatment [62].

Multidrug resistance happens when the drug molecule or therapeutic agents show resistance to tumour cells. MDR is also caused by a loss ineffectiveness of the drug [63].

The MDR develops with various intrinsic and acquired factors. Intrinsic factors are associated with degradation of the drug, alteration of prodrugs, modification of drug targets and receptors, and loss in drug–receptor interactions. And changes in the cell membrane, modifications in the metabolic process, cell cycle changes, DNA damage, and alterations in efflux pumps may associate to MDR. The acquired factors are involving with epigenetics. Patients with intrinsic factors do not respond to conventional treatments; patients with acquired factors resistance showed a reduced significance of the treatment for a longer time. [64].

The mechanism behind the resistance caused by chemotherapeutic agents towards cancer can be termed as cellular and non-cellular mechanisms. The cellular mechanism develops from the biochemical changes from the tumour cells. Non-cellular mechanisms are generated by internal characteristics like pH, that leads to aggressiveness of the tumour cells despite action of the cancer drugs [65]. The skin cancer is involved through a few of the cell signalling pathways and mechanisms, such as to circumvent of apoptosis pathways, changes in DNA repair, and P53 modifications [66].

11.4 Nanoparticles as Drug Carriers

Nanoparticles have been used as a drug carrier for a decade and hold a better potential for anticancer treatment. Nanocarriers prevent drugs from degradation, to enhance the stability and bioavailability, the drug is encapsulated through electrostatic force, hydrophilic and hydrophobic interactions, or the chemical moieties [67]. The foremost advantages are to the delivery of drug molecules through nanocarrier can effectively penetrate and enter tumour tissue through active or passive targeting, hence minimizing the adverse events in normal tissue. Different nanoparticles can be utilized as a nanocarrier for anticancer treatment, such as polymers, mesoporous silica, polymer micelles, dendrimers, carbon nanotubes, gold, silver, and other metal oxides. These nanocarriers should have low toxic effects upon treated with normal cells [68].

Skin cancer with nanotechnology has shown great potential for advanced therapeutics. The centre of attention has been on diagnosis and treating skin cancer. Various chemotherapeutic agents administered systemically showed toxic to healthy cells [69]. Engineered nanoparticles are directed for imaging, and specifically, deliver the drug molecule or small-interfering RNA to the most aggressive type of skin cancer [70]. Insolubility is the main disadvantage, fails clinically with many chemotherapeutic agents. Nanocarrier has overcome insolubility issues, as many drugs will be encapsulated into the nanoparticles [71].

11.4.1 Nanoparticles Technologies for Drug Delivery

There are different nanoparticles that have been developed, engineered, and used for applications of skin cancer. The nanoparticles involved are lipid nanoparticles, polymeric nanoparticles, nanoemulsions, and metallic nanoparticles. Many researchers have been extensively working on the nanotechnology with skin cancer using different nanoparticles. In this chapter, we briefed an overview of very commonly used systems in drug delivery [72].

11.4.1.1 Liposomes

Liposomes are a collection of cholesterol and phospholipids evolving in a hollow lipid bilayer, which encapsulates hydrophobic and hydrophilic entities with an aqueous core for solubilization. Liposomes enhance the drug's pharmacokinetics, specificity, and to improve efficacy with less toxicity [73]. In 1980, Mezei and Gulasekharan first identified the proposal for using liposomes for skin cancer. Consequently, there are numerous studies that have been undergone to use liposomes in combination with nanotechnology techniques for dermal delivery [74]. The most used phospholipids involving phosphatidylcholine take out from egg yolk, soybean, or other synthetic and hydrogenated forms. The composition of the liposomes allows adsorption on the surface of the skin and fusion with stratum corneum lipids, hence promoting drug release into the cells [75]. The electrostatic interaction between the positively charged liposomes and negatively charged SC benefits the adsorption and penetration in contrast with an anionic liposome. Researchers have designed liposomes attain an accumulation of the drug in different layers of the skin compared to the plain drug. Liposomes with 50 nm shown to penetrate deeply into the layers as compared to the larger particles that localized on the surface [76].

11.4.1.2 Natural Polymeric Nanoparticle

Among natural polymers, chitosan nanoparticles have been widely used for skin drug delivery. Chitosan, chitin are biodegradable, cationic, have antioxidant, anti-inflammatory, and antimicrobial properties thus utilized for skin cancer applications. The positive charge of the chitosan involving the polymer to attract with the negatively charged surface of the skin makes it possible to deliver the drugs and cross the barrier [77]. Chitosan nanoparticles have also been used because of its increased soluble property and delivery of retinol for the treatment of acne and wrinkles. Researchers also designed the ethylcellulose nanoparticles to initiate the deeper skin penetration and improve the retention of quercetin with sustained release of the drug [78].

11.4.1.3 Synthetic Polymeric Nanoparticle

Several synthetic biodegradable polymers, poly (lactide-co-glycolide) copolymers (PLGA), polylactic acid (PLA), and poly(ε-caprolactone) (PCL) have been used for skin cancer applications. Nanospheres created from tyrosine-derived polymers (TyroSpheres™) with a diameter of 70 nm have also been efficiently used for enhanced skin delivery of lipophilic drugs. These nanoparticles build by an ABA-type triblock copolymer. Therefore, block A shows the hydrophilic poly (ethylene glycol), and block B depicts the hydrophobic oligomers of suberic acid and tyrosine-derived diol [79]. TyroSpheres can encapsulate into hydrophobic drugs such as Paclitaxel or Cholecalciferol for enhanced delivery of skin cancer. Due to the small size of the nanoparticle, these polymeric nanoparticles tend to store by gathering inside the hair follicle and on the surface of the skin. The polymeric nanoparticle also integrates with paramagnetic metals, such as gadolinium (Gd) or manganese (Mn), for applications such as image contrast agents for live cell imaging [80].

11.4.1.4 Dendrimers

Dendrimers are the polymers, which are synthesized using unique methods as compared to other macromolecules. These nanoparticles have a central core that arises to symmetrically ordered replicated units. Dendrimers give unique advantages for tuning their biological relations and engineering functional properties. Dendrimer polymeric nanoparticles have become biocompatible, monodispersed, well-defined sized particles. Polyamidoamines (PAMAM), poly(L-lysine) (PLL) scaffold dendrimers, polyesters (PGLSA-OH), and polypropylenes (PPI) are most used drug delivery dendrimers [81]. The core-shell architecture of dendrimers promotes the integration of lipophilic and hydrophilic drugs, image contrast agents, and nucleic acids. The factors that contribute to penetrating the skin are surface charge, the hydrodynamic size, molecular weight, size of the generation, composition, and concentration. The physiochemical structure of the dendrimers are radial growth, well-defined molecular architecture, and spherical form of dendrimers converse the physicochemical properties [82].

Few studies have shown that (G0–G4), is a low generation of PAMAM dendrimers with hydrodynamic radii of less than 5 nm diameter transverse the intercellular lipid matrix. In contrast with neutral or anionic dendrimers, the cationic dendrimers can change the skin permeability via exchange with its lipids. Cationic dendrimers have been chosen as permeation enhancers accompanying skin pretreatment or co-administration with drugs [83]. Most of the studies have shown the achievable of using dendrimers for efficient skin delivery of non-steroidal anti-inflammatory drugs, antimicrobial, antiviral, anticancer, antihypertensive drugs, alpha-blockers, and peptides [84].

11.4.1.5 Nanofibres

Nanofibres have become a great interest in topical drug delivery systems, particularly for wound healing and antimicrobial activity. Nanofibres are not associated with the nanoparticles. The shape and structure of the nanofibres are with an average diameter of 100 nm. These nanofibres with potential properties such as tunable pore size, the surface-to-volume ratio, associated with hydrophilic and hydrophobic drugs [85]. A long ago, different polymers that are natural and synthetic polymers have been utilized for fabrication of nanofibre mats for drug delivery applications. Nanofibres evolved from collagen, hyaluronic acid polycaprolactone, PLA, PLGA, PGA, poly (vinyl pyrrolidone), polyurethane, poly (vinyl alcohol), tyrosine-derived polycarbonates, etc. Nanofibres have been investigated broadly for dermal drug delivery systems. Therefore, these nanofibres have been widely used for the delivery for anti-fungal, antioxidant, anti-proliferative for a controlled and sustained drug release [86].

11.4.1.6 Silica Nanoparticles

Mesoporous silica nanoparticles have shown potential advantages on cancer treatment because of its physiochemical properties such as particle size, morphology, tunable pore volume, ease of surface functionalization, chemical and mechanical stability, large surface area, and drug loading and releasing capacity [87]. Mesoporous silica nanoparticles have been transverse to both imaging and therapy, leading them to the theragnostic platform. In recent times, silica nanoparticles doped with dye are termed as Cornell dots (C dots), have been accepted for the application for targeted therapy and molecular diagnostics in the area of cancer.

11.4.1.7 Gold Nanoparticles

Gold nanoparticles (AuNP) are most widely used in drug and gene delivery systems. Gold nanoparticles are one among the metallic nanoparticles. The other metallic nanoparticles are Ag, Ni, Pt, and TiO_2. Gold nanoparticles are synthesized and prepared with different shapes and structure from 1 to 150 nm in size, such as spheres, cages, shells, and rods. The potential advantages of gold nanoparticles are ease of synthesis, surface functionalization, and capability to conjugate with other biomolecules without any change in biological properties [88]. Gold nanoparticles can cross the blood–brain barrier with an average size of 50 nm have been demonstrated. Several drugs, involving proteins and DNA and other anticancer drug molecules, associated with the surface chemistry gold nanoparticles, enhance therapeutic effect in different types of tumours, including melanoma. Moreover, gold nanoparticles are nontoxic, biocompatible. Therefore, gold nanoparticles do not produce an immune reaction [89].

11.5   Treatment Strategies

11.5.1 Chemotherapy

The chemotherapy treatment involving suppression of tumour cells and to kill the cancer cells. These chemotherapeutic drugs produce an adverse effect and also damage the healthy surrounding cells. Nanotechnology has been referred for the localization of the nanoparticles and drug delivery to the specific tumour sites without affecting the neighbour cells in contrast to molecular targeted drugs. Through obstructing the required cell signalling pathways which are essential for tumour growth [90].

11.5.2 Protein-Based-Therapy

(a) Protein transduction technology
    Synthetic and natural polymer peptides can transverse the lipid bilayer and enter into the cells. Peptides have been used to penetrate the lipid bilayer, protein transduction domains, and cell-penetrating peptides. The properties of peptides and proteins have been modified using recombinant technology with regard to cell permeability through protein transduction domains and cell-penetrating peptides. Which are utilized for transduction of nanoparticles, oligonucleotides on both in vitro and in vivo. Out of many protein transduction domains, R9-PTD-containing proteins to keep go on inflammatory cells in the injection area for a longer period and transduced into dermal cancer cells. These strategies could be termed as novel molecular targeting for skin cancer [91].
(b) Hsps chaperone-based therapies.
    Heat shock proteins are a class of proteins, which is stimulated by physical, chemical stress. The overexpression of heat shock proteins is overexpressed in a broad level of malignancies and associated with cell proliferation, differentiation, metastasis, and identification of the immune system. The mechanism behind the heat shock proteins towards progression and drug resistance for treatment is through the initiation of safeguarding the apoptosis created by therapy. Hence the heat shock proteins, a biomarker for carcinogenesis such as Hsp27, Hsp70, and 90 used as markers for differentiation of keratinocytes in the skin cancer. An anti-Hsp and circulating Hsp present in cancer patients may have opted for tumour diagnosis [92].

11.5.3 Biological Therapies

(a) Immunotherapies.
    It is said that the cancer cells are confessed by the immune system, which in turn may suppress the tumours. There are different immune therapy modalities had been undergoing for various cancer types. Recently few of the scientist had been

approached a novel immune stimulatory approach for skin cancer. Anti-CTLA4 agent's receptor CTLA-4) and PD-1/PD-L1 pathway blocking antibodies, which target a second co-inhibitory receptor PD-1, because of their recent trends in the clinical research and implementation.

The anti-CTLA-4 monoclonal antibodies such as Ipilimumab approved by FDA in 2011 and tremelimumab. Nivolumab and pembrolizumab are anti-PD1 agents, and pembrolizumab is approved by the FDA during 2014 termed as "checkpoint-blocking" antibodies. Therefore, involving in the down-modulation of CD8+ and CD4+ effector T cell function. CTLA-4 and PD-1 are negative regulators and take part in an inessential in regulating immune reaction. CLTA-4, associated with ligands such as CD80 and CD86, plays a vital role in the activation of T cells. PD-1 is associated with regulating T cell activation through coordination with other PD-L1 and PD-L2.

Moreover, the melanoma cells turn to express an elevated level for the PD-1 receptor, which is overexpressed in human tumours and circulating tumours with T cells with damaged T cell function. Hence, these data findings suggested that, the intrusion of the PD-1: PD-L1/PD-L2 would be potential for anticancer therapy through the hindrance of immune reaction in the tumour microenvironment [93].

(b) Laser therapy.

Photodynamic therapy is a widely used therapy upon laser irradiation. It has been broadly influenced by the scientific community and, in the clinic, included with other treatments. Photodynamic therapy is using of the photosensitizer with a specific wavelength, upon laser irradiation enhances the reactive oxygen species production and singlet oxygen molecules leading to cell death on biological, chemical, and physiological reactions [94]. Few of the studies showed that the using of nanoparticles such as lipid-based, polymer-based, and encapsulated with a wide range of photosensitizers upon laser light irradiation believed to be an ideal platform for enhancing the greater penetration and biological mechanisms of these photosensitizers loaded nanoparticles in skin cancer [95].

(c) Multifunctional delivery systems.

The multifunctional drug delivery systems have been developed for the progression and survival of cancer. The multifunctional drug delivery systems are carrying or loading with at least of two drug molecules with divergent pharmacological mechanisms against cancer for future cancer therapeutics [96]. In terms of skin cancer therapy, an advance in multifunctional drug delivery systems has been widely used through encapsulating at least two molecules dqawith a combination of chemo and radiation therapy or immunotherapy with the loading of siRNAs immunotherapeutic molecules has proven to be more advantageous than a single molecule. These multifunctional therapeutic strategies can be used in metastasis conditions [97].

11.6 Conclusion and Future Perspective

Nanoscience and technology have developed the technologies beyond conventional therapies and new challenges towards cancer therapy. Nanomedicine for skin tumour has launched a therapeutic strategy in recent times involving aggressive and invasive tumours through different administration routes. Initial tumour lesions can be treated using a topical way. Nanoparticles loaded with the drug molecules carrying to the tumour site to suppress the tumour mass and in combination therapy is the most attractive approach. The use of nanoparticles with specific and individualized treatments with lesser concentrations reduces the adverse effects in contrast with conventional therapies.

In summary, the utility of nanocarriers develops experimentally because of its cost-effectiveness, as their potential advantages direct to a better hope for diagnosis and treatments. The use of nanocarrier is also very effective for clinical setup. At the endpoint, the use of nanotechnology with several therapeutic strategies to destroy the illness called cancer is not still completed and more to come with effective and safeguarded therapy.

References

1. Naves LB, Dhand C, Venugopal JR, Rajamani L, Ramakrishna S, Almeida L (2017) Nanotechnology for the treatment of melanoma skin cancer. Prog Biomater 6:13–26
2. Allen DC (2013) Histopathology reporting: guidelines for surgical cancer. Springer, London, pp 197–206
3. Buczacki S (2016) In: Bradshaw RA, Stahl PD (eds) Encyclopedia of cell biology. Academic Press, Waltham, MA, pp 807–812
4. Jögi A, Vaapil M, Johansson M, Påhlman S (2012) Cancer cell differentiation heterogeneity and aggressive behavior in solid tumors. Ups J Med Sci 117:217–224
5. Yan M, Liu Q (2016) Differentiation therapy: a promising strategy for cancer treatment. Chin J Cancer 35:3
6. Cameron MC, Lee E, Hibler BP, Barker CA, Mori S, Cordova M, Nehal KS, Rossi AM (2019) Basal cell carcinoma: epidemiology; pathophysiology; clinical and histological subtypes; and disease associations. J Am Acad Dermatol 80:303–317
7. Li WW, Li VW, Hutnik M, Chiou AS (2012) Tumor angiogenesis as a target for dietary cancer prevention. J Oncol 2012:879623
8. Holtz C (2007) Global health care: issues and policies. Jones & Bartlett Learning, Burlington, MA
9. Lee JW, Ratnakumar K, Hung K-F, Rokunohe D, Kawasumi M (2020) Deciphering UV-induced DNA damage responses to prevent and treat skin cancer. Photochem Photobiol 96:478–499
10. Apalla Z, Lallas A, Sotiriou E, Lazaridou E, Ioannides D (2017) Epidemiological trends in skin cancer. Dermatol Pract Concept 7:1–6
11. Guy GP Jr, Machlin SR, Ekwueme DU, Yabroff KR (2015) Prevalence and costs of skin cancer treatment in the U.S., 2002-2006 and 2007-2011. Am J Prev Med 48:183–187
12. Ekwueme DU, Guy GPJ, Li C, Rim SH, Parelkar P, Chen SC (2011) The health burden and economic costs of cutaneous melanoma mortality by race/ethnicity-United States, 2000 to 2006. J Am Acad Dermatol 65:S133–S143
13. Leiter U, Keim U, Garbe C (2020) Epidemiology of skin cancer: update 2019. Adv Exp Med Biol 1268:123–139

14. Corona R (1996) Epidemiology of nonmelanoma skin cancer: a review. Ann Ist Super Sanita 32:37–42

15. Pesec M, Sherertz T (2015) Global health from a cancer care perspective. Future Oncol 11:2235–2245

16. Laikova KV, Oberemok VV, Krasnodubets AM, Gal'chinsky NV, Useinov RZ, Novikov IA, Temirova ZZ, Gorlov MV, Shved NA, Kumeiko VV, Makalish TP, Bessalova EY, Fomochkina II, Esin AS, Volkov ME, Kubyshkin AV (2019) Advances in the understanding of skin cancer: ultraviolet radiation, mutations, and antisense oligonucleotides as anticancer drugs. Molecules 24(8):1516. https://doi.org/10.3390/molecules24081516

17. Zadnik V, Primic Zakelj M, Lokar K, Jarm K, Ivanus U, Zagar T (2017) Cancer burden in slovenia with the time trends analysis. Radiol Oncol 51:47–55

18. Forsea AM, Del Marmol V, de Vries E, Bailey EE, Geller AC (2012) Melanoma incidence and mortality in Europe: new estimates, persistent disparities. Br J Dermatol 167:1124–1130

19. Bray F, Ferlay J, Soerjomataram I, Siegel RL, Torre LA, Jemal A (2018) Global cancer statistics 2018: GLOBOCAN estimates of incidence and mortality worldwide for 36 cancers in 185 countries. CA Cancer J Clin 68:394–424

20. Scoggins CR, Ross MI, Reintgen DS, Noyes RD, Goydos JS, Beitsch PD, Urist MM, Ariyan S, Sussman JJ, Edwards MJ, Chagpar AB, Martin RCG, Stromberg AJ, Hagendoorn L, McMasters KM (2006) The Sunbelt melanoma trial (2006) Gender-related differences in outcome for melanoma patients. Ann Surg 243:693–700

21. Sandru A, Voinea S, Panaitescu E, Blidaru A (2014) Survival rates of patients with metastatic malignant melanoma. J Med Life 7:572–576

22. Watson M, Holman DM, Maguire-Eisen M (2016) Ultraviolet radiation exposure and its impact on skin cancer risk. Semin Oncol Nurs 32:241–254

23. Xiang F, Lucas R, Hales S, Neale R (2014) Incidence of nonmelanoma skin cancer in relation to ambient UV radiation in white populations, 1978–2012: empirical relationships. JAMA Dermatology 150:1063–1071

24. Eide MJ, Krajenta R, Johnson D, Long JJ, Jacobsen G, Asgari MM, Lim HW, Johnson CC (2009) Providers' experiences with a melanoma web-based course: a discussion on barriers and intentions. Am J Epidemiol 171:123–128

25. Bauer A, Adam KE, Soyer PH, Adam KWJ (2020) In: John SM, Johansen JD, Rustemeyer T, Elsner P, Maibach HI (eds) Kanerva's occupational dermatology. Springer, Cham, pp 1685–1697

26. Tramutola A, Falcucci S, Brocco U, Triani F, Lanzillotta C, Donati M, Panetta C, Luzi F, Iavarone F, Vincenzoni F, Castagnola M, Perluigi M, Di Domenico F, De Marco F (2020) Protein oxidative damage in UV-related skin cancer and dysplastic lesions contributes to neoplastic promotion and progression. Cancers 12(1):110. https://doi.org/10.3390/cancers12010110

27. Khan I, Saeed K, Khan I (2019) Nanoparticles: properties, applications and toxicities. Arab J Chem 12:908–931

28. Chenthamara D, Subramaniam S, Ramakrishnan SG, Krishnaswamy S, Essa MM, Lin F-H, Qoronfleh MW (2019) Therapeutic efficacy of nanoparticles and routes of administration. Biomater Res 23:20

29. Patra JK, Das G, Fraceto LF, Campos EVR, Rodriguez-Torres MDP, Acosta-Torres LS, Diaz-Torres LA, Grillo R, Swamy MK, Sharma S, Habtemariam S, Shin H-S (2018) Nano based drug delivery systems: recent developments and future prospects. J Nanobiotechnology 16:71

30. Xin Y, Yin M, Zhao L, Meng F, Luo L (2017) Recent progress on nanoparticle-based drug delivery systems for cancer therapy. Cancer Biol Med 14:228–241

31. Senapati S, Mahanta AK, Kumar S, Maiti P (2018) Controlled drug delivery vehicles for cancer treatment and their performance. Signal Transduct Target Ther 3:7

32. Zhang H, Dong S, Li Z, Feng X, Xu W, Tulinao CMS, Jiang Y, Ding J (2020) Biointerface engineering nanoplatforms for cancer-targeted drug delivery. Asian J Pharm Sci 15:397–415

33. Ma L, Kohli M, Smith A (2013) Nanoparticles for combination drug therapy. ACS Nano 7:9518–9525
34. Gurunathan S, Kang M-H, Qasim M, Kim J-H (2018) Nanoparticle-mediated combination therapy: two-in-one approach for cancer. Int J Mol Sci 19(10):3264. https://doi.org/10.3390/ijms19103264
35. Zhao C-Y, Cheng R, Yang Z, Tian Z-M (2018) Nanotechnology for cancer therapy based on chemotherapy. Molecules 23(4):826. https://doi.org/10.3390/molecules23040826
36. Bertolotto C (2013) Melanoma: from melanocyte to genetic alterations and clinical options. Scientifica (Cairo) 2013:635203
37. Anna B, Blazej Z, Jacqueline G, Andrew CJ, Jeffrey R, Andrzej S (2007) Mechanism of UV-related carcinogenesis and its contribution to nevi/melanoma. Expert Rev Dermatol 2:451–469
38. Savoia P, Fava P, Casoni F, Cremona O (2019) Targeting the ERK signaling pathway in Melanoma. Int J Mol Sci 20(6):1483. https://doi.org/10.3390/ijms20061483
39. Agostinis P, Berg K, Cengel KA, Foster TH, Girotti AW, Gollnick SO, Hahn SM, Hamblin MR, Juzeniene A, Kessel D, Korbelik M, Moan J, Mroz P, Nowis D, Piette J, Wilson BC, Golab J (2011) Photodynamic therapy of cancer: an update. CA Cancer J Clin 61(4):250–281
40. Damsky WE, Rosenbaum LE, Bosenberg M (2010) Decoding melanoma metastasis. Cancers 3:126–163
41. Wernick BD, Goel N, Zih FS, Farma JM (2017) A surgical perspective report on melanoma management. Melanoma Manag 4:105–112
42. Puza CJ, Bressler ES, Terando AM, Howard JH, Brown MC, Hanks B, Salama AKS, Beasley GM (2019) The emerging role of surgery for patients with advanced melanoma treated with immunotherapy. J Surg Res 236:209–215
43. Hossen S, Hossain MK, Basher MK, Mia MNH, Rahman MT, Uddin MJ (2018) Smart nanocarrier-based drug delivery systems for cancer therapy and toxicity studies: a review. J Adv Res 15:1–18
44. Tanese K, Nakamura Y, Hirai I, Funakoshi T (2019) Updates on the systemic treatment of advanced non-melanoma skin cancer. Front Med 6:160
45. Peris K, Fargnoli MC, Garbe C, Kaufmann R, Bastholt L, Seguin NB, Bataille V, del Marmol V, Dummer R, Harwood CA, Hauschild A, Höller C, Haedersdal M, Malvehy J, Middleton MR, Morton CA, Nagore E, Stratigos AJ, Szeimies R-M, Tagliaferri L, Trakatelli M, Zalaudek I, Eggermont A, Grob JJ (2019) Diagnosis and treatment of basal cell carcinoma: European consensus-based interdisciplinary guidelines. Eur J Cancer 118:10–34
46. Cuomo MI (2012) A world without cancer: the making of a new cure and the real promise of prevention. Rodale Books, Pennsylvania, PA
47. Kallini JR, Hamed N, Khachemoune A (2015) Squamous cell carcinoma of the skin: epidemiology, classification, management, and novel trends. Int J Dermatol 54:130–140
48. Borgheti-Cardoso LN, Viegas JSR, Silvestrini AVP, Caron AL, Praça FG, Kravicz M, Bentley MVLB (2020) Adv Drug Deliv Rev 153:109–136
49. Thakor AS, Gambhir SS (2013) CA Cancer J Clin 63:395–418
50. Liu Q, Das M, Liu Y, Huang L (2018) Adv Drug Deliv Rev 127:208–221
51. Kahraman E, Kaykın M, Bektay HŞ, Güngör S (2019) Recent advances on topical application of ceramides to restore barrier function of skin. Cosmetics 6(3):52. https://doi.org/10.3390/cosmetics6030052
52. Norlén L (2006) Stratum corneum keratin structure, function and formation - a comprehensive review. Int J Cosmet Sci 28:397–425
53. Kabashima K, Honda T, Ginhoux F, Egawa G (2019) The immunological anatomy of the skin. Nat Rev Immunol 19:19–30
54. Alkilani AZ, McCrudden MTC, Donnelly RF (2015) Transdermal drug delivery: innovative pharmaceutical developments based on disruption of the barrier properties of the stratum corneum. Pharmaceutics 7:438–470

55. Barton JK, Gossage KW, Xu W, Ranger-Moore JR, Saboda K, Brooks CA, Duckett LD, Salasche SJ, Warneke JA, Alberts DS (2003) Investigating sun-damaged skin and actinic keratosis with optical coherence tomography: a pilot study. Technol Cancer Res Treat 2:525–535

56. Barua S, Mitragotri S (2014) Challenges associated with penetration of nanoparticles across cell and tissue barriers: a review of current status and future prospects. Nano Today 9:223–243

57. Zhao F, Zhao Y, Liu Y, Chang X, Chen C, Zhao Y (2011) Cellular uptake, intracellular trafficking, and cytotoxicity of nanomaterials. Small 7:1322–1337

58. Foroozandeh P, Aziz AA (2018) Insight into cellular uptake and intracellular trafficking of nanoparticles. Nanoscale Res Lett 13:339

59. Moghimi SM, Hunter AC, Murray JC (2005) Nanomedicine: current status and future prospects. FASEB J 19:311–330

60. Nakao S, Arai Y, Tasaki M, Yamashita M, Murakami R, Kawase T, Amino N, Nakatake M, Kurosaki H, Mori M, Takeuchi M, Nakamura T (2020) Intratumoral expression of IL-7 and IL-12 using an oncolytic virus increases systemic sensitivity to immune checkpoint blockade. Sci Transl Med 12(526):eaax7992. https://doi.org/10.1126/scitranslmed.aax7992

61. Mansoori B, Mohammadi A, Davudian S, Shirjang S, Baradaran B (2017) The different mechanisms of cancer drug resistance: a brief review. Adv Pharm Bull 7:339–348

62. Din FU, Aman W, Ullah I, Qureshi OS, Mustapha O, Shafique S, Zeb A (2017) Effective use of nanocarriers as drug delivery systems for the treatment of selected tumors. Int J Nanomed 12:7291–7309

63. Housman G, Byler S, Heerboth S, Lapinska K, Longacre M, Snyder N, Sarkar S (2014) Drug resistance in cancer: an overview. Cancers 6:1769–1792

64. Bukowski K, Kciuk M, Kontek R (2020) Mechanisms of multidrug resistance in cancer chemotherapy. Int J Mol Sci 21(9):3233

65. AL-Busairi W (2020) Cohen-Solal. IntechOpen, p 8

66. Sever R, Brugge JS (2015) Signal transduction in cancer. Cold Spring Harb Perspect Med 5: a006098

67. Singh R, Lillard JWJ (2009) Nanoparticle-based targeted drug delivery. Exp Mol Pathol 86:215–223

68. Navya PN, Kaphle A, Srinivas SP, Bhargava SK, Rotello VM, Daima HK (2019) Current trends and challenges in cancer management and therapy using designer nanomaterials. Nano Converg 6:23

69. Dianzani C, Zara GP, Maina G, Pettazzoni P, Pizzimenti S, Rossi F, Gigliotti CL, Ciamporcero ES, Daga M, Barrera G (2014) Biomed Res Int 2014:895986

70. Mihai MM, Holban AM, Călugăreanu A, Orzan OA (2017) In: Ficai A, Grumezescu AM (eds) Nanostructures for cancer therapy. Elsevier, Amsterdam, pp 285–306

71. Mundra V, Li W, Mahato RI (2015) Nanoparticle-mediated drug delivery for treating mela-noma. Nanomedicine 10:2613–2633

72. Youssef FS, El-Banna HA, Elzorba HY, Galal AM (2019) Application of some nanoparticles in the field of veterinary medicine. Int J Vet Sci Med 7:78–93

73. Bozzuto G, Molinari A (2015) Liposomes as nanomedical devices. Int J Nanomed 10:975–999

74. Hua S (2015) Lipid-based nano-delivery systems for skin delivery of drugs and bioactives. Front Pharmacol 6:219

75. Singh N, Joshi A, Verma G (2016) In: Grumezescu AM (ed) Engineering of nanobiomaterials. William Andrew Publishing, Amsterdam, pp 307–328

76. Blanco E, Shen H, Ferrari M (2015) Principles of nanoparticle design for overcoming biological barriers to drug delivery. Nat Biotechnol 33:941–951

77. Casadidio C, Peregrina DV, Gigliobianco MR, Deng S, Censi R, Di Martino P (2019) Chitin and chitosans: characteristics, eco-friendly processes, and applications in cosmetic science. Mar Drugs 17:369

78. Chaudhury A, Das S (2011) Recent advancement of chitosan-based nanoparticles for oral controlled delivery of insulin and other therapeutic agents. AAPS PharmSciTech 12:10–20

79. Elmowafy EM, Tiboni M, Soliman ME (2019) Biocompatibility, biodegradation and biomedical applications of poly(lactic acid)/poly(lactic-co-glycolic acid) micro and nanoparticles. J Pharm Investig 49:347–380
80. Pellico J, Ellis CM, Davis JJ (2019) Nanoparticle-based paramagnetic contrast agents for magnetic resonance imaging. Contrast Media Mol Imaging 2019:1845637
81. Madaan K, Kumar S, Poonia N, Lather V, Pandita D (2014) Dendrimers in drug delivery and targeting: drug-dendrimer interactions and toxicity issues. J Pharm Bioallied Sci 6:139–150
82. Abbasi E, Aval SF, Akbarzadeh A, Milani M, Nasrabadi HT, Joo SW, Hanifehpour Y, Nejati-Koshki K, Pashaei-Asl R (2014) Dendrimers: synthesis, applications, and properties. Nanoscale Res Lett 9:247
83. Venuganti VVK, Perumal OP (2009) Poly(amidoamine) dendrimers as skin penetration enhancers: Influence of charge, generation, and concentration. J Pharm Sci 98:2345–2356
84. Bar-Sela G, Epelbaum R, Schaffer M (2010) Curcumin as an anti-cancer agent: review of the gap between basic and clinical applications. Curr Med Chem 17:190–197
85. Croitoru A-M, Ficai D, Ficai A, Mihailescu N, Andronescu E, Turculet CF (2020) Nanostructured fibers containing natural or synthetic bioactive compounds in wound dressing applications. Materials 13:2407
86. Goyal R, Macri LK, Kaplan HM, Kohn J (2016) Nanoparticles and nanofibers for topical drug delivery. J Control Release 240:77–92
87. Murugan B, Narashimhan Ramana L, Gansdhi S, Sethuraman S, Krishnan UM (2013) Engineered chemoswitchable mesoporous silica for tumor-specific cytotoxicity. J Mater Chem B 1:3494
88. Murugan B, Krishnan UM (2018) Chemoresponsive smart mesoporous silica systems—An emerging paradigm for cancer therapy. Int J Pharm 553:310–326
89. Fratoddi I, Venditti I, Cametti C, Russo MV (2014) Gold nanoparticles and gold nanoparticle-conjugates for delivery of therapeutic molecules. Progress and challenges. J Mater Chem B 2:4204–4220
90. Bae KH, Chung HJ, Park TG (2011) Nanomaterials for cancer therapy and imaging. Mol Cells 31:295–302
91. Xie J, Bi Y, Zhang H, Dong S, Teng L, Lee RJ, Yang Z (2020) Cell-penetrating peptides in diagnosis and treatment of human diseases: from preclinical research to clinical application. Front Pharmacol 11:697
92. Ciocca DR, Calderwood SK (2005) Heat shock proteins in cancer: diagnostic, prognostic, predictive, and treatment implications. Cell Stress Chaperones 10:86–103
93. Han Y, Liu D, Li L (2020) PD-1/PD-L1 pathway: current researches in cancer. Am J Cancer Res 10:727–742
94. Sibata CH, Colussi VC, Oleinick NL, Kinsella TJ (2000) Photodynamic therapy: a new concept in medical treatment. Brazilian J Med Biol Res 33:869–880
95. Sivasubramanian M, Chuang YC, Lo L-W (2019) Evolution of nanoparticle-mediated photodynamic therapy: from superficial to deep-seated cancers. Molecules 24:520
96. El-Readi MZ, Althubiti MA (2019) Cancer nanomedicine: a new era of successful targeted therapy. J Nanomater 2019:4927312
97. Arruebo M, Vilaboa N, Sáez-Gutierrez B, Lambea J, Tres A, Valladares M, González-Fernández A (2011) Assessment of the evolution of cancer treatment therapies. Cancers 3:3279–3330

Non-Long Coding RNA and Role in Skin Cancer Diagnosis and Therapy

12

Anand Prakash Singh

Abstract

The exploration of genes responsible for cancer progression is needed for deeper understanding of molecular basis of the disease. Recent studies have shown critical role of protein-coding genes in malignancy and newly identified non-protein-coding genes have also depicted involvement in cancer development. These non-protein-coding genes are termed as non-coding RNAs (ncRNAs). The long non-coding RNAs (lncRNAs) are clearest example of ncRNAs, however, the identity and function of lncRNAs are largely unknown.

Herein, this chapter will detail the discovery and role of long non-coding RNAs (lncRNAs) in skin cancer (melanoma). In the USA, melanoma is one of the deadly skin cancers having moderately higher death rates. In 2020, more than 100,000 new cases of skin cancer have been predicted along with 11,000 estimated death. The early detection of melanoma and related treatments have shown better survival rates in patients. Hence, it is of utmost importance to develop novel diagnostic tools for early detection of melanoma and development of innovative anti-cancer therapies. To achieve this, in depth molecular mechanism of melanoma development is warranted.

Keywords

Melanoma · lncRNAs · HOTAIR · Metastasis

A. P. Singh (✉)
Division of Cardiovascular Disease, Department of Medicine, University of Alabama at Birmingham, Birmingham, AL, USA
e-mail: apsingh@uabmc.edu

211

12.1   Introduction

Recently, long non-coding RNAs (lncRNAs) have emerged as early biomarkers and attractive therapeutic targets in a variety of cancers, including melanoma. lncRNAs are mainly polyadenylated ncRNAs. They transcribed by RNA polymerase II and epigenetic signatures of protein-coding genes [1, 2]. There mature transcript display splicing of multiple exons. The transcription of lncRNAs involves independent gene promoter and is independent of transcription of associated parental gene [3–5]. Functional classifications of lncRNAs are still not well characterized. It is notable that subcellular localization of lncRNAs depicts specialized function in the cell. They act as epigenetic modifiers when localized in the nucleus while in the cytoplasm act as post-transcriptional modulators [6]. They differ from messenger RNA as they do not serve as template for protein synthesis, but they have significant role in protein-coding gene expression regulation.

12.2   Long ncRNAs in Melanoma

XIST, first discovered in 1990s, is well studied lncRNA [7]. However, its precise role in cancer remains unclear till date. Several elegant studies have suggested the role of XIST in breast cancer, mostly inherited BRCA1-deficient breast cancers [8, 9]. Before XIST discovery, importance of lncRNAs were completely disregarded. Later studies have defined their significant role gene expression regulation, nuclear to cytoplasmic trafficking, genomic imprinting, and organization of nuclear components which is very astonishing to scientific community [10, 11]. The following lncRNAs have shown their role in melanomas:

12.3   SPRY4-IT1

SPRY4-IT1 was found significantly upregulated in melanomas. In melanoma, higher expression of SPRY4-IT1 expression is primary localized in cytoplasm [12]. Its aberrant activation promotes melanoma as suggested by in vitro studies with melanoma cell line WM1552C and from real world patients having primary melanomas [12]. Gene knockdown studies have depicted that deletion of SPRY4-IT1 in melanoma cells caused apoptosis which subsequently halt the progression of melanoma [13]. At present, SPRY4-IT1 is used as biomarker melanoma pathogenesis in humans.

12.4   HOTAIR (HOX Transcript Antisense Intergenic RNA)

As per human genome studies there are 39 genes that encode for HOX transcription factors. HOX transcript antisense intergenic RNA (HOTAIR), is a best characterized lncRNA, located within the HOXC locus. HOTAIR overexpression has been stated in metastatic breast cancer [14], as supported overexpression studies of HOTAIR expression in cancer cell lines. Upregulation of HOTAIR lead to invasion of breast cancer cells and stimulates their proliferation.

In melanoma, HOTAIR overexpression plays a key role in lymph-node metastasis. An in vitro study which aimed to elucidate the beneficial effects of knocking down HOTAIR expression showed decrease motility and invasion of melanoma cells. This observation further suggests that HOTAIR might have a crucial role in melanoma cell invasiveness [15]. Since then, numerous studies have shown HOTAIR expression to melanoma, mainly metastasis and tumor invasion and proposed the use of HOTAIR as a diagnostic marker for metastatic melanoma.

12.5 ANRIL (Antisense Non-Coding RNA in the INK4 Locus)

ANRIL, a large antisense RNA localized at INK4b/ARF/INK4a locus [16] was initially identified in a melanoma-neural system tumor [17]. Concerning expression levels, studies suggested that oncogenic action of overexpressed ANRIL in melanoma cause enhanced progression of cancer cells [18]. Mechanically, ANRIL governs its oncogenic activity by regulation of tumor suppressors INK4A and INK4B.

12.6 BANCR (BRAF-Activated Non-Coding RNA)

BRAF-activated non-coding RNA (BANCR) is involved in a variety of human cancer, including lung carcinoma, colorectal cancer, melanoma, gastric cancer, and bladder cancer [19–21]. In melanoma, Flockhart and group showed upregulation of BANCR is connected with migration of melanoma cells [22]. Knockdown studies report that reduced.

BANCR expression is linked with reduced proliferation of melanoma cells by inhibition of prosurvival signaling pathway extracellular signal-regulated kinases 1/2 (ERK1/2) and c-Jun N-terminal kinase (JNK) [23]. Furthermore, experiments with nude mice having BANCR knockdown depicted perturb proliferation of melanoma [23]. These studies demonstrate that BANCR is highly upregulated in melanoma and can be potential therapeutic target to prevent malignancy.

In addition to above discussed lncRNA several others lncRNAs have also been studied in the context of progression of melanoma. They are MALAT1,Llme23, UCA1, SLNCR1 and SAMMSON (Fig. 12.1) [24–27]. Aberrant activation of these lncRNAs was found in melanoma and knockdown studies have suggested their inactivation has significant benefit to prevent cancer progression.

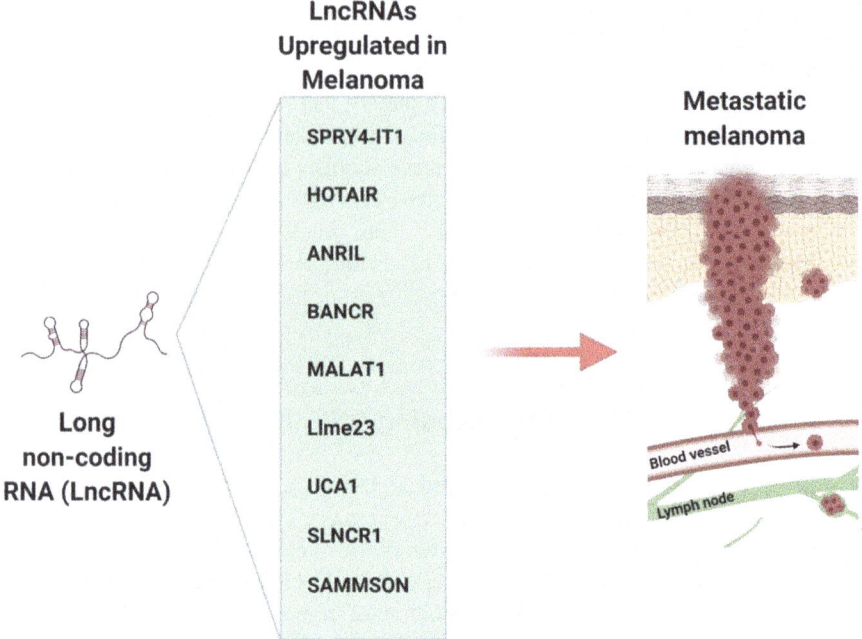

Fig. 12.1 Long coding RNAs upregulated in melanoma promoting metastasis

12.7 Conclusion

For the treatment of melanoma several drugs are already in the market but favorable clinical outcomes for cancer patients still remain poor and side effects of these therapies are very common. The advancement of biology of non-coding RNAs shows potential for the diagnosis, prognosis, and treatment of melanoma. Having said that, further research is warranted to utilize their therapeutic potential.

References

1. Faulkner GJ, Kimura Y, Daub CO, Wani S, Plessy C, Irvine KM, Schroder K, Cloonan N, Steptoe AL, Lassmann T, Waki K, Hornig N, Arakawa T, Takahashi H, Kawai J, Forrest AR, Suzuki H, Hayashizaki Y, Hume DA, Orlando V, Grimmond SM, Carninci P (2009) The regulated retrotransposon transcriptome of mammalian cells. Nat Genet 41:563–571
2. He Y, Vogelstein B, Velculescu VE, Papadopoulos N, Kinzler KW (2008) The antisense transcriptomes of human cells. Science 322:1855–1857
3. Kim TK, Hemberg M, Gray JM, Costa AM, Bear DM, Wu J, Harmin DA, Laptewicz M, Barbara-Haley K, Kuersten S, Markenscoff-Papadimitriou E, Kuhl D, Bito H, Worley PF, Kreiman G, Greenberg ME (2010) Widespread transcription at neuronal activity-regulated enhancers. Nature 465:182–187

4. Calin GA, Liu CG, Ferracin M, Hyslop T, Spizzo R, Sevignani C, Fabbri M, Cimmino A, Lee EJ, Wojcik SE, Shimizu M, Tili E, Rossi S, Taccioli C, Pichiorri F, Liu X, Zupo S, Herlea V, Gramantieri L, Lanza G, Alder H, Rassenti L, Volinia S, Schmittgen TD, Kipps TJ, Negrini M, Croce CM (2007) Ultraconserved regions encoding ncRNAs are altered in human leukemias and carcinomas. Cancer Cell 12:215–229

5. Braconi C, Valeri N, Kogure T, Gasparini P, Huang N, Nuovo GJ, Terracciano L, Croce CM, Patel T (2011) Expression and functional role of a transcribed noncoding RNA with an ultraconserved element in hepatocellular carcinoma. Proc Natl Acad Sci U S A 108:786–791

6. Carninci P, Kasukawa T, Katayama S, Gough J, Frith MC, Maeda N, Oyama R et al (2005) The transcriptional landscape of the mammalian genome. Science 309:1559–1563

7. Lee JT (2009) Lessons from X-chromosome inactivation: long ncRNA as guides and tethers to the epigenome. Genes Dev 23:1831–1842

8. Sirchia SM, Tabano S, Monti L, Recalcati MP, Gariboldi M, Grati FR, Porta G, Finelli P, Radice P, Miozzo M (2009) Misbehaviour of XIST RNA in breast cancer cells. PLoS One 4: e5559

9. Richardson AL, Wang ZC, De Nicolo A, Lu X, Brown M, Miron A, Liao X, Iglehart JD, Livingston DM, Ganesan S (2006) X chromosomal abnormalities in basal-like human breast cancer. Cancer Cell 9:121–132

10. Mercer TR, Dinger ME, Mattick JS (2009) Long non-coding RNAs: insights into functions. Nat Rev Genet 10:155–159

11. Moran VA, Perera RJ, Khalil AM (2012) Emerging functional and mechanistic paradigms of mammalian long non-coding RNAs. Nucleic Acids Res 40:6391–6400

12. Mazar J, Zhao W, Khalil AM, Lee B, Shelley J, Govindarajan SS, Yamamoto F, Ratnam M, Aftab MN, Collins S, Finck BN, Han X, Mattick JS, Dinger ME, Perera RJ (2014) The functional characterization of long noncoding RNA SPRY4-IT1 in human melanoma cells. Oncotarget 5:8959–8969

13. Khaitan D, Dinger ME, Mazar J, Crawford J, Smith MA, Mattick JS, Perera RJ (2011) The melanoma-upregulated long noncoding RNA SPRY4-IT1 modulates apoptosis and invasion. Cancer Res 71:3852–3862

14. Gupta RA, Shah N, Wang KC, Kim J, Horlings HM, Wong DJ, Tsai MC, Hung T, Argani P, Rinn JL, Wang Y, Brzoska P, Kong B, Li R, West RB, van de Vijver MJ, Sukumar S, Chang HY (2010) Long non-coding RNA HOTAIR reprograms chromatin state to promote cancer metastasis. Nature 464:1071–1076

15. Tang L, Zhang W, Su B, Yu B (2013) Long noncoding RNA HOTAIR is associated with motility, invasion, and metastatic potential of metastatic melanoma. Biomed Res Int 2013:251098

16. Popov N, Gil J (2010) Epigenetic regulation of the INK4b-ARF-INK4a locus: in sickness and in health. Epigenetics 5:685–690

17. Pasmant E, Laurendeau I, Heron D, Vidaud M, Vidaud D, Bieche I (2007) Characterization of a germ-line deletion, including the entire INK4/ARF locus, in a melanoma-neural system tumor family: identification of ANRIL, an antisense noncoding RNA whose expression coclusters with ARF. Cancer Res 67:3963–3969

18. Xu S, Wang H, Pan H, Shi Y, Li T, Ge S, Jia R, Zhang H, Fan X (2016) ANRIL lncRNA triggers efficient therapeutic efficacy by reprogramming the aberrant INK4-hub in melanoma. Cancer Lett 381:41–48

19. Jiang W, Zhang D, Xu B, Wu Z, Liu S, Zhang L, Tian Y, Han X, Tian D (2015) Long non-coding RNA BANCR promotes proliferation and migration of lung carcinoma via MAPK pathways. Biomed Pharmacother 69:90–95

20. Li L, Zhang L, Zhang Y, Zhou F (2015) Increased expression of LncRNA BANCR is associated with clinical progression and poor prognosis in gastric cancer. Biomed Pharmacother 72:109–112

21. Shi Y, Liu Y, Wang J, Jie D, Yun T, Li W, Yan L, Wang K, Feng J (2015) Downregulated long noncoding RNA BANCR promotes the proliferation of colorectal Cancer cells via Downregualtion of p21 expression. PLoS One 10:e0122679
22. Flockhart RJ, Webster DE, Qu K, Mascarenhas N, Kovalski J, Kretz M, Khavari PA (2012) BRAFV600E remodels the melanocyte transcriptome and induces BANCR to regulate melanoma cell migration. Genome Res 22:1006–1014
23. Li R, Zhang L, Jia L, Duan Y, Li Y, Bao L, Sha N (2014) Long non-coding RNA BANCR promotes proliferation in malignant melanoma by regulating MAPK pathway activation. PLoS One 9:e100893
24. Tian Y, Zhang X, Hao Y, Fang Z, He Y (2014) Potential roles of abnormally expressed long noncoding RNA UCA1 and Malat-1 in metastasis of melanoma. Melanoma Res 24:335–341
25. Wu CF, Tan GH, Ma CC, Li L (2013) The non-coding RNA llme23 drives the malignant property of human melanoma cells. J Genet Genomics 40:179–188
26. Shi X, Ma C, Zhu Q, Yuan D, Sun M, Gu X, Wu G, Lv T, Song Y (2016) Upregulation of long intergenic noncoding RNA 00673 promotes tumor proliferation via LSD1 interaction and repression of NCALD in non-small-cell lung cancer. Oncotarget 7:25558–25575
27. Leucci E, Vendramin R, Spinazzi M, Laurette P, Fiers M, Wouters J, Radaelli E, Eyckerman S, Leonelli C, Vanderheyden K, Rogiers A, Hermans E, Baatsen P, Aerts S, Amant F, Van Aelst S, van den Oord J, de Strooper B, Davidson I, Lafontaine DL, Gevaert K, Vandesompele J, Mestdagh P, Marine JC (2016) Melanoma addiction to the long non-coding RNA SAMMSON. Nature 531:518–522

Potential of Long Non-coding RNAs in the Diagnosis and Therapy of Melanoma Skin Cancer

Hitesh Singh Chaouhan, Vipin Rai, Sudarshan Kini,
Anusmita Shekher, Anurag Sharma, and Subash Chandra Gupta

Abstract

Skin carcinoma is categorized into melanoma and non-melanoma. Melanoma is among the highly aggressive and deadly forms of skin cancer. Melanoma is frequently associated with metastasis and therapeutic resistance. The combined immunotherapy and targeted therapies have emerged as attractive therapeutic options. However, the efficacy of these therapies is limited to advanced-stage melanoma and those who often acquire resistance. Over the years, the molecular bases of melanoma have been unraveled, which led to establishing specific and reliable biomarkers for the diagnosis, prognosis, and therapy. A good strategy in finding novel cancer targets could include shifting from the protein-translating regions to the genome's non-coding regions. The non-coding regions constitute approximately 98% of the genome. The microRNAs (miRNAs) and long

H. S. Chaouhan
Graduate Institute of Biomedical Sciences, China Medical University, Taichung, Taiwan

V. Rai · A. Shekher
Department of Biochemistry, Institute of Science, Banaras Hindu University, Varanasi, India

S. Kini
Nitte (Deemed to Be University), Nitte University Centre for Science Education and Research (NUCSER), Division of Nanobiotechnology, Kotekar-Beeri Road, Deralakatte, Mangaluru, India

A. Sharma
Nitte (Deemed to Be University), Nitte University Centre for Science Education and Research (NUCSER), Division of Environmental Health and Toxicology, Kotekar-Beeri Road, Deralakatte, Mangaluru, India

S. C. Gupta (✉)
Department of Biochemistry, Institute of Science, Banaras Hindu University, Varanasi, India

Department of Biochemistry, All India Institute of Medical Sciences, Guwahati, India
e-mail: sgupta@bhu.ac.in

© The Author(s), under exclusive license to Springer Nature Singapore Pte Ltd. 2021
A. Dwivedi et al. (eds.), *Skin Cancer: Pathogenesis and Diagnosis*,
https://doi.org/10.1007/978-981-16-0364-8_13

non-coding RNAs (lncRNAs) are two major classes of non-coding RNAs. Apart from coding RNA's, lncRNAs have also been attributed to exhibit proto-oncogenic and tumor suppressor roles in various cancers, including melanoma. This chapter summarizes the recent advancement of lncRNAs concerning diagnosis, prognosis, and therapy of melanoma.

Keywords

Biomarker · Immunotherapy · LncRNA · Melanoma · Metastasis

Abbreviations

AKT	Protein Kinase B
ANRIL	Antisense non-coding RNA in the INK4 locus
AR	Androgen receptor
ASOs	Antisense specific oligonucleotides
BANCR	v-raf murine sarcoma viral oncogene homolog B1 (BRAF)-activated non-coding RNA
Brn3a	Brain-specific homeobox protein 3a
BSC	Basal cell carcinoma
CASC15	Cancer susceptibility candidate 15
cSCC	Cutaneous squamous cell carcinoma
DIRC3	Disrupted in renal carcinoma 3
dsRNAs	Double-stranded RNAs
EMICERI	EQTN MOB3B IFNK C9orf72 enhancer RNA I
EMT	Epithelial-mesenchymal transition
ERK1/2	Extracellular signal-regulated protein kinases 1/2
FALEC	Focally amplified long non-coding RNA in epithelial cancer
FISH	Fluorescence in situ hybridization
GAS5	Growth arrest-specific 5
GEO	Gene expression omnibus
GO	Gene ontology
HOTAIR	HOX transcript antisense RNA
IGFBP5	Insulin-like growth factor binding protein 5
ISH	In situ hybridization
JNK	Jun N-terminal kinase
LNA	Locked nucleic acid
LncRNAs	Long non-coding RNAs
LNM	Lymph node metastasis
MALAT1	Metastasis associated lung adenocarcinoma transcript 1
MAPK	Mitogen-activated protein kinase
MEG3	Maternally expressed 3
MIFT	Microphthalmia-associated transcription factor
miRNAs	microRNAs

MMP	Matrix metalloproteinase
NB	Northern blotting
ncRNAs	Non-coding RNAs
NF-κB	Nuclear factor kappa light chain enhancer of activated B cells
NGS	Next-generation sequencing
NMCCs	Non-melanoma cutaneous carcinomas
OS	Overall survival
PCR	Polymerase chain reaction
PI3K	Phosphoinositol-3-kinase
PRC1/2	Polychrome repressive complex 1 and 2
PSF	Poly-pyrimidine tract-binding protein-associated splicing factor
PVT1	Plasmacytoma variant translocation 1
qRT-PCR	Quantitative reverse transcription PCR
RNAi	RNA interference
RNA-seq	RNA-sequencing
RTK	Receptor tyrosine kinase
SAMMSON	Survival associated mitochondrial-melanoma specific oncogenic non-coding RNA
shRNA	Short hairpin RNA
siRNA	Short interference RNA
SLNCR1	SRA-like non-coding RNA1
SNHG5	SnoRNA host gene 5
SPRY4-IT1	Sprouty4-intronic transcript 1
ssRNAs	Single-stranded RNAs
STAT3	Signal transducer and activator of transcription 3
TCGA	The cancer genome atlas
UCA1	Urothelial carcinoma associated 1
WNT	Wingless-related integration site
XIST	X-inactive specific transcript

13.1 Introduction

Cutaneous (skin) carcinoma is a common type of malignancy with a constant increase globally [1, 2]. There are mainly two types: melanoma and non-melanoma cutaneous carcinomas (NMCCs). The subtypes include basal cell carcinoma (BSC) and cutaneous squamous cell carcinoma (cSCC). The melanoma derived from melanocytes is an aggressive cutaneous carcinoma. It accounts for the majority of skin cancer-associated mortality worldwide. Higher death rates are mostly because of its fast growth and high metastatic potential to distant organs such as the liver, brain, and lung, making it lethal. According to Globocan, an estimated 132,000 new cases and 50,000 melanoma-related deaths worldwide and the number of cases has rapidly increased in recent years [3, 4]. Accumulating epidemiological data from the USA and Europe show a constant and dramatic rise in incidence during the last decades [5]. UV-radiation (UVR) is a major risk factor for melanoma. Other risk factors for melanoma include old age, immunosuppression, genetic factors, and exposure to toxic agents. Generally, cancer therapies such as surgery, histopathologic diagnosis, and embolization are often treated to control tumor progression in melanoma patients. Still, they are mostly palliative approaches without much success rate. Chemotherapy and radiotherapy remain the mainstay for melanoma treatment with a high success rate [6]. Unfortunately, most advanced melanoma types develop resistance against chemotherapy and radiotherapy and proceed to the lethal stage [7–10]. Although combined immunotherapy and targeted drug delivery have emerged as new promising therapeutic approaches, their efficacy is limited to those who often acquire resistance to conventional therapy, and therapeutic options are very limited to end-stage melanoma [11]. Therefore, understanding the molecular mechanisms of melanoma progression and tumorigenesis would facilitate the novel biomarkers identification for early melanoma prognosis and effective therapeutic strategies for metastatic melanoma.

In the last two decades, high-throughput deep sequencing technology and ENCODE project have shown that roughly 2% of the total genome is translated into proteins, whereas a considerable portion ($\geq$90%) is transcribed into non-coding RNAs (ncRNAs) [12, 13]. Earlier, ncRNAs were considered as transcriptional noises. However, ncRNAs are now known to play a crucial function in gene regulation and are recurrently dysregulated in several cancer types [14]. Based on the transcript length, ncRNAs are categorized into two major classes: short ncRNAs (miRNAs; <200 nucleotides) and long ncRNAs (lncRNAs, $\geq$200 nucleotides). Earlier studies have described that lncRNAs can modulate a complex network of cancer signaling in different types of malignancies through numerous mechanisms such as chromatin modification, miRNA sequestration, transcriptional activation/repression, and translational regulation [15, 16]. Previously, lncRNAs were considered as wastage or junk in various biological processes. Recent data have shown the functional role of lncRNAs in several malignancies, including melanoma. However, only a few lncRNAs have been studied in melanoma. The expression of lncRNAs such as survival associated mitochondrial-melanoma specific oncogenic non-coding RNA (*SAMMSON*), metastasis associated lung adenocarcinoma transcript-1 (*MALAT1*), HOX transcript antisense RNA (*HOTAIR*), Plasmacytoma Variant Translocation 1 (*PVT1*), v-raf murine sarcoma viral oncogene homolog B1 (BRAF)-activated non-coding RNA (*BANCR*), Antisense non-coding RNA in the INK4 locus (*ANRIL*), Urothelial carcinoma associated 1 (*UCA1*), Focally amplified lncRNA on chromosome 1 (*FALEC1*), and *Llme23* is increased in melanomas and serves as a pro-oncogenic player. In contrast, growth arrest-specific 5 (*GAS5*), Maternally Expressed 3 (*MEG3*), and Disrupted in Renal Carcinoma 3 (*DIRC3*) lncRNAs are suppressed and exhibit tumor suppressor functions in melanomas [17–28].

This chapter summarizes the recent information on functions of lncRNAs in melanomas, focusing on the interplay with prominent cancer signaling, and define their role in the acquisition of resistance to molecular targeted therapy. We also emphasize the potential of lncRNAs as a promising biomarker in the diagnosis, prognosis, and therapy of melanoma.

13.2 Experimental Methods and Tools for Analyzing lncRNAs in Melanoma

An abnormal expression of lncRNAs is reported in several cancer types [29, 30]. LncRNAs exhibit high similarities with mRNAs concerning length, RNA polymerase II-mediated transcription, splicing, 5′-capping, and poly(A)tail. Therefore, elucidating the functions of lncRNAs in cancer initiation, progression, and metastasis is still challenging. Here, we describe various in vitro and in silico methods that have been employed to examine differences in gene expression profiling between normal and cancer cells for elucidating the lncRNAs functions in cancer pathogenesis (Table 13.1).

13.2.1 LncRNAs Expression Profiling Techniques

The expression of lncRNAs has been examined by high-throughput techniques such as arrays and next-generation sequencing (NGS).

13.2.1.1 Microarray

Initially developed for protein-coding mRNAs, microarray has also been used for examining the expression profile of lncRNAs. In this technique, nucleic acid hybridization is achieved between fluorescent target RNA sequence and their specific complementary DNA sequences (also known as probes) immobilized on a grid. Expression of multiple lncRNAs analyzed through this technique displays high sensitivity and specificity at relatively low cost and can also detect few RNA molecules without any post Polymerase Chain Reaction (PCR) setups. Khaitan et al. [31] first studied melanoma-associated lncRNA using custom-made microarray. The group observed an increase in the expression of 77 lncRNAs in the WM1552C stage III melanoma compared to control cells. Another study identified a group of 39 known lncRNAs and 70 new intergenic lncRNAs in BRAF^{V600E} mutated melanoma cells and found that their expression was regulated through oncogenic signaling [21]. Several platforms for lncRNA profiling are based on in vitro transcription amplification and are specified by fewer technical differences than miRNA platforms. For instance, the *Agilent SurePrint G3 Gene Expression v3 microarray*, the *Arraystar LncRNA microarray* labeled 39,317 lncRNAs, *Clariom D human array* targeting >55,900 lncRNAs transcripts are widely used [32]. However, limitations include the applicability of known probe (lncRNAs) sequences, nucleic acid hybridization, non-specificity, higher variability for low expressing genes, and restricted linear lncRNAs sequence variants.

Table 13.1 A list of lncRNAs with potential in the diagnosis and prognosis of malignant melanoma

LncRNA	Preclinical/clinical samples	Tools/techniques	Diagnostic/ prognostic markers	References
MALAT1 (oncogene)	• Human melanoma cell line A375, C32, EDMEL3, G361, HBL, WM1115, SK-MEL-1, M14, MV3, A875, M21 and normal cell lines Hermes1, Hermes4, HEK293T, TE353. SK, Hacat. • 50 primary lymph node metastases melanoma tissues and 14 paired adjacent normal tissue • Three primary samples and matched lymph node metastases	RNA-Seq, q-RT-PCR	Prognostic marker (higher expression related with lymph node metastasis)	[78, 77]
HOTAIR (oncogene)	• Three pairs of primary melanoma samples along with matched lymph node metastases • Primary melanoma samples (7 with pT1a stage, 30 with pT3/4 stage) and 32 visceral metastases. • 28 primary and 38 metastatic tissues and matched normal tissues • Serum samples of 34 patients, • Human metastatic melanoma cell line (A875, A375, SK-MEL-5, SK-MEL-1, SK-MEL-2), • 63 melanoma and paired normal adjacent tissue	q-RT-PCR, ISH, GEO database analysis	Non-invasive circulating prognostic/ diagnostic marker	[17, 37, 61, 64]

(continued)

Table 13.1 (continued)

LncRNA	Preclinical/clinical samples	Tools/techniques	Diagnostic/ prognostic markers	References
BANCR (oncogene)	• 48 melanoma tumor tissues and adjacent normal tissues • Two mutant primary melanoma samples • Advanced-stage melanoma and normal samples from 69 patients • Human melanoma cell lines	q-RT-PCR, RNA-Seq, microarray, DIANA tools	Prognostic marker (negative correlation between BANCR expression and survival)	[21, 59, 84, 85]
ANRIL (oncogene)	• A375 (cutaneous melanoma) and OM431 (uveal melanoma) cell line. • 174 melanoma cell lines from 134 metastasized melanoma patients • 18 cutaneous, 10 uveal primary melanoma, and 9 benign tissue samples	q-RT-PCR, aCGH, GEO database	Early diagnostic marker	[25, 86, 88]
UCA1 (oncogene)	• Five melanoma cell lines • 52 primary melanoma tumor and adjacent matched normal tissue • 18 primary cutaneous melanoma metastatic tissue and 20 benign samples	q-RT-PCR, microarray, miRcode, TargetScan, miRDB tools	Prognostic marker	[19, 93, 94]
SPRY4-IT1 (oncogene)	• Eight human melanoma cell lines, normal melanocytes and keratinocytes • 25 metastatic (primary, nodal, regional, and distant) melanoma	RNA-Seq, q-RT-PCR, FISH, ENSEMBL database	Independent negative prognostic marker in plasma samples by multivariate survival analysis	[31, 39, 99, 100]

(continued)

Table 13.1 (continued)

LncRNA	Preclinical/clinical samples	Tools/techniques	Diagnostic/ prognostic markers	References
	patient and 20 normal melanocyte samples • Plasma (70 patients, 79 healthy controls).			
SLNCR1 (oncogene)	• Melanoma cell lines (A375, WM), • 29 melanoma and normal skin samples	RNA-Seq, q-RT-PCR, FISH, microarray, TCGA database, MiTranscriptome, MOTTIF search tool	Prognostic marker	[97, 98]
SAMMSON (oncogene)	• Early-stage samples from human melanoma patients • Patient derived melanoma xenograft model • Human melanoma cell lines	RNA-Seq, q-RT-PCR, FISH, microarray, TCGA database	Early diagnostic marker	[22]
Llme23 (oncogene)	• Melanoma cell lines, • Tumor nude mice model	RNA-SELEX affinity chromatography	Unknown	[26]
FALEC (oncogene)	• 78 human melanoma tissues • Human melanoma cell lines (M21, B16, MEL-RM) and normal cell lines (HEMn)	q-RT-PCR	Prognosis marker (increased expression associated with lymph node metastasis and poor survival outcomes)	[24]
GAS5 (tumor suppressor)	• 94 melanoma tissue samples • Nine melanoma cell lines	q-RT-PCR, FISH, RNA Vienna tool	Unknown	[68, 102]

aCGH array comparative genomic hybridization, *ANRIL* antisense non coding RNA in the INK4 locus, *BANCR* v-raf murine sarcoma viral oncogene homolog B1 (BRAF) activated non-coding RNA, *FALEC* focally amplified long non-coding RNA in epithelial cancer, *FISH* fluorescence in situ hybridization, *GAS5* growth arrest-specific 5, *GEO* gene expression omnibus, *HOTAIR* HOX transcript antisense RNA, *ISH* in situ hybridization, *LNM* lymph node metastases, *MALAT1* metastasis associated lung adenocarcinoma transcript 1, *qRT-PCR* quantitative reverse transcription PCR, *RNA-Seq* RNA-sequencing, *SAMMSON* survival associated mitochondrial-melanoma specific oncogenic non-coding RNA, *SLNCR1* SRA-like non-coding RNA1, *SPRY4-IT1* sprouty4-intronic transcript 1, *TCGA* the cancer genome atlas, *UCA1* urothelial carcinoma associated 1

13.2.1.2 RNA-Sequencing

RNA-sequencing (RNA-seq) is the most precise method for the quantification of lncRNAs in biological samples. In this method, the preparation of a cDNA library is followed by sequencing of transcripts of interest. The small RNA-seq is mainly used for ncRNAs such as miRNA, whereas the total RNA-seq is employed for lncRNAs. As compared to the microarray, the main advantage of RNA-seq is independent of previous sequence information. Moreover, it shows a high dynamic range, detecting several isoforms of lncRNAs that differ, even by a single nucleotide sequence. It offers complete profiling of whole transcriptomes. Besides, the major limitations of RNA-seq are the high cost, complexity in data analysis, and higher depth reads required to analyze a low quantity of the targets. In one study, 339 lncRNA transcripts were dysregulated in clinical melanoma samples than standard cell lines and tissue samples [33]. In another study, Siena et al. [34] identified that lncRNA Zinc finger E-box binding homeobox 1 antisense 1 (*ZEB1-AS1*) was associated with metastatic melanoma as alternative therapeutic targets and/or biomarkers using RNA-seq methods. Coe et al. [20] identified two novel tumor suppressor genes *DIRC3* and Insulin-Like Growth Factor Binding Protein 5 (*IGFBP5*) in human melanoma cells by using data from RNA-seq and Chromatin immunoprecipitation (ChIP)-seq.

13.2.2 Validation of Arrays and RNA-Seq Data

The data obtained from the arrays, RNA-seq, and related databases should be further validated. For this purpose, techniques such as northern blotting (NB), quantitative reverse transcription PCR (qRT-PCR), in situ hybridization (ISH), and fluorescence in situ hybridization (FISH) are successfully being used.

13.2.2.1 Quantitative Reverse Transcription PCR (qRT-PCR)

The qRT-PCR is a fluorescence-based standard method for the quantification of lncRNAs in biological samples. TaqMan and SYBR green are used in the majority of the qRT-PCR techniques. In this method, RNAs are reverse transcribed using random or sequence-specific stem-loop primers. Using qRT-PCR, the lncRNAs such as RMEL3, SAMMSON, LLME23, and HOTAIR have been identified as an independent predictor of melanoma-associated metastasis [17, 22, 26, 35–37].

13.2.2.2 Northern Blot (NB) Analysis

Northern blot (NB) is the most primitive technique for the analysis of mRNA expression. NB can also be used to analyze the expression pattern of lncRNAs. This technology is based on gel electrophoresis to separate RNA samples by size and detection through RNA-probe hybridization that complements the part of or the entire target sequence [38]. Mazar et al. [39] demonstrated lncRNA SPRY4-IT1 as a new predictive marker and therapeutic target in melanoma cancer based on its expression levels. This technique's major pitfalls are high risk of degradation of the sample by RNases, low sensitivity and time consumption, increased quantity of total RNA in samples, and use of hazardous chemicals such as radiolabeling, formaldehyde, and ethidium bromide. Some non-radioactive labeling probes, such as digoxigenin or biotin-labeled probes, are used for NB analysis to increase their affinity and sensitivity [40].

13.2.2.3 In Situ Hybridization (ISH) or Fluorescence In Situ Hybridization (FISH)

ISH and FISH techniques have improved the visualization and examination of lncRNAs expression. These fluorescent-based techniques are used to investigate the subcellular localization of specific lncRNAs and their binding partners. Using FISH and confocal microscopy, LINC00518 was identified to be localized in the cytoplasm preventing anti-metastatic effects by sponging miR-204-5p and regulating AP1S2 expression in melanoma cells [41]. The technique becomes highly challenging due to short and repetitive sequences in fluorescence-labeled DNA or RNA probes. Recently, modified probes such as 2'-O-methyl (2OMe) or hapten-labeled locked nucleic acids (LNA) oligos have been used to increase the affinity and sensitivity to RNA targets. Thus it reduces the chance of cross-hybridization [42, 43].

13.3 Datasets and Bioinformatics Tools for Analyzing lncRNAs in Skin Cancer

The lncRNAs expression data generated through microarray and NGS technologies have also been analyzed using various bioinformatics tools.

13.3.1 Bioinformatic Analysis

Bioinformatics analysis include: (a) examining the differentially expressed genes between control and cancer samples; (b) gene clustering; (c) classification; (d) gene enrichment pathways and interaction analysis. Several methods/tools are available to identify and interpret gene expression data from microarray and NGS technologies. Tools such as Cluster 3.0 software and Tree View are used for clustering analysis and hierarchical heat map visualization. Genes function enrichment and pathway analysis is performed with Gene Ontology (GO), Kyoto Encyclopedia of Genes and Genomes (KEGG), Reactome, PANTHER, BioCyc, and WikiPathways. Candidate target gene analysis requires lncRNA2Target, ENCORI, DIANA, UCSC genome browser, and RNAplex 0.2. lncRNAs structure analysis is performed through RNAfold, RMDB, and LncFinder. Further, the co-expression network analysis uses Cytoscape MCODE plug-in 3.4.0, WGCNA, and NEED [44–48].

13.3.2 Data Analysis

Many computational datasets have been developed and used to precisely and fast investigate lncRNAs in cancer subsets. MiTranscriptome is an RNA-seq data set consisting of a large-scale of lncRNAs from cell lines, tissues, and clinical samples [33]. OncoLnc database is based on the information from The Cancer Genome Atlas (TCGA) database to link the lncRNAs expression with patient survival [49]. The Cancer LncRNome Atlas provides comprehensive details on lncRNAs expression, DNA methylation, Single Nucleotide Polymorphism (SNP), and somatic copy number aberration (SCNA) from diverse types of cancers using the National Cancer Institute (NCI) Cancer Genomics web source and TCGA [50]. Besides, many databases are also available for LncRNAs investigation in cancer, including TCGA, which characterize genetic mutations in 20,000 human tumors representing 33 different cancer types. It also provides molecular profile data linked to genomic expression, miRNA expression, protein profiling, DNA methylation, and somatic mutation. Gene Expression Omnibus (GEO), a public repository database, contains genome expression, genome methylation, protein expression, chromatin conformation, and genome–protein binding. NONCODE 4.0 comprises a total 4,87,164 lncRNAs transcripts and 3,24,646 lncRNAs genes from 16 different species. GEO allows searching of sequences, orthologs, expression, functions, and related diseases to a given input gene or transcript. LncRNA Map consists of 23,355 lncRNAs sequences from Ensembl 65 to study lncRNAs expression in the human genome. LncRNAdb provides comprehensive information about eukaryotic lncRNAs sequences, expression, structure, molecular functions, and genomic context. LNCipedia 3.0 contains 1,27,802 human lncRNAs transcripts, provides information such as sequences, expression, annotations, and manually curated lncRNAs articles. Lnc2cancer contains resource for lncRNAs expression associated to human cancers. TANRIC provides the platforms for the functional and clinical investigations of lncRNAs in cancer. The lncRNA base 2.0 predicts lncRNA–target interaction network. LncRNAtor determines interactions of lncRNA with miRNA and protein and their expression profiling analysis. NPInter determines functional interactions between lncRNAs and other molecules (DNA, RNA, transcription factors, and protein) based on regularly updated literatures, high-throughput techniques, and computational predictions [32, 44, 48, 51–53].

13.4 Modulation of Cell Signaling Pathways by lncRNAs in Melanoma Skin Cancer

In *E. coli* and yeast, lncRNAs have been associated with protein modules in the cell membrane, suggesting that lncRNAs can also function within functionally distinct non-cytoplasmic parts [54]. As a result, lncRNA–chaperone protein interactions are further involved in modulating cellular signaling cascades via a specific receptor tyrosine kinase (RTK).

About 90% of melanoma cases exhibit abnormal activation of two core signaling: mitogen-activated protein kinase (MAPK) signaling and the phosphoinositol-3-kinase/Protein kinase B (PI3K)/AKT signaling. These pathways are critically involved in the melanoma growth and progression through cell cycle deregulation and apoptosis inhibition. In another 8–10% of cases, other signaling cascades such as the wingless-related integration site (WNT)/β-catenin, Nuclear factor kappa light chain enhancer of activated B cells (NF-κB), Notch, and Hippo pathways are associated with metastasis [55–57]. Interestingly, these dysregulated pathways have been linked with the impaired expression of lncRNAs. Earlier studies identified lncRNAs that were modulated in melanoma cells. These lncRNAs were reported as a positive modulator of cell proliferation and migration. For example, BANCR and RMEL3 lncRNAs overexpression in BRAF^{V600E} mutated malignant melanoma induces cell proliferation as well as cell migration through regulating Matrix metalloproteinases (MMP)2 and MMP9 via activation of extracellular signal-regulated protein kinases 1/2 (ERK1/2)-Jun N-terminal kinases (JNK)/MAPK signaling pathways in the absence of growth factors [21, 58]. In another study, upregulation of BANCR significantly induced melanoma growth and migration through activation of Notch2 signaling cascades by sponging mir-204 expression [59]. In melanoma cells, cell proliferation is also enhanced by the SAMMSON lncRNA, through its interaction with p32, which is a key regulator of mitochondrial homeostasis and metabolism [22].

Besides, overexpressed OR3A4 significantly induces melanoma cells' tumorigenesis by activating PI3K/AKT signaling pathway [60]. The overexpression in HOTAIR was found to increase cell growth and metastatic activity of melanoma cells significantly mediated through an increase in the expression of c-MET (a growth factor receptor) and activation of PI3K/AKT/mTOR pathway [61, 62]. In another study, overexpression of HOTAIR and H19 promoted migration and invasion of melanoma cells through the degradation of inhibitor of nuclear factor kappa B (IκBα) facilitated through PI3K/AKT pathway activation, which consequently leads to activation of NF-κB signaling [63, 64]. Overexpression of Myocardial Infarction Associated Transcript (MIAT) promotes melanoma growth, migration, and invasion through increased PI3K and AKT phosphorylation and induced cMyc and cyclin-D1 protein expression [65]. The higher expression of X-inactive specific transcript (XIST) significantly promoted cell proliferation and migration in the malignant melanoma cells through the activation of PI3K/AKT signaling, leading to inhibition of intrinsic apoptosis signaling [66].

Elevated expression of lncRNA LHFPL3 antisense RNA 1 (LHFPL3-AS1), like a sponge of miR-580-3p augmented signal transducer and activator of transcription 3 (STAT3) expression and subsequently activated Janus Kinase 2 (JAK2)/STAT3 signaling leading to malignancy in melanoma cells [67]. In contrast, overexpressed lncRNA MEG3 suppressed melanoma cell growth and migration through inhibition of WNT/β-catenin pathway. Specifically, it reduced the β-catenin and cyclin-D1 level while increasing Glycogen synthase kinase (GSK)-3β level [23]. In another study, overexpression of lncRNA, Gas5 inhibited MMP2 expression that in turn inhibited migration and invasion in SK-Mel-110 cells [68].

13.5 Long Non-Coding RNAs as a Predictive Marker for Melanoma Skin Cancer

Numerous therapeutic approaches have been developed for the eradication of cancer cells. However, most cancer cells show higher relapse rates, primarily due to the acquisition of resistance mechanisms. Therefore, the emergence of novel therapeutic strategies calls for searching biomarkers that help stratify patients according to tumor recurrence. From this perception, lncRNAs could stand as a potential biomarker involved in oncogenic signaling, malignant transformation, and apoptosis-resistance. It has been observed that lncRNAs expression and dysregulation in particular cells, tissue, and disease conditions in contrast to protein-coding genes, makes them a suitable predictor of tumor status [69–73]. Recently, the development of advanced biological techniques such as microarray and RNA-seq has identified several lncRNAs, which could play a crucial role in melanoma pathogenesis. Here, we discuss the role of lncRNAs as a potential biomarker in skin melanoma cancer (Table 13.2).

13.5.1 MALAT1

Metastasis associated lung adenocarcinoma transcript-1 (MALAT1) is a nuclear-enriched intergenic lncRNA with 8302 bp in length. It was first recognized as a candidate marker for lung cancer migration and metastasis [74]. MALAT1 is abnormally dysregulated in various human malignancies, including breast, liver, gastric, lung, bladder, and neuroblastoma cancers [75]. An increase in MALAT1 expression is associated with proliferation, migration, and invasion by inhibiting tumor suppressor genes, the activation of MAPK, WNT/β-catenin, and anti-apoptotic signaling cascades. Specifically, upregulation of MALAT1 enhanced integrin β1 by sponging miR-183 in SK-MEL-1 and HBL melanoma cell lines [76, 77]. Luan et al. [78] found that MALAT1 potently regulated melanoma cell migration and metastasis by modulating MMP14 and SNAIL via silencing miR-22 expression.

13.5.2 HOTAIR

HOX transcript antisense RNA (HOTAIR) is a prominent nuclear-enriched lncRNA in the human HOXC gene cluster with 2364 bp in length. The elevated level of HOTAIR correlates to primary and metastatic lesions of breast cancers [79]. HOTAIR is believed to promote epithelial–mesenchymal transition (EMT) and cancer metastasis by recruiting Polycomb Repressive Complex 2 (PRC2) and lysine-specific demethylase 1 (LSD1). Further, it leads to suppression and silencing of the transcription of tumor suppressor genes through histone tail methylation. Accumulating evidence suggests that the aberrant expression of HOTAIR is found in diverse types of human cancers, including hepatocellular, lung, colorectal,

Table 13.2 LncRNAs as a potential regulator of melanoma development

LncRNAs	Classification	Size (bp)	Location	Expression	Molecular targets	Effects	References
MALAT1	Intergenic	8302	Nucleus	Up-regulated	miR-140, miR-183, miR-22, integrin-β1, slug, snail, ADAM10, MMP14	Induction of melanoma cells proliferation, migration, and metastasis	[77, 78]
HOTAIR	Antisense	2364	Nucleus and cytoplasm	Up-regulated	miR-152-3p	Enhanced cell motility, invasiveness, and metastasis potentially by increasing gelatin matrix degradation	[37, 61, 64]
BANCR	Intergenic	693	Cytoplasm	Up-regulated	miR-204, miR-206, miR-571, CXCL11,	Promoted cell survival, proliferation, and migration	[59, 85]
ANRIL	Antisense	2659	Nucleus and cytoplasm	Up-regulated	miR-204, miR-377, p15INK4B, p16INK4A	Increased colony formation and migration	[25, 87–89]
UCA1	Intergenic	1410	Nucleus and cytoplasm	Up-regulated	miR-185, miR-507, miR-28-5p, FOXM1, HOXB3	Induced cell proliferation and migration	[19, 93, 94]
SPRY4-IT1	Intergenic	708	Cytoplasm	Up-regulated	Lipin2, diacylglycerol O-acyltransferase 2	Promoted cell growth, differentiation, migration, invasion; inhibited apoptosis	[31]
SLNCR1	Intergenic	2257	Nucleus	Up-regulated	MMP9, Brn3a, AR	Degraded ECM components and increased invasiveness	[97]
SAMMSON	Intergenic	2027	Cytoplasm	Up-regulated	p32, MITF	Promotes melanoma survival and growth, and regulated tumor metabolism	[22]
LIme23	Intergenic	1609	Nucleus	Up-regulated	PSF, Rab23	Increased colony growth and migration	[26]
FALEC	Intergenic	566	Nucleus	Up-regulated	EZH2/p21	Enhanced cell proliferation	[24]

GAS5	Antisense	656	Nucleus and cytoplasm	Down-regulated	MMP2, miR-137	Inhibits melanoma growth, migration, and invasion	[68, 102]

ADAM10 a disintegrin and metalloproteinase domain-containing protein 10, *ANRIL* antisense non-coding RNA in the INK4 locus, *AR* androgen receptor, *BANCR* v-raf murine sarcoma viral oncogene homolog B1 (BRAF)-activated non-coding RNA, *Brn3a* brain-specific homeobox protein 3a, *ECM* extracellular matrix, *EZH2* enhancer of zeste homolog 2, *FALEC* focally amplified long non-coding RNA in epithelial cancer, *FOXM1* forkhead box protein M1, *GAS5* growth arrest-specific 5, *HOTAIR* HOX transcript antisense RNA, *MALAT1* metastasis associated lung adenocarcinoma transcript 1, *MITF* microphthalmia-associated transcription factor, *MMP* matrix metalloproteinase, *PSF* poly-pyrimidine tract-binding protein-associated splicing factor, *SAMMSON* survival associated mitochondrial-melanoma specific oncogenic non-coding RNA, *SLNCR1* SRA-like non-coding RNA1, *SPRY4-IT1* Sprouty4-intronic transcript 1, *UCA1* urothelial carcinoma associated 1

pancreatic, gastric, and nasopharyngeal carcinomas, wherein higher expression of HOTAIR acts as an oncogenic player which is positively correlated with cancer metastasis and poor prognosis [27, 80–83]. In melanoma, HOTAIR was also exclusively expressed in the metastatic phase compared with primary melanoma lesions and was linked to increased cell migration and invasiveness [17, 37]. Besides, knockdown of HOTAIR accompanied by repressed gelatine matrix degradation in vitro suggested that HOTAIR might promote melanoma cells invasiveness by increasing the gelatinase activity in the A375 melanoma cell line [37]. Luan et al. [61] have shown that HOTAIR acts as a competing endogenous RNA for miR-152-3p to enhance melanoma cell proliferation, invasion, and migration by modulating EMT in A375 and A875 melanoma cell lines. Wang et al. [64] reported that short interference RNA (siRNA)-mediated HOTAIR downregulation remarkably suppressed melanoma cell proliferation and migration, accompanied by increased apoptosis, and inhibited the NF-κB signaling in the A375 cell line. Overall, these observations suggest the role of HOTAIR in melanoma pathogenesis and thus could be a potential candidate biomarker.

13.5.3 BANCR

BRAF-activated non-coding RNA (BANCR) is 693 bp in length. It is primarily identified in V600E BRAF mutated human melanoma cells. It is abnormally expressed in melanoma cell lines and tissues. Through RNA-seq analysis, BANCR was identified as one of the activated genes downstream of BRAF^{V600E} in melanocytes by Flockhart et al. [21]. BANCR is recurrently overexpressed in the melanoma cell lines and primary metastatic tissues. The increased level of BANCR correlated with poor survival outcomes in human patients, suggesting its oncogenic role [84]. Moreover, siRNA-mediated BANCR downregulation reduced melanoma cell proliferation and migration that could be rescued by the overexpression of CXCL11 [21]. Besides, overexpression of BANCR stimulates the melanoma cell proliferation and migration via MAPK signaling pathways (ERK1/2 and c-JUN components) and the Notch cascades via sponging miR-204 in A375, A875, and M14 human melanoma cell lines [59]. BANCR was found to suppress miR-206 and miR-571 and facilitated melanoma cell proliferation, migration, and invasion by inducing Glucose-6-phosphate dehydrogenase (G6PD) expression Yang et al. [85]. Overall, these data indicated that BANCR is positively correlated with metastatic progression and thus could be a predictive marker for melanoma.

13.5.4 ANRIL

Antisense non-coding RNA in the INK4 locus (ANRIL) is a prominent nuclear- and perinuclear-enriched lncRNA with 3834 bp in length. It is co-expressed with p15/CDKN2B-p16/CDKN2A-p14/ARF cluster in an antisense direction. ANRIL interacts with polychrome repressive complex 1 and 2 (PRC1/2) and decreases the expression of p15INK4B/p16INK4A in melanoma cell lines and cutaneous tissues [25, 86]. The function of ANRIL has been reported in cell cycle regulation. It inhibits cellular senescence by sequestering miR-204 and miR-377 and decreasing inhibitors of CD**K4B** (INK4B) and inhibitors of CD**K4A** (INK4A) expression to the recruitment of E2F transcription factors into its cell cycle-related genes locus [87–89]. Interestingly, chromosome 9p21, a gene locus of ANRIL, is usually deactivated in both uveal and cutaneous melanoma metastatic tissues [90–92]. These findings suggested that ANRIL acts as an oncogene in melanoma by recruiting chromatin remodeling factors or recurrent fusion transcripts of ANRIL and tumor suppressor genes to its gene locus.

13.5.5 UCA1

Urothelial carcinoma associated 1 (UCA1) is a lncRNA with 1400 bp in length. It was first identified as highly expressed in bladder cell carcinoma. The lncRNA was up-regulated in the melanoma tissues compared to the adjacent normal tissues. Further, UCA1 was reported mostly in more advanced melanomas stages (stages III/IV). Moreover, UCA1 expression could increase melanoma cells' tumorigenic features by suppressing miR-185, leading to an upregulation in the Wnt/β-catenin signaling pathway [19]. UCA1 can also reverse the miR-507 mediated suppression of forkhead box protein M1 (FOXM1) expression, a key transcription factor of G2-M phase transition and even a direct target miR-507, which contributes to melanoma cells proliferation, invasion, and migration via G2/M cell cycle phase progression [93]. Han et al. [94] reported that enhanced expression of UCA1 markedly increased the growth and invasion of melanoma cells by regulating the miR-28-5p-HOXB3 (homeobox-B3) axis.

13.5.6 LLME23

Llme23 is 1600 bp in length discovered as a poly-pyrimidine tract-binding protein-associated splicing factor (PSF) in the human melanoma cell line YUSAC [26]. Llme23 interacts with PSF and consequently blocks its RNA binding domain. As a result, Llme23 dissociates from the repressed genes and reverses the transcriptional repression of proto-oncogene *Rab23* [26]. Because Llme23 is solely expressed in human melanoma cells, it could serve as a specific biomarker.

13.5.7 SAMMSON

Survival associated mitochondrial-melanoma specific oncogenic non-coding RNA (SAMMSON) is a cytoplasmic-enriched intergenic lncRNA with 2000 bp in length. It is co-expressed with microphthalmia-associated transcription factor (MITF) [22]. TCGA and RNA-seq data set analysis showed that SAMMSON is co-amplified with MITF in only 10% of melanoma cases. In contrast, SAMMSON itself was amplified in 90% of human melanoma samples. Functional assays reported that SAMMSON binds to p32 to assist its mitochondrial localization and thus regulate tumor metabolism by balancing glycolysis, oxidative phosphorylation, and mitochondrial dynamics in a cancer-cell-specific manner [22]. Mechanistically, exogenously driven SAMMSON expression stimulates the lineage-specific onco-genic potential of melanoma cells, while knockdown of SAMMSON reduced the cell viability and increased apoptosis by enhancing the sensitivity to MAPK-targeting therapeutics [95]. The above findings suggested that SAMMSON silencing might provide highly efficient anti-melanoma treatments.

13.5.8 SLNCR1

SRA-like non-coding RNA1 (SLNCR1) is a nuclear-enriched intergenic lncRNA associated with melanoma invasion, poor prognosis, and inferior survival outcomes in melanoma patients [96]. Using the RNA-associated transcription factor array (RATA) technique, studies have shown that SLNCR1 co-expressed with brain-specific homeobox protein 3a (Brn3a) and the androgen receptor (AR). SLNCR1 increases melanoma invasion via upregulating MMP9, leading to the degradation of extracellular matrix components for invasion and EMT-like phenotypes [97, 98]. These findings provide a direct link of AR to melanomas invasion and a probable explanation of why males showed higher features of melanoma metastases and exhibited poor survival outcomes than females.

13.5.9 SPRY4-IT1

SPRY4-IT1 is a 708 bp cytoplasmic-enriched lncRNA localized in the intron of the Sprouty 4 (SPRY4) gene. Its secondary structure contains several long-hairpin-like conformations. By analyzing lncRNA microarray data sets, Khaitan et al. [31] demonstrated that SPRY4-IT is significantly up-regulated in melanoma cell lines compared to the normal melanocytes and keratinocytes. A study found that SPRY4-IT1 is involved in melanoma recurrence, metastasis and progression, and apoptosis inhibition [39, 99, 100]. The pathways wherein SPRY4-IT1 executes its roles as an oncogene in melanoma involve the following: (a) by direct binding with lipin2 (a lipid phosphatase) and suppressing the generation of several free fatty acyl chains, acylcarnitine, and diacylglycerol; (b) through direct interaction with diacylglycerol O-acyltransferase 2 and silencing its enzymatic activity that involved in the conver-sion of diacylglycerol to triacylglycerol. These observations indicated that abnormal upregulation of SPRY4-IT1 might be associated with lipid synthesis and apoptosis inhibition that arisen from lipid metabolism and lipid toxicity. Additionally, SPRY4-IT1 acts as a tumor suppressor through the inhibition of MAPK signaling [31].

13.5.10 FALEC1

Focally amplified lncRNA on chromosome 1 (FALEC1) is a nuclear-enriched intergenic lncRNA with 566 bp length and exerts an oncogenic potential in various human cancers [96]. Functional assays demonstrated that silencing of FALEC inhibited the proliferation and invasion in melanoma cell lines and melanoma tissues, resulting in the arrest of cell cycle and cell death [24]. Mechanistically, the former study identified that FALEC heightened melanoma cell proliferation through direct recruitment of Enhancer of zeste homolog 2 enhancers on p21 promoter region and derepress p21-targeted inhibition of cyclin-D1 gene expression.

13.5.11 GAS5

GAS5 is a tumor suppressor lncRNA that is generally induced under stress responses such as serum starvation and cell–cell contact inhibition [27]. The lower GAS5 level was significantly associated with lymph node metastasis (LNM) in multiple malignancies, leading to evasion of apoptosis [101]. Chen et al. [68] demonstrated that lentiviral-mediated GAS5 overexpression significantly suppressed the migratory and invasive potential in SK-MEL-110 cell lines through diminished MMP2 expression. Moreover, GAS5 expression drastically reduced the melanoma progression via epigenetic silencing of miR-137 [102].

13.6   Diagnostic and Prognostic Potential of lncRNAs in Melanoma

The disease and tissue specificity of lncRNAs make them valuable tools for diagnostics. Furthermore, various sensitive molecular methods are available to detect tumor-specific ncRNAs in plasma or serum. Among them, liquid biopsy is used as the first line of diagnostic tools. Nevertheless, it is clinically expensive and invasive. Diagnosis using circulating lncRNAs could provide an additional advantage over tumor biopsies [103]. Being minimally invasive and inexpensive, these can be employed for high-risk patients. Moreover, lncRNAs with increased plasma or serum expression could also provide important prognostic information, including early tumor detection, staging, and tumor size.

All 11 lncRNAs, except GAS5, are significantly up-regulated in melanoma in comparison to normal tissue. Among them, HOTAIR, LLME23, and SAMMSON are considered to be melanoma specific. GAS5 is significantly suppressed in melanoma and other malignancies [68, 104–106]. In one of the studies, ANRIL was significantly higher in 10 uveal and 18 cutaneous primary melanoma samples than nine healthy tissue samples, including choroid, retina, and benign nevi [88]. In the serum, SNHG5 is significantly increased in 24 melanoma patients than 15 healthy controls and five cSCC patients. In five melanoma patients, SNHG5 level in the serum was significantly decreased after surgery. Out of the five patients, two patients exhibited an increased level of SNHG5 in the serum at the time of recurrence [107]. Moreover, SNHG5 was also observed in 36 primary melanoma tissues and four nevi samples [35]. Besides their application in the diagnosis, lncRNAs could also be used in the prognosis of melanoma skin disorder. Prognosis is an estimate or prediction of a disease's likely outcome and the chances of successful recovery or survival from cancer. Dysregulated lncRNAs, such as FALEC, HOTAIR, SLNCR1, SPRY4-IT, MALAT1, UCA1, and CASC15, predict poor survival in melanoma patients [24, 31, 61, 98, 108, 109].

The level of SPRY4-IT in the plasma was significantly increased in 70 melanoma patients compared to 79 healthy individuals [99]. SPRY4-IT was reported to be a prognostic marker for the overall survival (OS) of melanoma patients. Cantile et al. [17] observed a significant increase in HOTAIR in both tumor and serum at different melanoma stages (pT1 to pT4). Tang et al. [37] found overexpression of HOTAIR in the LNM tissue compared to matched primary melanoma. An analysis from the publicly available GEO database revealed a high level of HOTAIR in the melanoma samples than normal tissue samples [37]. Overall, these studies suggest a substantial implication of HOTAIR in melanoma carcinogenesis.

Earlier studies revealed that expression levels of BANCR and SLNCR1 in melanoma samples associate with poor survival outcomes [84, 98]. Li et al. [84] reported higher expression of BANCR in 103 primary melanoma samples than 12 melanocytic samples. An analysis in 72 patients found that patients with an increased BANCR in the primary tumor associate with lower OS rates than patients with a lower BANCR expression. It can be concluded that BANCR expression associates with the clinical stage of melanoma. Further, an analysis from the TCGA dataset showed dysregulation of SLNCR1 in 150 randomly selected primary melanoma samples. Its higher expression was linked with shorter OS [98]. Studies found that CASC15, MALAT1, and UCA1 are correlated with LNM in malignant melanoma. The higher level of CASC15 was associated with lower survival as detected by RNA in situ hybridization [109]. Tian et al. [110] found a high level of MALAT1 in 63 LNM tissues compared to paired primary melanomas samples. Moreover, patients with LNM displayed a high UCA1 expression in the primary tumor than those without LNM [93, 110].

13.7   Therapeutic Potential of lncRNAs in Melanoma Cancer

LncRNAs exhibit the following characteristics that make them promising therapeutic targets in cancer cells: (1) easily identified in the plasma, serum, saliva, urine, and the other tissues of cancer patients; (2) precise expression of lncRNAs in selected cancer tissues/cells provides a therapeutic target for cancer eradication; (3) their low expression might allow the clinicians to use low therapeutic doses, which can alleviate some kinds of toxicities observed with oligonucleotide therapies; (4) since the localization of several lncRNAs are found to be specific in the nucleus and regulates the expression of Cis-regulatory elements, targeting lncRNAs may be an alternative approach to modulate the expression of such genes. The therapeutic potential of lncRNAs has been demonstrated through molecular approaches such as RNA interference (RNAi), antisense specific oligonucleotides (ASOs), CRISPR/Cas9-mediated gene editing, lncRNAs replacements, LNA, or by use of small molecules inhibitors [32].

13.7.1 Targeted Silencing of lncRNAs with Oncogenic Features

Short interference RNA (siRNA) is the most currently used knockdown strategy for lncRNAs. siRNAs are the small double-stranded RNAs (dsRNAs) with a targeted mRNA sequence. DICER processing is converted into single-stranded RNAs (ssRNAs) and attaches with RNA-induced silencing complex (RISC). Further, based on complementarity, the processed ssRNAs bind to their targeted mRNA, resulting in gene silencing either transcriptionally or post-transcriptionally [111]. Another form of silencing is a short hairpin RNA (shRNA) expressed endogenously in the cell. shRNAs mediated knockdown responses may be stable or transient and gives a higher off-target effect than siRNAs. For efficient silencing in cancer cells, transfection is mainly achieved by siRNAs or shRNAs plasmid vectors [112].

siRNA-based silencing of lncRNA, SPRY4-IT1 suppressed tumor cell growth, and invasion leads to apoptosis in human melanoma cell lines WM1552C and A375 [31, 39, 99, 104, 100]. Similarly, knocking down HOTAIR inhibited the melanoma cell migration and invasion in vitro, accompanied by repressed gelatine matrix degradation, NF-κB inhibition, and apoptosis induction [37, 64]. MALAT1 knockdown in human melanoma cell lines suppressed the cell proliferation and migration, wherein its function as a molecular sponge to inhibit miRNA expressions was reduced [78, 110, 113, 114]. ANRIL silencing in the A375 cells leads to the reprogramming of tumor suppressor genes, p15INK4B and p16INK4A and an observed decrease in colony formation suggesting the inhibition of metastasis [88]. UCA1 silencing in A375 and SK-MEL2 cell lines significantly decreased the migration and invasion by deactivating Wnt/β-catenin signaling leading to G0/G1 phase cell arrest [93]. Besides, Han et al. [94] reported that the downregulation of UCA1 in A375 cells suppressed the growth and invasion of melanoma cells through miR-28-5p/HOXB3 axis. SLNCR1 knockdown in WM1976 cell lines was associated with decreased melanoma invasion [98]. However, cell proliferation and migration were not affected. RNAi-mediated silencing of SAMMSON reduced the cell viability and induced apoptosis in MAPK-targeting therapeutics treated SAMMSON-expressing melanoma cell cultures [95]. LLME23-deficient YUSAC melanoma cells exhibited a significant reduction in clonogenicity in soft agar due to decreased expression of *Rab23*, and the same cells after injection into the nude mice demonstrated a 75% smaller tumor volume at 38 days [26]. shRNA-mediated BANCR knockdown in SK-MEL-5 cell lines impaired melanoma cell migration via down-regulated CXCL11 expression [21] (Table 13.3).

Antisense specific oligonucleotides (ASOs) are short (13 mer) nucleic acid sequences that specifically bind through complementary base pairing. ASOs degrade

RNA by recruiting RNase H to the DNA/RNA heteroduplex [115, 116]. ASOs do not interfere with RNAi machinery and target those lncRNAs localized to subcellular compartments [50]. Thus, ASOs have recently been added as a promising therapeutic molecule to knockdown lncRNAs. Leucci et al. [22] demonstrated that intravenously delivering a SAMMSON-specific ASOs in a tumor xenograft derived from melanoma patients significantly reduced tumor growth. Using SAMMSON-specific ASOs with dabrafenib, a BRAF inhibitor, significantly induced apoptosis in melanoma tumor xenograft compared to dabrafenib alone restrain only the tumor growth. Moreover, no significant signs of toxicity were observed when used in combination of SAMMSON-specific ASOs and dabrafenib compared to administration of MEK or BRAF inhibitors alone. Amodio et al. [29] reported that the administration of a MALAT1-specific LNA GapmeR ASO remarkably antagonized the cell proliferation and triggered apoptosis in the multiple human myelomas. Thus, the above study would provide us with new anticipation to target the MALAT1 lncRNAs via LNA gapmeR ASO (Table 13.3).

13.7.2 LncRNAs Replacements and Overexpression of Tumor Suppressor lncRNAs.

Many lncRNAs in cancer are genomically deleted or exhibit loss of function due to mutations in their transcribed sequences acting as tumor suppressors. Thus, the reactivation of these lncRNAs might produce anti-cancer activity. Thus, replacement approaches are usually applied to reactivation of the tumor suppressor lncRNAs using a short (22-mer) synthetic dsRNA that share the same sequence of mature lncRNAs or its precursor. These are called mimics. An example is GAS5, a well-known tumor suppressor lncRNAs in melanoma. Chen et al. [117] reported that short oligonucleotides mimic the GAS5 mutated sequence in melanoma cells, showing increased apoptotic activity and a decline in tumor growth in vivo. An overexpression of GAS5 in the SK-MEL 110 cells exhibited a reduction in the migration and invasion due to decreased MMP2 expression and, administration of the same cells in nude mice significantly restrains the tumor growth [68]. Li et al. [23] found that overexpression in MEG3 significantly suppressed melanoma cell growth and migration by inhibiting WNT/β-catenin signaling. Besides, Coe et al. [20] showed that upregulation of the *DIRC3* tumor suppressor lncRNAs activated expression of its adjacent *IGFBP5* tumor suppressor. Further, it modulated the chromatin structure and suppressed the SOX10 binding to putative regulatory regions within *DIRC3* locus. As a result, the melanoma cell proliferation was inhibited. However, more work is required to fully explore the therapeutic potential of GAS5, MEG3, and DIRC3 in melanoma and skin cancers (Table 13.3).

Table 13.3 LncRNAs as promising therapeutic target with a potential for clinical applications

LncRNAs	Experimental models	Functional inactivation/activation techniques	Therapeutic effect(s)	References
SPRY4-IT1	Malignant melanoma cell lines	siRNA-mediated knockdown	Inhibited cell growth, differentiation, invasion, and induced apoptosis	[31, 39, 99, 100, 104]
HOTAIR			Impaired cell motility, invasion, and migration	[37, 64]
MALAT1			Prevented cell proliferation and migration	[77, 78, 110, 113]
UCA1			Impaired proliferation and metastasis; induced cell cycle arrest	[93, 94]
SLNCR1			Reduced invasiveness of melanoma cells	[98]
ANRIL			Decreased colony growth and metastatic ability of melanoma cells	[88]
Llme23			Diminished clonogenicity and migration	[26]
FALEC			Hinders cell proliferation by suppressing cell cycle progression and induction of apoptosis	[24]
BANCR	–	shRNA-mediated knockdown	Impaired cell proliferation and migration	[21]
SAMMSON	Tumor xenograft derived from melanoma patients	Locked nucleic acid (LNA)-modified antisense specific oligonucleotide (GapmeR3) and siRNA-mediated knockdown	Reduced tumor growth and induced apoptosis; produced significant effects with dabrafenib	[22]
GAS5	In vitro and in vivo models	Lentiviral mediated-overexpression	Impaired melanoma growth, migration, and invasion; enhanced apoptosis	[68, 117]
MEG3 (tumor suppressor)				[23]

(continued)

Table 13.3 (continued)

LncRNAs	Experimental models	Functional inactivation/activation techniques	Therapeutic effect(s)	References
DIRC3 (tumor suppressor)				[20]
PTENP1 (tumor suppressor)				[127]

ANRIL antisense non-coding RNA in the INK4 locus, *BANCR* v-raf murine sarcoma viral oncogene homolog B1 (BRAF)-activated non-coding RNA, *DIRC3* disrupted in renal carcinoma 3, *FALEC* focally amplified long non-coding RNA in epithelial cancer, *GAS5* growth arrest-specific 5, *HOTAIR* HOX transcript antisense RNA, *LNA* locked nucleic acid, *MALAT1* metastasis associated lung adenocarcinoma transcript 1, *MEG3* maternally expressed 3, *PTENP1* phosphatase and tensin homolog pseudogene 1, *SAMMSON* survival associated mitochondrial-melanoma specific oncogenic non-coding RNA, *SLNCR1* SRA-like non-coding RNA 1, *SPRY4-IT1* sprouty4-intronic transcript 1, *UCA1* urothelial carcinoma associated 1

13.8 Potential of lncRNAs in Predicting Chemoresistance and Radioresistance in Melanoma Skin Cancer

Unfortunately, in melanoma, long-term treatment with targeted-based chemotherapeutic agents is discouraged due to drug-resistance acquisition that causes melanoma recurrence within a short-period after therapy. The United States Food and Drug Administration approved alkylating agents with cytostatic (Temozolomide and Decarbazine) and BRAF inhibitors or combination with MEK inhibitors (trametinib) for patients with BRAF V600E-mutated metastatic melanoma. However, these are not able to prevent disease recurrence [118–120]. Development of resistance to chemotherapeutic drugs in melanomas is frequently associated with the higher expression of multi-drug resistance proteins, MITF, a melanoma specific transcription factor, and O6-alkylguanine DNA alkyl-transferase (MGMT, a DNA repair protein), which reduces sensitivity to treatments with clinically approved therapeutic agents [121–123].

The role of miRNAs in the melanomas drug resistance has been reported. However, studies on the role of lncRNAs in drug resistance are limited. Sanlorenzo et al. [124] found that MAPK Inhibitor Resistance Associated Transcript (MIRAT) is significantly up-regulated in MAPKi resistant melanoma cells. The silencing of SAMMSON was shown to limit melanoma resistance to MAPKi-based therapeutics, but the underlying mechanism remains to be elucidated [22]. The lncRNA, EMICERI (EQTN MOB3B IFNK C9orf72 enhancer RNA I) was identified through a genome-scale activation screening analysis by Joung et al. [125]. EMICERI can promote melanoma cells' resistance to vemurafenib due to the higher expression of MOB3B (MOB kinase activator 3B) and activation of the Hippo signaling pathway. A functional study by Pan et al. [66] demonstrated that overexpression of XIST promotes tumor progression and oxaliplatin-resistance in malignant melanoma cells and tissues. LINC00518 can promote radioresistance by regulating the Hypoxia-inducible factor-1α/lactate dehydrogenase-glycolysis axis in malignant melanoma cells and tissues [126].

13.9   Conclusion

Melanoma is a highly aggressive malignant skin cancer with metastatic phenotypes. The advanced-stage melanomas do not respond to conventional therapies and are associated with poor survival outcomes. Early diagnosis is essential for the management of melanoma. Initially, lncRNAs were described as junk or garbage and therefore regarded as dark matter and transcriptional genome noise. However, growing studies have elucidated their functional roles in various physiological processes and are frequently dysfunctional in several diseases. Several lncRNAs are now significantly associated with many types of malignancies, including skin cancer. However, only small numbers have been functionally studied in melanoma cancer. In this chapter, we described the functions of several lncRNAs in melanoma cancer. In melanoma, SAMMSON, MALAT1, HOTAIR, BANCR, ANRIL1, UCA1, FALEC1, SLNCR1, SPRY-IT1, and Llme23 lncRNAs are differentially expressed and serve as potent regulators of melanoma growth and metastasis. In contrast, GAS5, MEG3, and DIRC3 lncRNAs expression are decreased and function as a tumor suppressor in melanoma. Therefore, lncRNAs show broad potential in rising new diagnostic and clinical utilities. Along with conventional molecular markers, the specific expression signature of lncRNAs can offer superior diagnostic accuracy of the disease. However, there are some limitations in using lncRNAs as predictive biomarkers. For example, generally, the lncRNAs present in plasma are low in quantity. Thus, unlike miRNAs, most lncRNAs are not easily detected in plasma through standard techniques such as qRT-PCR and microarray. Besides, the exact molecular mechanism by which lncRNAs modulate skin cancer pathogenesis has not been elucidated. Therefore, more studies are required to elucidate the upstream and downstream molecular mechanisms and the therapeutic efficacy of tumorigenic lncRNAs in melanoma.

Acknowledgments The study was supported in part from Indian Council of Medical Research, New Delhi (5/13/51/2020/NCD-III) in the SCG's laboratory. The work was also supported by Nitte Research Grant (NU/DR/NUFR1/NUCSER/2019-20/01) to A Sharma. The support from Nitte Research (N/RG/NUSR2/NUCSER/2020/16 and N/RG/NUSR2/NUCSER/2020/14) to SK is thankfully acknowledged. VR is supported from Indian Council of Medical Research, New Delhi in the form of Senior Research Fellowship (3/2/2/43/2018/Online Onco Fship/NCD-III).

References

1. Asgari MM, Moffet HH, Ray GT, Quesenberry CP (2015) Trends in basal cell carcinoma incidence and identification of high-risk subgroups, 1998–2012. JAMA Dermatol 151 (9):976–981. https://doi.org/10.1001/jamadermatol.2015.1188
2. Rogers HW, Weinstock MA, Feldman SR, Coldiron BM (2015) Incidence estimate of nonmelanoma skin Cancer (keratinocyte carcinomas) in the U.S. population, 2012. JAMA Dermatol 151(10):1081–1086. https://doi.org/10.1001/jamadermatol.2015.1187
3. Siegel RL, Miller KD, Jemal A (2017) Cancer statistics, 2017. CA Cancer J Clin 67(1):7–30. https://doi.org/10.3322/caac.21387
4. Torre LA, Bray F, Siegel RL, Ferlay J, Lortet-Tieulent J, Jemal A (2015) Global cancer statistics, 2012. CA Cancer J Clin 65(2):87–108. https://doi.org/10.3322/caac.21262
5. Apalla Z, Lallas A, Sotiriou E, Lazaridou E, Ioannides D (2017) Epidemiological trends in skin cancer. Dermatol Pract Concept 7(2):1–6. https://doi.org/10.5826/dpc.0702a01
6. Singh BP, Salama AK (2016) Updates in therapy for advanced melanoma. Cancers 8(1):17. https://doi.org/10.3390/cancers8010017
7. Alcala AM, Flaherty KT (2012) BRAF inhibitors for the treatment of metastatic melanoma: clinical trials and mechanisms of resistance. Clin Cancer Res 18(1):33–39. https://doi.org/10. 1158/1078-0432.CCR-11-0997
8. Kugel CH 3rd, Aplin AE (2014) Adaptive resistance to RAF inhibitors in melanoma. Pigment Cell Melanoma Res 27(6):1032–1038. https://doi.org/10.1111/pcmr.12264
9. Roesch A (2015) Tumor heterogeneity and plasticity as elusive drivers for resistance to MAPK pathway inhibition in melanoma. Oncogene 34(23):2951–2957. https://doi.org/10.1038/onc. 2014.249
10. Wellbrock C (2014) MAPK pathway inhibition in melanoma: resistance three ways. Biochem Soc Trans 42(4):727–732. https://doi.org/10.1042/BST20140020
11. Reddy SM, Reuben A, Wargo JA (2016) Influences of BRAF inhibitors on the immune microenvironment and the rationale for combined molecular and immune targeted therapy. Curr Oncol Rep 18(7):42. https://doi.org/10.1007/s11912-016-0531-z
12. Harrow J, Frankish A, Gonzalez JM, Tapanari E, Diekhans M, Kokocinski F, Aken BL, Barrell D, Zadissa A, Searle S, Barnes I, Bignell A, Boychenko V, Hunt T, Kay M, Mukherjee G, Rajan J, Despacio-Reyes G, Saunders G, Steward C, Harte R, Lin M, Howald C, Tanzer A, Derrien T, Chrast J, Walters N, Balasubramanian S, Pei B, Tress M, Rodriguez JM, Ezkurdia I, van Baren J, Brent M, Haussler D, Kellis M, Valencia A, Reymond A, Gerstein M, Guigo R, Hubbard TJ (2012) GENCODE: the reference human genome annotation for the ENCODE project. Genome Res 22(9):1760–1774. https://doi.org/ 10.1101/gr.135350.111
13. Miller DFB, Yan PX, Fang F, Buechlein A, Ford JB, Tang H, Huang TH, Burow ME, Liu Y, Rusch DB, Nephew KP (2015) Stranded whole transcriptome RNA-Seq for all RNA types. Curr Protoc Hum Genet 84:11. https://doi.org/10.1002/0471142905.hg1114s84
14. Ponjavic J, Ponting CP, Lunter G (2007) Functionality or transcriptional noise? Evidence for selection within long non-coding RNAs. Genome Res 17(5):556–565. https://doi.org/10.1101/ gr.6036807
15. Mercer TR, Dinger ME, Mattick JS (2009) Long non-coding RNAs: insights into functions. Nat Rev Genet 10(3):155–159. https://doi.org/10.1038/nrg2521
16. Moran VA, Perera RJ, Khalil AM (2012) Emerging functional and mechanistic paradigms of mammalian long non-coding RNAs. Nucleic Acids Res 40(14):6391–6400. https://doi.org/10. 1093/nar/gks296
17. Cantile M, Scognamiglio G, Marra L, Aquino G, Botti C, Falcone MR, Malzone MG, Liguori G, Di Bonito M, Franco R, Ascierto PA, Botti G (2017) HOTAIR role in melanoma progression and its identification in the blood of patients with advanced disease. J Cell Physiol 232(12):3422–3432. https://doi.org/10.1002/jcp.25789

18. Chen X, Gao G, Liu S, Yu L, Yan D, Yao X, Sun W, Han D, Dong H (2017) Long noncoding RNA PVT1 as a novel diagnostic biomarker and therapeutic target for melanoma. Biomed Res Int 2017:7038579. https://doi.org/10.1155/2017/7038579

19. Chen X, Gao J, Yu Y, Zhao Z, Pan Y (2018) Long non-coding RNA UCA1 targets miR-185-5p and regulates cell mobility by affecting epithelial-mesenchymal transition in melanoma via Wnt/beta-catenin signaling pathway. Gene 676:298–305. https://doi.org/10.1016/j.gene.2018.08.065

20. Coe EA, Tan JY, Shapiro M, Louphrasitthiphol P, Bassett AR, Marques AC, Goding CR, Vance KW (2019) The MITF-SOX10 regulated long non-coding RNA DIRC3 is a melanoma tumour suppressor. PLoS Genet 15(12):e1008501. https://doi.org/10.1371/journal.pgen.1008501

21. Flockhart RJ, Webster DE, Qu K, Mascarenhas N, Kovalski J, Kretz M, Khavari PA (2012) BRAFV600E remodels the melanocyte transcriptome and induces BANCR to regulate melanoma cell migration. Genome Res 22(6):1006–1014. https://doi.org/10.1101/gr.140061.112

22. Leucci E, Vendramin R, Spinazzi M, Laurette P, Fiers M, Wouters J, Radaelli E, Eyckerman S, Leonelli C, Vanderheyden K, Rogiers A, Hermans E, Baatsen P, Aerts S, Amant F, Van Aelst S, van den Oord J, de Strooper B, Davidson I, Lafontaine DL, Gevaert K, Vandesompele J, Mestdagh P, Marine JC (2016) Melanoma addiction to the long non-coding RNA SAMMSON. Nature 531(7595):518–522. https://doi.org/10.1038/nature17161

23. Li P, Gao Y, Li J, Zhou Y, Yuan J, Guan H, Yao P (2018) LncRNA MEG3 repressed malignant melanoma progression via inactivating Wnt signaling pathway. J Cell Biochem 119(9):7498–7505. https://doi.org/10.1002/jcb.27061

24. Ni N, Song H, Wang X, Xu X, Jiang Y, Sun J (2017) Up-regulation of long non-coding RNA FALEC predicts poor prognosis and promotes melanoma cell proliferation through epigenetically silencing p21. Biomed Pharmacother 96:1371–1379. https://doi.org/10.1016/j.biopha.2017.11.060

25. Pasmant E, Laurendeau I, Heron D, Vidaud M, Vidaud D, Bieche I (2007) Characterization of a germ-line deletion, including the entire INK4/ARF locus, in a melanoma-neural system tumor family: identification of ANRIL, an antisense non-coding RNA whose expression coclusters with ARF. Cancer Res 67(8):3963–3969. https://doi.org/10.1158/0008-5472.CAN-06-2004

26. Wu CF, Tan GH, Ma CC, Li L (2013) The non-coding RNA llme23 drives the malignant property of human melanoma cells. J Genet Genomics 40(4):179–188. https://doi.org/10.1016/j.jgg.2013.03.001

27. Yu X, Li Z (2015) Long non-coding RNA growth arrest-specific transcript 5 in tumor biology. Oncol Lett 10(4):1953–1958. https://doi.org/10.3892/ol.2015.3553

28. Zhao H, Xing G, Wang Y, Luo Z, Liu G, Meng H (2017) Long non-coding RNA HEIH promotes melanoma cell proliferation, migration and invasion via inhibition of miR-200b/a/429. Biosci Rep 37(3):BSR20170682. https://doi.org/10.1042/BSR20170682

29. Amodio N, Stamato MA, Juli G, Morelli E, Fulciniti M, Manzoni M, Taiana E, Agnelli L, Cantafio MEG, Romeo E, Raimondi L, Caracciolo D, Zuccala V, Rossi M, Neri A, Munshi NC, Tagliaferri P, Tassone P (2018) Drugging the lncRNA MALAT1 via LNA gapmeR ASO inhibits gene expression of proteasome subunits and triggers anti-multiple myeloma activity. Leukemia 32(9):1948–1957. https://doi.org/10.1038/s41375-018-0067-3

30. Tang Q, Zheng F, Liu Z, Wu J, Chai X, He C, Li L, Hann SS (2019) Novel reciprocal interaction of lncRNA HOTAIR and miR-214-3p contribute to the solamargine-inhibited PDPK1 gene expression in human lung cancer. J Cell Mol Med 23(11):7749–7761. https://doi.org/10.1111/jcmm.14649

31. Khaitan D, Dinger ME, Mazar J, Crawford J, Smith MA, Mattick JS, Perera RJ (2011) The melanoma-upregulated long non-coding RNA SPRY4-IT1 modulates apoptosis and invasion. Cancer Res 71(11):3852–3862. https://doi.org/10.1158/0008-5472.CAN-10-4460

32. Grillone K, Riillo C, Scionti F, Rocca R, Tradigo G, Guzzi PH, Alcaro S, Di Martino MT, Tagliaferri P, Tassone P (2020) Non-coding RNAs in cancer: platforms and strategies for investigating the genomic "dark matter". J Exp Clin Cancer Res 39(1):117. https://doi.org/10.1186/s13046-020-01622-x

33. Iyer MK, Niknafs YS, Malik R, Singhal U, Sahu A, Hosono Y, Barrette TR, Prensner JR, Evans JR, Zhao S, Poliakov A, Cao X, Dhanasekaran SM, Wu YM, Robinson DR, Beer DG, Feng FY, Iyer HK, Chinnaiyan AM (2015) The landscape of long non-coding RNAs in the human transcriptome. Nat Genet 47(3):199–208. https://doi.org/10.1038/ng.3192

34. Siena ADD, Placa JR, Araujo LF, de Barros II, Peronni K, Molfetta G, de Biagi CAO Jr, Espreafico EM, Sousa JF, Silva WA Jr (2019) Whole transcriptome analysis reveals correlation of long non-coding RNA ZEB1-AS1 with invasive profile in melanoma. Sci Rep 9 (1):11350. https://doi.org/10.1038/s41598-019-47363-6

35. Hulstaert E, Brochez L, Volders PJ, Vandesompele J, Mestdagh P (2017) Long non-coding RNAs in cutaneous melanoma: clinical perspectives. Oncotarget 8(26):43470–43480. https://doi.org/10.18632/oncotarget.16478

36. Safa A, Gholipour M, Dinger ME, Taheri M, Ghafouri-Fard S (2020) The critical roles of lncRNAs in the pathogenesis of melanoma. Exp Mol Pathol 117:104558. https://doi.org/10.1016/j.yexmp.2020.104558

37. Tang L, Zhang W, Su B, Yu B (2013) Long non-coding RNA HOTAIR is associated with motility, invasion, and metastatic potential of metastatic melanoma. Biomed Res Int 2013:251098. https://doi.org/10.1155/2013/251098

38. Zhu J, Fu H, Wu Y, Zheng X (2013) Function of lncRNAs and approaches to lncRNA-protein interactions. Sci China Life Sci 56(10):876–885. https://doi.org/10.1007/s11427-013-4553-6

39. Mazar J, Zhao W, Khalil AM, Lee B, Shelley J, Govindarajan SS, Yamamoto F, Ratnam M, Aftab MN, Collins S, Finck BN, Han X, Mattick JS, Dinger ME, Perera RJ (2014) The functional characterization of long non-coding RNA SPRY4-IT1 in human melanoma cells. Oncotarget 5(19):8959–8969. https://doi.org/10.18632/oncotarget.1863

40. Huang Q, Mao Z, Li S, Hu J, Zhu Y (2014) A non-radioactive method for small RNA detection by northern blotting. Rice 7(1):26. https://doi.org/10.1186/s12284-014-0026-1

41. Luan W, Ding Y, Ma S, Ruan H, Wang J, Lu F (2019) Long non-coding RNA LINC00518 acts as a competing endogenous RNA to promote the metastasis of malignant melanoma via miR-204-5p/AP1S2 axis. Cell Death Dis 10(11):855. https://doi.org/10.1038/s41419-019-2090-3

42. Jorgensen S, Baker A, Moller S, Nielsen BS (2010) Robust one-day in situ hybridization protocol for detection of microRNAs in paraffin samples using LNA probes. Methods 52 (4):375–381. https://doi.org/10.1016/j.ymeth.2010.07.002

43. Zhang A, Zhao JC, Kim J, Fong KW, Yang YA, Chakravarti D, Mo YY, Yu J (2015) LncRNA HOTAIR enhances the androgen-receptor-mediated transcriptional program and drives castration-resistant prostate Cancer. Cell Rep 13(1):209–221. https://doi.org/10.1016/j.celrep.2015.08.069

44. Da Sacco L, Baldassarre A, Masotti A (2012) Bioinformatics tools and novel challenges in long non-coding RNAs (lncRNAs) functional analysis. Int J Mol Sci 13(1):97–114. https://doi.org/10.3390/ijms13010097

45. Olson NE (2006) The microarray data analysis process: from raw data to biological significance. NeuroRx 3(3):373–383. https://doi.org/10.1016/j.nurx.2006.05.005

46. Pinkney HR, Wright BM, Diermeier SD (2020) The lncRNA toolkit: databases and in silico tools for lncRNA analysis. Non-Coding RNA 6(4):49. https://doi.org/10.3390/ncrna6040049

47. Pirim H, Eksioglu B, Perkins A, Yuceer C (2012) Clustering of high throughput gene expression data. Comput Oper Res 39(12):3046–3061. https://doi.org/10.1016/j.cor.2012.03.008

48. Yotsukura S, duVerle D, Hancock T, Natsume-Kitatani Y, Mamitsuka H (2017) Computational recognition for long non-coding RNA (lncRNA): software and databases. Brief Bioinform 18(1):9–27. https://doi.org/10.1093/bib/bbv114

49. Anaya J (2016) OncoLnc: linking TCGA survival data to mRNAs, miRNAs, and lncRNAs. PeerJ Computer Science 2:e67

50. Leucci E, Coe EA, Marine JC, Vance KW (2016) The emerging role of long non-coding RNAs in cutaneous melanoma. Pigment Cell Melanoma Res 29(6):619–626. https://doi.org/10.1111/pcmr.12537

51. Iwakiri J, Hamada M, Asai K (2016) Bioinformatics tools for lncRNA research. Biochim Biophys Acta 1859(1):23–30. https://doi.org/10.1016/j.bbagrm.2015.07.014

52. Li JH, Liu S, Zheng LL, Wu J, Sun WJ, Wang ZL, Zhou H, Qu LH, Yang JH (2014) Discovery of protein-lncRNA interactions by integrating large-scale CLIP-Seq and RNA-Seq datasets. Front Bioeng Biotechnol 2:88. https://doi.org/10.3389/fbioe.2014.00088

53. Ning S, Zhang J, Wang P, Zhi H, Wang J, Liu Y, Gao Y, Guo M, Yue M, Wang L, Li X (2016) Lnc2Cancer: a manually curated database of experimentally supported lncRNAs associated with various human cancers. Nucleic Acids Res 44(D1):D980–D985. https://doi.org/10.1093/nar/gkv1094

54. Ala U, Karreth FA, Bosia C, Pagnani A, Taulli R, Leopold V, Tay Y, Provero P, Zecchina R, Pandolfi PP (2013) Integrated transcriptional and competitive endogenous RNA networks are cross-regulated in permissive molecular environments. Proc Natl Acad Sci U S A 110 (18):7154–7159. https://doi.org/10.1073/pnas.1222509110

55. Cohen C, Zavala-Pompa A, Sequeira JH, Shoji M, Sexton DG, Cotsonis G, Cerimele F, Govindarajan B, Macaron N, Arbiser JL (2002) Mitogen-acted protein kinase activation is an early event in melanoma progression. Clin Cancer Res 8(12):3728–3733

56. Wang YF, Jiang CC, Kiejda KA, Gillespie S, Zhang XD, Hersey P (2007) Apoptosis induction in human melanoma cells by inhibition of MEK is caspase-independent and mediated by the Bcl-2 family members PUMA, Bim, and Mcl-1. Clin Cancer Res 13(16):4934–4942. https://doi.org/10.1158/1078-0432.CCR-07-0665

57. Wellbrock C, Karasarides M, Marais R (2004) The RAF proteins take Centre stage. Nat Rev Mol Cell Biol 5(11):875–885. https://doi.org/10.1038/nrm1498

58. Hombach S, Kretz M (2013) The non-coding skin: exploring the roles of long non-coding RNAs in epidermal homeostasis and disease. BioEssays 35(12):1093–1100. https://doi.org/10.1002/bies.201300068

59. Cai B, Zheng Y, Ma S, Xing Q, Wang X, Yang B, Yin G, Guan F (2017) BANCR contributes to the growth and invasion of melanoma by functioning as a competing endogenous RNA to upregulate Notch2 expression by sponging miR204. Int J Oncol 51(6):1941–1951. https://doi.org/10.3892/ijo.2017.4173

60. Wu J, Zhou MY, Yu XP, Wu Y, Xie PL (2019) Long non-coding RNA OR3A4 promotes the migration and invasion of melanoma through the PI3K/AKT signaling pathway. Eur Rev Med Pharmacol Sci 23(16):6991–6996. https://doi.org/10.26355/eurrev_201908_18739

61. Luan W, Li R, Liu L, Ni X, Shi Y, Xia Y, Wang J, Lu F, Xu B (2017) Long non-coding RNA HOTAIR acts as a competing endogenous RNA to promote malignant melanoma progression by sponging miR-152-3p. Oncotarget 8(49):85401–85414. https://doi.org/10.18632/oncotarget.19910

62. Shang Z, Feng H, Cui L, Wang W, Fu H (2018) Propofol promotes apoptosis and suppresses the HOTAIR-mediated mTOR/p70S6K signaling pathway in melanoma cells. Oncol Lett 15 (1):630–634. https://doi.org/10.3892/ol.2017.7297

63. Liao Z, Zhao J, Yang Y (2018) Downregulation of lncRNA H19 inhibits the migration and invasion of melanoma cells by inactivating the NFkappaB and PI3K/Akt signaling pathways. Mol Med Rep 17(5):7313–7318. https://doi.org/10.3892/mmr.2018.8782

64. Wang J, Chen J, Jing G, Dong D (2020) LncRNA HOTAIR promotes proliferation of malignant melanoma cells through NF-varkappaB pathway. Iran J Public Health 49 (10):1931–1939. https://doi.org/10.18502/ijph.v49i10.4696

65. Yang Y, Zhang Z, Wu Z, Lin W, Yu M (2019) Downregulation of the expression of the lncRNA MIAT inhibits melanoma migration and invasion through the PI3K/AKT signaling pathway. Cancer Biomark 24(2):203–211. https://doi.org/10.3233/CBM-181869

66. Pan B, Lin X, Zhang L, Hong W, Zhang Y (2019) Long non-coding RNA X-inactive specific transcript promotes malignant melanoma progression and oxaliplatin resistance. Melanoma Res 29(3):254–262. https://doi.org/10.1097/CMR.0000000000000560

67. Peng Q, Liu L, Pei H, Zhang J, Chen M, Zhai X (2020) A LHFPL3-AS1/miR-580-3p/STAT3 feedback loop promotes the malignancy in melanoma via activation of JAK2/STAT3 signaling. Mol Cancer Res 18(11):1724–1734. https://doi.org/10.1158/1541-7786.MCR-19-1046

68. Chen L, Yang H, Xiao Y, Tang X, Li Y, Han Q, Fu J, Yang Y, Zhu Y (2016) Lentiviral-mediated overexpression of long non-coding RNA GAS5 reduces invasion by mediating MMP2 expression and activity in human melanoma cells. Int J Oncol 48(4):1509–1518. https://doi.org/10.3892/ijo.2016.3377

69. Bao S, Zhao H, Yuan J, Fan D, Zhang Z, Su J, Zhou M (2020) Computational identification of mutator-derived lncRNA signatures of genome instability for improving the clinical outcome of cancers: a case study in breast cancer. Brief Bioinform 21(5):1742–1755. https://doi.org/10.1093/bib/bbz118

70. Hauptman N, Glavac D (2013) Long non-coding RNA in cancer. Int J Mol Sci 14 (3):4655–4669. https://doi.org/10.3390/ijms14034655

71. Salviano-Silva A, Lobo-Alves SC, Almeida RC, Malheiros D, Petzl-Erler ML (2018) Besides pathology: long non-coding RNA in cell and tissue homeostasis. Non-coding RNA 4(1):3. https://doi.org/10.3390/ncrna4010003

72. Zhou M, Zhao H, Wang Z, Cheng L, Yang L, Shi H, Yang H, Sun J (2015) Identification and validation of potential prognostic lncRNA biomarkers for predicting survival in patients with multiple myeloma. J Exp Clin Cancer Res 34:102. https://doi.org/10.1186/s13046-015-0219-5

73. Zhou M, Zhao H, Xu W, Bao S, Cheng L, Sun J (2017) Discovery and validation of immune-associated long non-coding RNA biomarkers associated with clinically molecular subtype and prognosis in diffuse large B cell lymphoma. Mol Cancer 16(1):16. https://doi.org/10.1186/s12943-017-0580-4

74. Carninci P, Kasukawa T, Katayama S, Gough J, Frith MC, Maeda N, Oyama R, Ravasi T, Lenhard B, Wells C, Kodzius R, Shimokawa K, Bajic VB, Brenner SE, Batalov S, Forrest AR, Zavolan M, Davis MJ, Wilming LG, Aidinis V, Allen JE, Ambesi-Impiombato A, Apweiler R, Aturaliya RN, Bailey TL, Bansal M, Baxter L, Beisel KW, Bersano T, Bono H, Chalk AM, Chiu KP, Choudhary V, Christoffels A, Clutterbuck DR, Crowe ML, Dalla E, Dalrymple BP, de Bono B, Della Gatta G, di Bernardo D, Down T, Engstrom P, Fagiolini M, Faulkner G, Fletcher CF, Fukushima T, Furuno M, Futaki S, Gariboldi M, Georgii-Hemming P, Gingeras TR, Gojobori T, Green RE, Gustincich S, Harbers M, Hayashi Y, Hensch TK, Hirokawa N, Hill D, Huminiecki L, Iacono M, Ikeo K, Iwama A, Ishikawa T, Jakt M, Kanapin A, Katoh M, Kawasawa Y, Kelso J, Kitamura H, Kitano H, Kollias G, Krishnan SP, Kruger A, Kummerfeld SK, Kurochkin IV, Lareau LF, Lazarevic D, Lipovich L, Liu J, Liuni S, McWilliam S, Madan Babu M, Madera M, Marchionni L, Matsuda H, Matsuzawa S, Miki H, Mignone F, Miyake S, Morris K, Mottagui-Tabar S, Mulder N, Nakano N, Nakauchi H, Ng P, Nilsson R, Nishiguchi S, Nishikawa S, Nori F, Ohara O, Okazaki Y, Orlando V, Pang KC, Pavan WJ, Pavesi G, Pesole G, Petrovsky N, Piazza S, Reed J, Reid JF, Ring BZ, Ringwald M, Rost B, Ruan Y, Salzberg SL, Sandelin A, Schneider C, Schonbach C, Sekiguchi K, Semple CA, Seno S, Sessa L, Sheng Y, Shibata Y, Shimada H, Shimada K, Silva D, Sinclair B, Sperling S, Stupka E, Sugiura K, Sultana R, Takenaka Y, Taki K, Tammoja K, Tan SL, Tang S, Taylor MS, Tegner J, Teichmann SA, Ueda HR, van Nimwegen E, Verardo R, Wei CL, Yagi K, Yamanishi H, Zabarovsky E, Zhu S, Zimmer A, Hide W, Bult C, Grimmond SM, Teasdale RD, Liu ET, Brusic V, Quackenbush J, Wahlestedt C, Mattick JS, Hume DA, Kai C, Sasaki D, Tomaru Y, Fukuda S, Kanamori-Katayama M, Suzuki M, Aoki J, Arakawa T, Iida J, Imamura K, Itoh M, Kato T, Kawaji H, Kawagashira N, Kawashima T, Kojima M, Kondo S, Konno H, Nakano K, Ninomiya N, Nishio T, Okada M, Plessy C, Shibata K, Shiraki T, Suzuki S, Tagami M, Waki K, Watahiki A, Okamura-Oho Y, Suzuki H, Kawai J, Hayashizaki Y, Consortium F, Group RGER, Genome Science G (2005) The transcriptional

landscape of the mammalian genome. Science 309(5740):1559–1563. https://doi.org/10.1126/science.1112014

75. Yoshimoto R, Mayeda A, Yoshida M, Nakagawa S (2016) MALAT1 long non-coding RNA in cancer. Biochim Biophys Acta 1859(1):192–199. https://doi.org/10.1016/j.bbagrm.2015.09.012

76. Virginie V, Delphine F (2018) Non-coding RNAs in cutaneous melanoma development, progression and dissemination. OBM Genetics 2(2):20

77. Sun Y, Cheng H, Wang G, Yu G, Zhang D, Wang Y, Fan W, Yang W (2017) Deregulation of miR-183 promotes melanoma development via lncRNA MALAT1 regulation and ITGB1 signal activation. Oncotarget 8(2):3509–3518. https://doi.org/10.18632/oncotarget.13862

78. Luan W, Li L, Shi Y, Bu X, Xia Y, Wang J, Djangmah HS, Liu X, You Y, Xu B (2016) Long non-coding RNA MALAT1 acts as a competing endogenous RNA to promote malignant melanoma growth and metastasis by sponging miR-22. Oncotarget 7(39):63901–63912. https://doi.org/10.18632/oncotarget.11564

79. Gupta RA, Shah N, Wang KC, Kim J, Horlings HM, Wong DJ, Tsai MC, Hung T, Argani P, Rinn JL, Wang Y, Brzoska P, Kong B, Li R, West RB, van de Vijver MJ, Sukumar S, Chang HY (2010) Long non-coding RNA HOTAIR reprograms chromatin state to promote cancer metastasis. Nature 464(7291):1071–1076. https://doi.org/10.1038/nature08975

80. Geng YJ, Xie SL, Li Q, Ma J, Wang GY (2011) Large intervening non-coding RNA HOTAIR is associated with hepatocellular carcinoma progression. J Int Med Res 39(6):2119–2128. https://doi.org/10.1177/147323001103900608

81. Kim K, Jutooru I, Chadalapaka G, Johnson G, Frank J, Burghardt R, Kim S, Safe S (2013) HOTAIR is a negative prognostic factor and exhibits pro-oncogenic activity in pancreatic cancer. Oncogene 32(13):1616–1625. https://doi.org/10.1038/onc.2012.193

82. Nie Y, Liu X, Qu S, Song E, Zou H, Gong C (2013) Long non-coding RNA HOTAIR is an independent prognostic marker for nasopharyngeal carcinoma progression and survival. Cancer Sci 104(4):458–464. https://doi.org/10.1111/cas.12092

83. Svoboda M, Slyskova J, Schneiderova M, Makovicky P, Bielik L, Levy M, Lipska L, Hemmelova B, Kala Z, Protivankova M, Vycital O, Liska V, Schwarzova L, Vodickova L, Vodicka P (2014) HOTAIR long non-coding RNA is a negative prognostic factor not only in primary tumors, but also in the blood of colorectal cancer patients. Carcinogenesis 35 (7):1510–1515. https://doi.org/10.1093/carcin/bgu055

84. Li R, Zhang L, Jia L, Duan Y, Li Y, Bao L, Sha N (2014) Long non-coding RNA BANCR promotes proliferation in malignant melanoma by regulating MAPK pathway activation. PLoS One 9(6):e100893. https://doi.org/10.1371/journal.pone.0100893

85. Yang Y, Yang H, Yi Z, Yang L, Ni Y, Zhou M, Xiong G, Agbrana Y, Zhao L, Yang Z, Zhang Q, Kuang Y, Zhu Y (2020) LncRNA BANCR facilitates melanoma cells growth, migration and invasion by inhibiting miR-206 and miR-571 to induce G6PD expression. Res Sq. https://doi.org/10.21203/rs.3.rs-31582/v1.

86. Xie H, Rachakonda PS, Heidenreich B, Nagore E, Sucker A, Hemminki K, Schadendorf D, Kumar R (2016) Mapping of deletion breakpoints at the CDKN2A locus in melanoma: detection of MTAP-ANRIL fusion transcripts. Oncotarget 7(13):16490 16504. https://doi.org/10.18632/oncotarget.7503

87. Dar AA, Majid S, de Semir D, Nosrati M, Bezrookove V, Kashani-Sabet M (2011) miRNA-205 suppresses melanoma cell proliferation and induces senescence via regulation of E2F1 protein. J Biol Chem 286(19):16606–16614. https://doi.org/10.1074/jbc.M111.227611

88. Xu S, Wang H, Pan H, Shi Y, Li T, Ge S, Jia R, Zhang H, Fan X (2016) ANRIL lncRNA triggers efficient therapeutic efficacy by reprogramming the aberrant INK4-hub in melanoma. Cancer Lett 381(1):41–48. https://doi.org/10.1016/j.canlet.2016.07.024

89. Zehavi L, Schayek H, Jacob-Hirsch J, Sidi Y, Leibowitz-Amit R, Avni D (2015) MiR-377 targets E2F3 and alters the NF-kB signaling pathway through MAP 3K7 in malignant melanoma. Mol Cancer 14:68. https://doi.org/10.1186/s12943-015-0338-9

90. Amos CI, Wang LE, Lee JE, Gershenwald JE, Chen WV, Fang S, Kosoy R, Zhang M, Qureshi AA, Vattathil S, Schacherer CW, Gardner JM, Wang Y, Bishop DT, Barrett JH, Geno MELI, MacGregor S, Hayward NK, Martin NG, Duffy DL, Investigators QM, Mann GJ, Cust A, Hopper J, Investigators A, Brown KM, Grimm EA, Xu Y, Han Y, Jing K, McHugh C, Laurie CC, Doheny KF, Pugh EW, Seldin MF, Han J, Wei Q (2011) Genome-wide association study identifies novel loci predisposing to cutaneous melanoma. Hum Mol Genet 20 (24):5012–5023. https://doi.org/10.1093/hmg/ddr415

91. Baker MJ, Goldstein AM, Gordon PL, Harbaugh KS, Mackley HB, Glantz MJ, Drabick JJ (2016) An interstitial deletion within 9p21.3 and extending beyond CDKN2A predisposes to melanoma, neural system tumours and possible haematological malignancies. J Med Genet 53 (11):721–727. https://doi.org/10.1136/jmedgenet-2015-103446

92. Maccioni L, Rachakonda PS, Bermejo JL, Planelles D, Requena C, Hemminki K, Nagore E, Kumar R (2013) Variants at the 9p21 locus and melanoma risk. BMC Cancer 13:325. https://doi.org/10.1186/1471-2407-13-325

93. Wei Y, Sun Q, Zhao L, Wu J, Chen X, Wang Y, Zang W, Zhao G (2016) LncRNA UCA1-miR-507-FOXM1 axis is involved in cell proliferation, invasion and G0/G1 cell cycle arrest in melanoma. Med Oncol 33(8):88. https://doi.org/10.1007/s12032-016-0804-2

94. Han C, Tang F, Chen J, Xu D, Li X, Xu Y, Wang S, Zhou J (2019) Knockdown of lncRNA-UCA1 inhibits the proliferation and migration of melanoma cells through modulating the miR-28-5p/HOXB3 axis. Exp Ther Med 17(5):4294–4302. https://doi.org/10.3892/etm.2019.7421

95. Yu X, Zheng H, Tse G, Chan MT, Wu WK (2018) Long non-coding RNAs in melanoma. Cell Prolif 51(4):e12457. https://doi.org/10.1111/cpr.12457

96. Tang L, Liang Y, Xie H, Yang X, Zheng G (2020) Long non-coding RNAs in cutaneous biology and proliferative skin diseases: advances and perspectives. Cell Prolif 53(1):e12698. https://doi.org/10.1111/cpr.12698

97. Aubuchon MM, Bolt LJ, Janssen-Heijnen ML, Verleisdonk-Bolhaar ST, van Marion A, van Berlo CL (2017) Epidemiology, management and survival outcomes of primary cutaneous melanoma: a ten-year overview. Acta Chir Belg 117(1):29–35. https://doi.org/10.1080/00015458.2016.1242214

98. Schmidt K, Joyce CE, Buquicchio F, Brown A, Ritz J, Distel RJ, Yoon CH, Novina CD (2016) The lncRNA SLNCR1 mediates melanoma invasion through a conserved SRA1-like region. Cell Rep 15(9):2025–2037. https://doi.org/10.1016/j.celrep.2016.04.018

99. Liu T, Shen SK, Xiong JG, Xu Y, Zhang HQ, Liu HJ, Lu ZG (2016) Clinical significance of long non-coding RNA SPRY4-IT1 in melanoma patients. FEBS Open Bio 6(2):147–154. https://doi.org/10.1002/2211-5463.12030

100. Zhao W, Mazar J, Lee B, Sawada J, Li JL, Shelley J, Govindarajan S, Towler D, Mattick JS, Komatsu M, Dinger ME, Perera RJ (2016) The long noncoding RNA SPRIGHTLY regulates cell proliferation in primary human melanocytes. J Invest Dermatol 136(4):819–828. https://doi.org/10.1016/j.jid.2016.01.018

101. Song W, Wang K, Zhang RJ, Dai QX, Zou SB (2016) Long non-coding RNA GAS5 can predict metastasis and poor prognosis: a meta-analysis. Minerva Med 107(1):70–76

102. Bian D, Shi W, Shao Y, Li P, Song G (2017) Long non-coding RNA GAS5 inhibits tumorigenesis via miR-137 in melanoma. Am J Transl Res 9(3):1509–1520

103. Shain AH, Bastian BC (2016) From melanocytes to melanomas. Nat Rev Cancer 16 (6):345–358. https://doi.org/10.1038/nrc.2016.37

104. Aftab MN, Dinger ME, Perera RJ (2014) The role of microRNAs and long non-coding RNAs in the pathology, diagnosis, and management of melanoma. Arch Biochem Biophys 563:60–70. https://doi.org/10.1016/j.abb.2014.07.022

105. Smedley D, Sidhar S, Birdsall S, Bennett D, Herlyn M, Cooper C, Shipley J (2000) Characterization of chromosome 1 abnormalities in malignant melanomas. Genes Chromosomes Cancer 28(1):121–125. https://doi.org/10.1002/(sici)1098-2264(200005)28:1

106. Thorenoor N, Faltejskova-Vychytilova P, Hombach S, Mlcochova J, Kretz M, Svoboda M, Slaby O (2016) Long non-coding RNA ZFAS1 interacts with CDK1 and is involved in p53-dependent cell cycle control and apoptosis in colorectal cancer. Oncotarget 7 (1):622–637. https://doi.org/10.18632/oncotarget.5807
107. Ichigozaki Y, Fukushima S, Jinnin M, Miyashita A, Nakahara S, Tokuzumi A, Yamashita J, Kajihara I, Aoi J, Masuguchi S, Zhongzhi W, Ihn H (2016) Serum long non-coding RNA, snoRNA host gene 5 level as a new tumor marker of malignant melanoma. Exp Dermatol 25 (1):67–69. https://doi.org/10.1111/exd.12868
108. Guo L, Yao L, Jiang Y (2016) A novel integrative approach to identify lncRNAs associated with the survival of melanoma patients. Gene 585(2):216–220. https://doi.org/10.1016/j.gene. 2016.03.036
109. Lessard L, Liu M, Marzese DM, Wang H, Chong K, Kawas N, Donovan NC, Kiyohara E, Hsu S, Nelson N, Izraely S, Sagi-Assif O, Witz IP, Ma XJ, Luo Y, Hoon DSB (2015) The CASC15 long intergenic noncoding RNA locus is involved in melanoma progression and phenotype switching. J Invest Dermatol 135(10):2464–2474. https://doi.org/10.1038/jid.2015. 200
110. Tian Y, Zhang X, Hao Y, Fang Z, He Y (2014) Potential roles of abnormally expressed long non-coding RNA UCA1 and Malat-1 in metastasis of melanoma. Melanoma Res 24 (4):335–341. https://doi.org/10.1097/CMR.0000000000000080
111. Martinez J, Patkaniowska A, Urlaub H, Luhrmann R, Tuschl T (2002) Single-stranded antisense siRNAs guide target RNA cleavage in RNAi. Cell 110(5):563–574. https://doi. org/10.1016/s0092-8674(02)00908-x
112. Buchholz F, Kittler R, Slabicki M, Theis M (2006) Enzymatically prepared RNAi libraries. Nat Methods 3(9):696–700. https://doi.org/10.1038/nmeth912
113. Li F, Li X, Qiao L, Liu W, Xu C, Wang X (2019) MALAT1 regulates miR-34a expression in melanoma cells. Cell Death Dis 10(6):389. https://doi.org/10.1038/s41419-019-1620-3
114. Sun L, Sun P, Zhou QY, Gao X, Han Q (2016) Long non-coding RNA MALAT1 promotes uveal melanoma cell growth and invasion by silencing of miR-140. Am J Transl Res 8 (9):3939–3946
115. Walder RY, Walder JA (1988) Role of RNase H in hybrid-arrested translation by antisense oligonucleotides. Proc Natl Acad Sci U S A 85(14):5011–5015. https://doi.org/10.1073/pnas. 85.14.5011
116. Zamecnik PC, Stephenson ML (1978) Inhibition of Rous sarcoma virus replication and cell transformation by a specific oligodeoxynucleotide. Proc Natl Acad Sci U S A 75(1):280–284. https://doi.org/10.1073/pnas.75.1.280
117. Chen L, Yang H, Xiao Y, Tang X, Li Y, Han Q, Fu J, Yang Y, Zhu Y (2016) LncRNA GAS5 is a critical regulator of metastasis phenotype of melanoma cells and inhibits tumor growth in vivo. Onco Targets Ther 9:4075–4087. https://doi.org/10.2147/OTT.S98203
118. Maverakis E, Cornelius LA, Bowen GM, Phan T, Patel FB, Fitzmaurice S, He Y, Burrall B, Duong C, Kloxin AM, Sultani H, Wilken R, Martinez SR, Patel F (2015) Metastatic melanoma - a review of current and future treatment options. Acta Derm Venereol 95(5):516–524. https:// doi.org/10.2340/00015555-2035
119. Nazarian R, Shi H, Wang Q, Kong X, Koya RC, Lee H, Chen Z, Lee MK, Attar N, Sazegar H, Chodon T, Nelson SF, McArthur G, Sosman JA, Ribas A, Lo RS (2010) Melanomas acquire resistance to B-RAF(V600E) inhibition by RTK or N-RAS upregulation. Nature 468 (7326):973–977. https://doi.org/10.1038/nature09626
120. Robert C, Thomas L, Bondarenko I, O'Day S, Weber J, Garbe C, Lebbe C, Baurain JF, Testori A, Grob JJ, Davidson N, Richards J, Maio M, Hauschild A, Miller WH Jr, Gascon P, Lotem M, Harmankaya K, Ibrahim R, Francis S, Chen TT, Humphrey R, Hoos A, Wolchok JD (2011) Ipilimumab plus dacarbazine for previously untreated metastatic melanoma. N Engl J Med 364(26):2517–2526. https://doi.org/10.1056/NEJMoa1104621

121. Ji Z, Erin Chen Y, Kumar R, Taylor M, Jenny Njauw CN, Miao B, Frederick DT, Wargo JA, Flaherty KT, Jonsson G, Tsao H (2015) MITF modulates therapeutic resistance through EGFR signaling. J Invest Dermatol 135(7):1863–1872. https://doi.org/10.1038/jid.2015.105

122. Van Allen EM, Wagle N, Sucker A, Treacy DJ, Johannessen CM, Goetz EM, Place CS, Taylor-Weiner A, Whittaker S, Kryukov GV, Hodis E, Rosenberg M, McKenna A, Cibulskis K, Farlow D, Zimmer L, Hillen U, Gutzmer R, Goldinger SM, Ugurel S, Gogas HJ, Egberts F, Berking C, Trefzer U, Loquai C, Weide B, Hassel JC, Gabriel SB, Carter SL, Getz G, Garraway LA, Schadendorf D, Dermatologic Cooperative Oncology Group of G (2014) The genetic landscape of clinical resistance to RAF inhibition in metastatic melanoma. Cancer Discov 4(1):94–109. https://doi.org/10.1158/2159-8290.CD-13-0617

123. Zheng M, Bocangel D, Ramesh R, Ekmekcioglu S, Poindexter N, Grimm EA, Chada S (2008) Interleukin-24 overcomes temozolomide resistance and enhances cell death by down-regulation of O6-methylguanine-DNA methyltransferase in human melanoma cells. Mol Cancer Ther 7(12):3842–3851. https://doi.org/10.1158/1535-7163.MCT-08-0516

124. Sanlorenzo M, Vujic I, Esteve-Puig R, Lai K, Vujic M, Lin K, Posch C, Dimon M, Moy A, Zekhtser M, Johnston K, Gho D, Ho W, Gajjala A, Oses Prieto J, Burlingame A, Daud A, Rappersberger K, Ortiz-Urda S (2018) The lincRNA MIRAT binds to IQGAP1 and modulates the MAPK pathway in NRAS mutant melanoma. Sci Rep 8(1):10902. https://doi.org/10.1038/s41598-018-27643-3

125. Joung J, Engreitz JM, Konermann S, Abudayyeh OO, Verdine VK, Aguet F, Gootenberg JS, Sanjana NE, Wright JB, Fulco CP, Tseng YY, Yoon CH, Boehm JS, Lander ES, Zhang F (2017) Genome-scale activation screen identifies a lncRNA locus regulating a gene neighbourhood. Nature 548(7667):343–346. https://doi.org/10.1038/nature23451

126. Cao K, Yan L, Dong H, Mengqin X, Liang X, Yuxing Z (2020) Long non-coding RNA LINC00518 induces Radioresistance by regulating glycolysis through an miR-33a-3p/HIF-1α negative feedback loop in melanoma. Cell Death Disease 12:245

127. Poliseno L, Haimovic A, Christos PJ, YSDMEC V, Shapiro R, Pavlick A, Berman RS, Darvishian F, Osman I (2011) Deletion of PTENP1 pseudogene in human melanoma. J Invest Dermatol 131(12):2497–2500. https://doi.org/10.1038/jid.2011.232

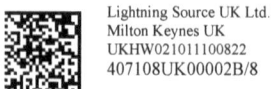

Lightning Source UK Ltd.
Milton Keynes UK
UKHW021011100822
407108UK00002B/8